Voices

Lincoln Hospital School of Nursing,
Durham, North Carolina, 1903 . . .

LINCOLN HOSPITAL SCHOOL OF NURSING

School Song

Dear Alma Mater, though we stray from thy side,
Dear Alma Mater, we will be your bride.
In Thy walls of learning, which we've grown to love so well
Dreams of fondest yearning, hold us in their spell.
Lincoln, dear old Lincoln,
With thy colors white and blue,
Lincoln, dear old Lincoln,
To Thee we'll be true.

(set to the tune of "Juanita")

Voices

Lincoln Hospital School of Nursing, Durham, North Carolina, 1903 . . .

EVELYN PEARL BOOKER WICKER

To Clinmie Hilliard

Enjoy reading

Evelyn Pearl Booker Wicker EdD RN

April 2018

JONES BOOKER PUBLISHING

Fuquay Varina, North Carolina

Photographs from North Carolina Central University have been reproduced
    courtesy of the James E. Shepard Memorial Library University Archives
    and Records.
Unless otherwise noted, images are from the Lincoln Hospital School of Nursing
    archives. Every effort has been made to locate the copyright owner of all
    images; please send information about image ownership to the publisher so
    that corrected information may be included in future editions of this book.

First edition, second printing
Design & production by BW&A Books, Inc., Durham, North Carolina
Printed in the United States of America

Library of Congress Control Number: 2013940357
ISBN 978-0-9894208-0-8 (paper)
ISBN 978-0-9894208-1-5 (cloth)

Dedicated to

Ruby Jewel Bell Borden

*for her unwavering commitment and dedication
to this project during her lifetime*

(1938–2010)

RUBY BELL BORDEN was born in 1938 in Shamrock, Florida. She grew up in the town of Bayboro, North Carolina, with her great uncle and aunt, Jake and Lula Mae Hamilton. Following her completion of high school in Bayboro in 1956, she entered Lincoln Hospital School of Nursing in Durham, North Carolina, and graduated in 1959. Upon passing the Board of Nursing licensure examination she received the registered nurse license for professional practice. In 1972 she received the bachelor of science degree in nursing from North Carolina Central University in Durham, North Carolina.

Ruby began her career at Duke University Hospital in Durham, North Carolina, as a Registered Nurse and later transitioned into Medical Informatics, which historically was a male-dominated field. She was a risk taker with a pioneering spirit. Ruby had a vision for the future of informatics in health care and the role that nurses could play in charting the course for this innovation to improve the quality and efficiency of patient care. She had over thirty years of experience as an administrator, analyst, and project manager in medical informatics. Her expertise in the area created opportunities for career advancement, including her assumption of an executive role as the Director of Information Systems at Vanderbilt University Medi-

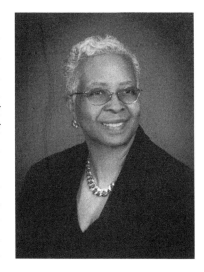

cal Center in Nashville, Tennessee. Ruby wrote and presented several papers on topics related to the use of technology in patient-care delivery. She received certifications in Project Management, Facilitative Leadership, and Work Redesign.

Ruby was passionate about nursing and was the epitome of a Lincoln nurse. As both a nursing student and a professional nurse she was involved in the community and in leadership roles, especially in the Central Carolina Black Nurses Council, Inc. She was one of the first Lincoln students to attend the State and National Student Nurses Associations representing the district after the desegregation of the association. Ruby idealized this book project as a way of "keeping the spirit of Lincoln alive" and wanted all to view it as an extension of the Lincoln Hospital School of Nursing legacy, of which she was a vital part.

Contents

Foreword   ix
Preface   xiii
Introduction   xv

CHAPTER ONE   1
Evolution of the Hospital-Based Nurse Training School, 1903–1924

CHAPTER TWO   35
Period of Growth and Development, 1924–1944

CHAPTER THREE   93
The Changing Tide, 1945–1971

CHAPTER FOUR   183
Continuing the Legacy

EPILOGUE   253
Reflections

APPENDICES
1. Leadership and Service Contributors   259
2. Historical Roster   281

List of Supporters   293
References   301
Index   307
About the Author   321

Foreword

THIS informative volume is about the many women who somewhere between the ages of seventeen and thirty-five entered Lincoln Hospital School of Nursing between 1903 and 1969. These gifted women left this magnificent center of knowledge with the skills to practice excellent nursing and to provide much-needed health care in their communities and in the world. Lincoln Hospital School of Nursing (LHSN) became a place of learning for Negro women who wanted to become nurses. Because of the times in which they lived, they entered its hallowed halls unsure of what they would find; in time, LHSN became a home and a haven for many of them for two or three years. Lincoln Hospital as a community agency existed because there was a need for health-care services for members of the Negro community. It provided a necessary service—although, for many of its consumers, it became synonymous with death and dying.

In the early years of institutionalized health care, many Negroes equated the need for hospitalization with being very close to death. Too often those entering the hospital did not return home to their loved ones. No wonder Lincoln had difficulty keeping its daily patient census above seventy-five. However, we know that African Americans have historically lacked access to sufficient health-care services and the hospital did fulfill a need in the Negro community. I grew up in Goldsboro, North Carolina, in the 1940s and coming to Lincoln Hospital in Durham, North Carolina, was nearly on par with coming to "Dukes," as many locals referred to Duke Hospital at the time.

The writers of this history of Lincoln Hospital School of Nursing, Evelyn Pearl Booker Wicker and Ruby Jewell Bell Borden [before her death], remind us that Lincoln Hospital opened in 1901. With a gift from the philanthropist Washington Duke, Lincoln Hospital saw its first patients on the corner of Cozart Street and Procter Avenue. While Mr. Duke had planned to erect a monument commemorating Negro slaves for their loyalty during the dark days of the American Civil War, more farsighted members of the Negro community had another vision. Why not build a hospital that would provide care to the descendants of that bloody war?

Dr. Aaron Moore (the first Negro physician in Durham), Mr. John Merrick, Dr. Stanford Lee Warren, and others managed to convince the bene-factor that a hospital would make a more fitting tribute, especially in light of the fact that the monument was to be raised on the campus of Duke University, which at the time did not admit Negroes except as employees. The Negro community greatly needed a hospital where they could enter and be treated with the respect and dignity they deserved, be it for the purpose of dying or of recovering from a serious illness. For seventy-two years, Lincoln Hospital (1901–1973) lived out its purpose.

All across North Carolina Lincoln Hospital was known to provide medical services to the citizenry of Durham. It was indeed a place where Negro citizens requiring care could find that care delivered with respect and dignity. It is a productive legacy.

A vital part of Lincoln Hospital was the School of Nursing, which is the focus of this book. Given the mission of the hospital, a nursing school was essential. Good nurses were needed to provide the basic hygienic care necessary to ensure that patients could recover and return to their communities. This commemorative volume describes the triumph of building a facility for the descendants of the descendants of the enslaved who helped to build this great country and state of ours. Many young Negro women also found a career path here, in nursing, the noblest of professions. Lincoln Hospital was a source of both training and employment for many who would find their life's work in providing medical services. X-ray and laboratory technicians, anesthesiologists, nursing assistants, physical therapists, nurses (who at the time were considered physicians' handmaidens) and medical doctors all got their start at Lincoln Hospital. From those roots have grown a small nation of dedicated women who know how to work hard while remaining caring and compassionate.

In 2003 the graduates of Lincoln Hospital School of Nursing came together to celebrate 100 years of service and contributions to the Durham community. They also celebrated the contributions of those descendants of the enslaved who had dedicated their lives to caring for their own communities. Lincoln Hospital School of Nursing graduates have spread far and wide doing what they were trained to do best: provide the best care they could to their patients. A debt of gratitude is owed to those who had the wisdom to ask for more in order to remember their ancestors and their descendants. Today, those graduates are that living monument. For more than seventy years, young women entered Lincoln Hospital School of Nursing and two to three years later graduated with the skills and abilities to pass the licensing exam and thus declare themselves Registered Nurses. From 1961 to 1963 this writer had the pleasure of teaching a cohort of these young women. Little did I know that I would return to Durham some fifteen years later and find those same young women occupying some of the loftiest positions in the Durham Medical Community. Such is the legacy of a vision. From modest beginnings, a multitude of health-care providers, some of them still practicing, are fulfilling the legacy of the founders of Lincoln Hospital. We have yet to fully comprehend the impact of this group of dynamic women who set out on an unknown path to become members of one of the greatest and most honored professions on earth, even though much of the work we do was once frowned upon by the masses. Where indeed would Durham be without the influence of this mighty movement that began in 1903? Lincoln Hospital School of Nursing alumni, this book salutes you. It forever preserves what you contributed in your youth to your adopted communities and to your own successful lives. You indeed make all of us proud and should yourselves be proud. You have fulfilled a God-given purpose on this earth. May your descendants and others never forget the contribution made by each of you. We salute you.

God Bless!

Written by E. Joyce Simmons Roland, RN, PhD,
Lincoln Hospital School of Nursing,
medical-surgical instructor, 1961–1963

Special Thanks

SPECIAL AND HEART-FELT THANKS go to the "Committee:" Diann Johnson, Patricia Martin Blue, Dorothy Esta Dennis Segars and Gwendolyn Cooper Jones Parham. They gave countless hours of their time and talents in editorial support, compiling art, researching sources, reading drafts, typing, and participating in many meetings. Had Ruby lived to see the completion of this book, she would have been as grateful as I am for this extraordinary committee who stepped up to fill her shoes. And Ruby would be so proud of her Lincoln Sisters.

Preface

I N 1971, while enrolled in an undergraduate research course in the Department of Nursing at North Carolina Central University, Ruby Jewel Bell
Borden and I drafted a brief history of Lincoln Hospital School of Nursing
for a class project. While conducting the preliminary research, we realized
how little information was available. We felt strongly that our school and its
graduates should be a part of recorded nursing history and that the struggles and contributions of this group of African American nurses should be
acknowledged. We believed this was a part of our proud heritage and could
provide inspiration for others who aspired to become registered nurses. We
committed to each other then that later in our nursing careers we would
revisit this idea and do a more in-depth project on our alma mater. In December 2009 the idea resurfaced and the planning for this adventure began.

Ruby, intelligent, strong-willed, and fun-loving, had little tolerance for
nonsense. Throughout our work together, she was a stickler for staying on
track. Once the plan and timelines were developed, there was no wavering—
she was committed to the deadlines. I, on the other hand, believed there
would always be another deadline.

In April 2010, Ruby was diagnosed with an aggressive terminal illness.
Still, her enduring spirit, mental toughness, and tenacity gave her the physical strength to push ahead. Although burdened with failing health, her
commitment, dedication, and loyalty to the project never wavered. That September, six weeks before her death, she sent me her handwritten notes of
suggestions for the manuscript because she was too weak to sit at the computer. Her final handwritten notes were comforting and encouraged me to
keep pressing toward our goal. Ruby and I shared a sisterly bond and this
experience strengthened it even more.

In October 2010, Ruby left her family and alumni sisters for a place with
the Master. Ruby lives on in all our hearts. Sometimes when I was struck
with writer's block I could hear her saying, "Evelyn, just cut through all that
and get it done." I missed Ruby's ability to keep the project on schedule.

Producing this manuscript has been an arduous task filled with sadness,
frustration, joy, and unpredictability. I am grateful that, with the support

and help of many people, I have been able to see it through to completion. I want to thank all of my sources, named and unnamed. I am also thankful to everyone at BW&A Books, Inc., for their expert advice and counsel; to Floyd Wicker, my husband, for his semi-technical expertise; to my son, Rev. Floyd Wicker Jr., who provided continuous spiritual support; to my daughter, Dr. Ingrid Wicker McCree, as well as Phyllon Jackson and my goddaughter, Tiffany Deana Johnson, all of whom provided administrative support; to my early reviewers, Rosa Steele and Evelyn Smith Booker; to Andre Vann, the Archivist at NCCU; and to R. Kelly Bryant, Phoebe Pollitt, Mary Richardson Baldwin, Carolyn Evangeline Henderson, Lynn Richardson, Dr. Howard Fitts, Lois Clements Brown Thorpe, Julia Oliver, and everyone else who helped to make this possible. I wish to give a special acknowledgement to Marion Jean Tucker, my sounding board and grounding force; Gloria Taylor Cheek King, who also contributed ideas for the title of this book; and to all the people who supplied pictures, yearbooks, letters, and so on. Lastly, I thank each contributor for providing readers with a window into the historical legacy of Lincoln Hospital School of Nursing and the contributions of its graduates locally, nationally, and internationally.

This work has been financed by the author, the LHSN Alumni Association, Inc., many Lincoln graduates, and friends of Lincoln including the Mary Duke Biddle Foundation. A list of supporters is included in the back of the book. This history of the Lincoln Hospital School of Nursing is not exhaustive; rather, it is an attempt to acknowledge the role that LHSN and some of its graduates have played in the nursing profession and the health-care community.

Introduction

THROUGHOUT the history of modern nursing, Colored, Negro, or Black nurses have made their contributions. However, they also have struggled for acceptance as professionals, quality healthcare for Negro citizens, equality in education, career mobility, and employee rights.

Hospitals and schools of nursing were a microcosm of the social and political climate in which they operated. In North Carolina, many nursing schools, from their beginnings in the late 1800s through the 1960s, were hospital-based and segregated. In 1903, when Lincoln Hospital School of Nursing (LHSN) was established, there were two other Negro nursing schools in North Carolina; St. Agnes, in Raleigh, and Good Samaritan, in Charlotte. These were followed by two more: Kate Biting Reynolds Hospital, in Winston-Salem, and L. Richardson Memorial Hospital, in Greensboro.

As nursing advanced to become a profession, the education and preparation of future nurses transitioned to colleges, universities, and technical community colleges. This change in status was directed toward enhancing the preparation of nurses for leadership and management roles. Hospital-based nursing programs were being phased out.

By the late 1960s all the Negro hospital-based nursing schools in North Carolina had closed with the exception of Kate Biting and LHSN. However, three predominately Negro baccalaureate nursing programs now existed in colleges and universities: North Carolina Agricultural and Technical University (A&T), in Greensboro, Winston-Salem State University School of Nursing (WSSU), in Winston-Salem, and North Carolina Central University (NCCU) Department of Nursing, in Durham. These three collegiate programs continue today. Many of the African American students in these programs, and in other programs throughout the educational system, were the products of poor primary and secondary education systems throughout the South. They struggled to pass the Board of Nursing licensure examination (the standard by which nursing schools are evaluated). Many failed their first attempt but were successful upon subsequent tries. These programs—A&T, WSSU, and NCCU—in spite of the obstacles, have produced graduate nurses who went on to make phenomenal contributions to the nursing profession and health care.

During the early years of nursing organizations in North Carolina, Negro nurses were prohibited from participating in professional organizations that governed nursing standards and practice. However, they were held accountable to the rules the Board of Nursing established. In 1923 Negro nurses in North Carolina started the North Carolina State Association of Colored Registered Nurses, Inc. The Lincoln Hospital nursing administration leadership participated in this organization.

In 1903 Lincoln Hospital Nurse Training School (later Lincoln Hospital School of Nursing, or LHSN) was established and incorporated into Lincoln Hospital. The school was a very important part of Durham. In North Carolina, especially in Durham, you need only mention LHSN to a person over fifty years of age and a sparkle comes into their eyes; in all probability their lives have been touched by Lincoln Hospital or by a Lincoln nurse. On the other hand, people under fifty may have no idea that LHSN even existed.

From their inceptions in 1901 and 1903, respectively, Lincoln Hospital and the Nurse Training School struggled for existence. The School of Nursing became the cornerstone for most of the nurses who trained there, marking the beginnings of their professional nursing careers. The school became a family and a home away from home that fostered a spirit of community and a closeness that permeated the lives of all who studied and labored there.

This book is designed to reflect on the rich heritage and legacy of a nurses' training school, and its association with a Negro hospital, in the segregated South. It records a partial history of Lincoln Hospital Nurse Training School as well as narratives by some of the leaders who made it happen and by students who completed the nurse training program. As of this writing, the oldest living graduate of the Lincoln Hospital School of Nursing, Mrs. Josephine Demmons McBride, is 104 years old. Just imagine her life—the struggles, obstacles, challenges, and joys she witnessed and experienced. We hope this book will inspire young men and women, especially people of color, to choose professional careers in nursing. Cultural and racial identity is fundamental to promoting individual wholeness and healing and to minimizing racial disparity in health care.

Writing this book in a way that reflects the context of the times has been challenging. The changes in racial designations over the years from Colored, to Negro, to Black, to African American are indicative of changing sociological perspectives. The Articles of Incorporation of Lincoln Hospital, written in 1901, used the term "Colored"; this designation was used interchangeably with "Negro" in the early years. The term "Black" was popularized in the 1960s during the height of the Civil Rights Movement. The 1980s gave rise to the term "African American," which continues to be used today.

Writing this book has been a soulful journey that allowed me to learn about and appreciate LHSN and the powerful Negro women who studied and worked there. It is written from a developmental perspective. I believe institutions are like people; they move through different phases as they evolve and develop to achieve their goals. There are the very early establishing years, the years of transition, the years of growth and expansion of the institution, and the changing tide of the sunset years, which bought the closure of the school. The book is divided into four parts, which cover sixty-eight years of the school's existence and end with the alumni today. Its story, set within the context of the times, chronicles: 1) why and how Lincoln Hospital and Lincoln Hospital School of Nursing started; 2) the leaders who were instrumental in the history of the school; 3) the school's operation, student life, admission requirements, curriculum, and classes and the external forces (economic, cultural, and political, including the North Carolina Board of Nursing and other professional associations) that shaped it; and 4) the perspectives and reflections of some of the alumni, who describe how LHSN affected their personal and professional lives and the Alumni Association (past and present), including a roster of about 90 percent of the school's 614 graduates, beginning with the class of 1907 and ending with the class of 1971. Finally, this book captures the "voices" of some Lincoln graduates. Lincoln nurses have always exhibited strength, intelligence, resilience, and a passion for their careers. Their "voices" will continue to illuminate the spirit of LHSN, which lives on in our hearts and souls.

Nurse's Prayer

Because the day that stretches out for me
Is full of busy hours, I come to Thee
To ask Thee, Lord, that Thou wilt see me through
The many things that I have to do.

Help me to make my bed the smoothest way
Help me to make more tempting every tray
Help me to sense when pain must have relief
Help me to deal with those borne down by grief.

Help me to take to every patient's room
The light of life to brighten up the gloom;
Help me to bring to every soul in fear
The sure and steadfast thought that Thou art near.

Help me to live throughout the live-long day
As one who loves Thee well, dear Lord I pray;
And when the day is done and evening stars
Shine through the dark above the sunset bars,
When weary quite, I turn to see my rest
Lord, may I truly know I've done my best.

—Author Unknown

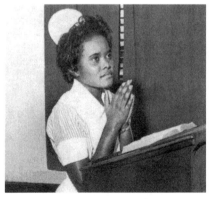

JoAnn Moore, RN '65

Chapter One

Evolution of the Hospital-Based Nurse Training School, 1903–1924

LOOKING BACK TO MOVE FORWARD

It's Sunday, August 22, 1971, at two in the afternoon. The last graduation ceremony of Lincoln Hospital School of Nursing (LHSN) is about to begin. The sanctuary at St. Mark A.M.E. Zion Church in Durham, North Carolina, is filled with five hundred parents, spouses, family members, community personalities, and friends anxiously awaiting the arrival of fourteen young ladies who are about to end one phase of their lives and begin another. There is a tremendous sense of accomplishment, pride, and sadness as this omega class of LHSN prepares to proceed into the sanctuary. Also in the procession are proud alumni, immaculately dressed in their white uniforms and nursing caps to display their Lincoln "dignity." Ruby and I are present on this historical occasion: she is mistress of ceremony and I am one of the proud alumni. The graduation speaker is one of our very own, the nationally and internationally renowned Captain Mary Lee Mills, a 1933 graduate of LHSN. On this day, she is challenging members of the graduating class to take their places in society in order to experience and help to remedy the inequities under which many Black students were "crippled, stymied and impoverished during educational pursuits." This day, the graduates will begin their nursing careers with many of the same challenges but also with new opportunities for growth in the recently integrated society legislated by the federal government where health care is a right for all and not a privilege. In addition, these graduates will have access to leadership, employment, and educational opportunities as never before, and they are prepared to face the challenge. As Lincoln alumni, they will always be prepared to uphold the traditional values, the family bonds, and the legacy of Lincoln Hospital School of Nursing.

(continues on page 6)

1

Commencement Marks Ending And Beginning

The 66th commencement exercise for the 1971 class of Lincoln Hospital's School of Nursing marked the ending of the school which was started in 1903 and a beginning for the 14 members of the graduating class (left). Miss Mary L. Mills (right), a nurse consultant, Comprehensive Health Service Branch, Division of Health Care Service, told the graduating class about a national revolution for requirements for nurses and for health care. Miss Mills was a member of the 1933 graduating class. From *Durham Morning Herald*, August 23, 1971, courtesy of Carolyn Evangeline Henderson.

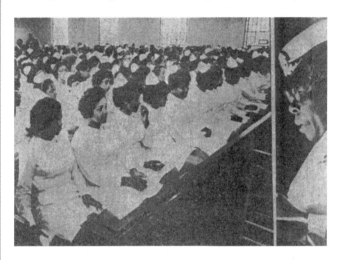

This portrait of Miss Mary Mills by Betsy Graves Reyneau is included in the Smithsonian Institution's Harmon Foundation collection of portraits of notable African Americans. The institution calls her 'one of the finest ambassadors for America's nurses.' Reproduced from a feature article on Mary L. Mills, September 5, 1998, *The Carolina Times*, courtesy of Phoebe Pollit.

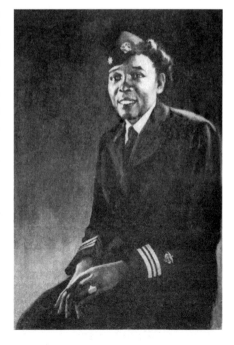

Captain Mary Lee Mills, RN '34
August 23, 1912–February 02, 2010

Captain Mary Lee Mills, the oldest child of Jack Dallas Mills and Margaret Ann Mills, was born on August 23, 1912, in Wallace, North Carolina. She was raised outside Watha, a rural area, and in the course of her life traveled from her native North Carolina to Africa, South Asia, the Middle East, and more as a nurse in the U.S. Public Health Service. A nursing pioneer, Mary blazed a truly international trail as a leader in public health. One of the most inspiring yet little-known facts about Mary is that she was one of eleven children and the granddaughter of slaves. Through education and determination—Mary went on to earn her RN, MSN, MPH, and CNM— Mary had an international nursing career that brought health and hope to medically underserved people around the world.

Mary received her early education in a one-teacher schoolhouse at a time when racial segregation was the law of the land and educational opportunities for African American children in rural North Carolina were deplorable. She was an exceptional student and soon completed the limited public schooling that was available to her as a young, Black female in the Jim Crow South of the early twentieth century.

At the height of the Great Depression, Mary made her way to Durham, where in 1934 she graduated from the Lincoln Hospital School of Nursing and became a registered nurse. She worked as a public health nurse and then in advanced practice as a nurse-midwife while she completed additional education. She earned a certificate in public health nursing from the Medical College of Virginia, a certificate in midwifery from the Lobenstein School of Midwifery in New York City, bachelor's and master's degrees in nursing from New York University, and a graduate certificate in health-care administration from George Washington University in Washington, D.C. In 1946, Mary returned to North Carolina to direct the public health nursing certificate program at the historically Black North Carolina College (now North Carolina Central University) in Durham, North Carolina. Also that year, she was commissioned as an officer in the U.S. Public Health Service (USPHS).

Going Global

Mary Mills began her distinguished career in global and transcultural nursing in February 1946, when she joined the Office of International Health and was assigned to the USPHS mission in Monrovia, Liberia. While in Liberia she created some of that country's first health-education campaigns, initiated a national public health library, and advocated for legislation to strengthen nursing as a profession. A 1956 article in the *American Journal of Nursing* describes her work in Liberia this way:

From 1946 until 1952 she served as chief nursing officer for the USPHS in Liberia, West Africa. In addition to trips into the interior with her colleagues to set up immunization stations and health centers, she helped organize and establish the Franklin D. Roosevelt Memorial Children's Ward at the government hospital in Monrovia and she was instrumental in organizing the Tubman National School of Nursing. Liberia invested her as Knight Official of the Liberian Humane Order of African Redemption.

After a short period back in the United States for study, rest, and family visits, Mary, who had been promoted from the USPHS rank of Major to that of Lieutenant Colonel, then Colonel, and finally Captain—received her next international assignment, to Beirut, Lebanon, in January 1952.

On her way from North Carolina to the Middle East, Captain Mills represented the United States at conferences of the International Council of Nurses and the World Health Organization. In Beirut, she worked hard to establish Lebanon's first school of nursing. These efforts earned her the Order of the Cedars, one of Lebanon's highest awards for service. A nursing dormitory at the school was named in her honor.

Throughout her twenty-year career with the Office of International Health, Captain Mills was an ambassador of good will, representing both North Carolina and the United States around the globe. In addition to her work in Liberia and Lebanon, she provided health education, nursing care, and midwifery services to countless individuals and families in South Vietnam, Cambodia, and Chad. In those countries, Captain Mills worked on campaigns to eradicate smallpox and malaria; improve sanitation, hygiene, and nutrition; and establish health-education programs and maternal-and-child health clinics. She was proficient in multiple languages: Arabic, French, Cambodian, and several African dialects.

Captain Mills was also instrumental in initiating or expanding schools of nursing in many countries. Leaders of every nation in which she worked honored her untiring efforts to improve their citizens' quality of life and health.

Accolades at Home

In 1966, Captain Mills returned permanently to the United States and took a job with the Department of Health Education and Welfare (HEW), the predecessor of today's Department of Health and Human Services. In her new position as a nursing consultant in the migrant health program, she advised the Secretary of Health, Education, and Welfare, a cabinet member who in turn advised the president, on political, policy, and program matters relating to migrant-worker health care and other public health problems.

In this capacity, she went to Finland, Germany, and Denmark to study their national health-care systems and brought back ideas that might be put to use in the United States. She also represented the United States at international nursing, midwifery, and public health conferences in Mexico, Canada, Germany, Australia, Italy, and Sweden.

In addition, Captain Mills was an active member and officer of many professional associations, including the American College of Nurse-Midwives, the National League for Nursing, the Frontier Nursing Service, the American Public Health Association, the American Nurses Association, the North Carolina Nurses Association (District 11), and the National Association for the Advancement of Colored People.

During her ten years at HEW, Mary received many awards honoring her contributions to improving public health at both the national and international levels. These honors include a USPHS Distinguished Service Award, Princeton University's Rockefeller Public Service Award, the American Nurses Association's Mary Mahoney Award, and North Carolina's highest honor, the Long Leaf Pine Award. Tuskegee University awarded her an Honorary Doctor of Science Degree, and Seton Hall University awarded her a Honorary Doctor of Laws Degree. For her distinguished service in public health, Captain Mary L. Mills was chosen by the Harmon Foundation to have her portrait painted by Betsy Graves Reyneau as one of a series of thirty-three oil paintings of outstanding African Americans, including Marian Anderson, Mary McCloud Bethune, and Ralph Bunche. That portrait is now a permanent part of the Harmon Collection at the Smithsonian Institution in Washington, D.C.

Captain Mary L. Mills retired from government service in 1976 to her beloved Pender County, in North Carolina. Although her story is summarized briefly in Dr. M. Elizabeth Carnegie's classic history book *The Path We Tread: Blacks in Nursing Worldwide*, her contributions to the nursing profession are still relatively unknown. Mary L. Mills was an extraordinary role model who overcame barriers of race, gender, class, and geography to become an international leader in nursing and an outstanding humanitarian. Her life story is an inspiration to all, and shows us that we too can expand our horizons and be of service not just at home but to people all over the world.

(Mrs. Mills' obituary was compiled from the article "Nursing Ambassador to the World." Author, Phoebe Pollitt, PhD, RN, C)

History defines our past, informs our present, and helps us to prepare for the future. Knowing the history of nursing provides a solid foundation upon which to build the profession. Nursing is an art and a science. But where did it all begin?

When we contemplate the profession of nursing, our thoughts commonly flow to Florence Nightingale. However, scholars of nursing know that the profession's history begins about 330–400 AD in Italy with Fabiola, the first person to make nursing a vocation. In 390 AD she founded the first general hospital in Rome, which on a daily basis provided care for the poor and infirm. She is reported to have personally sought out the sick and carried them to the hospital. She "nursed the unhappy, emaciated victims of hunger and disease, dressed their wounds and bathed them with her own hands." She was, at various times, praised, ridiculed, and ostracized for her deeds, but those deeds formed the roots of the nursing tradition. From this beginning through the early 1800s, individuals, both male and female, worked alone and in concert with others in religious orders, on battlefields, during epidemics and plagues, and in hospitals and homes, untiringly and unselfishly administering care to the poor, the humble, the weak, and the outcast.

Then came Florence Nightingale (1820–1860) and the beginning of modern nursing. She is remembered for nursing British soldiers in 1854 during the Crimean War. Her values included the ethical treatment of patients, the prevention of illness, the provision of clean air and water and good nutrition, and the universal right of all to health care. These values continue today as the foundation for nursing practice. One can see the influence of Florence Nightingale in the organization of nursing schools, both in their philosophy and principles and in the courses that make up their curriculum. Her behavior exemplified courage, compassion, dedication, untiring work, and high standards of performance. These principles and values were embraced by early nursing schools. Although other heroic personalities preceded her, Florence Nightingale "wove the threads of Nursing into a composite, beautiful and effective pattern." She is widely recognized as the mother of modern nursing. Many nurses consider the contributions of Florence Nightingale to mark the beginning of the science of nursing.

Negro nurses were early advocates for professional nursing even though the paths they trod were filled with obstacles. Although not as recognized, Mary Seacole, a Black nurse from Jamaica, worked as a volunteer alongside Florence Nightingale during the Crimean War. Gaining acceptance was a challenge at the time, and yet she persisted in her efforts. In later years Mary Secole was honored and recognized as the most outstanding Black person in Britain.

Negro women have been nurses since slavery. Perhaps their role as caretakers and wet nurses for the families of slave owners prevented Negro women from being recognized for their knowledge and intellect. Negro nurses have advocated for equality and participated in matters of nursing related to securing educational opportunities in nursing and quality care for Negro citizens. We proudly salute and pay tribute to Mary Eliza Mahoney, the first formally educated Negro nurse, who graduated from the New England Hospital for Women and Children, Boston, Massachusetts, in 1879. In 1908 she co-founded the National Association for Colored Graduate Nurses (NACGN) with Adah B. Thoms. She has been nationally recognized for her significant contributions to the advancement of equal opportunities in nursing for members of minority groups. In 1936 the NACGN established the Mary Mahoney Award, which is awarded biannually by the American Nurses Association. She has also been honored with a United States commemorative postage stamp.

Training of Negro Nurses In North Carolina

Training schools for Negro nurses were borne out of necessity: hospitals needed staff for providing health care to Negro citizens. This societal need gave rise to hospital-based nurse training schools.

There were two hospitals in Raleigh, North Carolina: Rex for the White citizens, which also had a nursing school exclusively for White women, and Leonard Hospital for the Negro citizens, which had no nursing school. Leonard Hospital, established by the Shaw University Medical Department in 1885, has the distinction of being the first Negro hospital in North Carolina as well as the first hospital in the state to employ Colored nurses.

The need for Negro hospitals and nurse training schools was recognized in North Carolina as early as 1886. Several movements throughout the state led to their establishment. In 1886, the General Convention of the Episcopal Church, under the auspices of St. Augustine College (now St. Augustine University), established St. Agnes Hospital in Raleigh to care for sick Negroes. As was the tradition with hospitals, St. Agnes opened the St. Agnes School of Nursing the same year, becoming the first professional nurse training school for Negroes in North Carolina. The first head or chief nurse of St. Agnes Hospital was Marie Louise Burgess, a graduate of New England

Hospital for Women and Children, in Boston, Massachusetts. The school opened with two students, who from the beginning were taught through lectures, recitations, and the regular observation of surgical operations that were a scheduled part of their day. The records of their early days were primitive, but they persisted and in 1888 two students graduated, Anna A. Groves and Effie Wortham. At first, the school required one and one-half years of training, but the training was extended to three years in 1915 as required by law. The school closed in 1961.

Following the opening of St. Agnes School of Nursing, other nurse training schools for Negroes opened. Good Samaritan Hospital and Training School for Nurses, for example, opened in Charlotte, North Carolina, in 1888. Lincoln Hospital Nurse Training School followed in 1903, and in 1920 Community Hospital and the Nurse Training School were established in Wilmington. The Nurse Training School continued through 1936, and twenty-two nurses graduated during that time. Salome Taylor, a graduate of Lincoln Hospital Nurse Training School in New York City, was the superintendent of Community Hospital. There was no relationship between Lincoln Hospital Training School in New York and Lincoln Hospital Nurse Training School in Durham, N.C.

In October 1923 the Negro Division of the North Carolina State Sanatorium was opened for the care of Negroes with tuberculosis. In 1926, Carrie Early Broadfoot, as the head nurse in charge, organized the training school for Negro nurses in the Sanatorium. Two nurses graduated in the first class, Claretta Redding and Mary Elliott.

L. Richardson Memorial Hospital in Greensboro opened on May 18, 1927, for the care of sick Negroes. The training school for Negro nurses opened in the same year, and a home for the nursing students was added in 1929. Ms. Geneva Sitrena Collins, a graduate of St. Agnes Hospital School of Nursing in Raleigh, was the director of the school. Seven students graduated from the school in 1930. The school of nursing closed in 1954.

Kate Biting Reynolds Memorial School of Nursing opened in Winston-Salem in 1938, closing thirty-four years later in 1972. The school was associated with Kate Biting Reynolds Hospital, and during the first ten years of its operation the administration of the hospital and of the school of nursing was White. Later Negro nurse administrators provided leadership until the closure of the nursing school and hospital. The last two classes graduated from Forsyth School of Nursing, which was the White school of nursing in Winston-Salem, N.C. The alumni of Kate Biting continue to meet frequently.

Jubilee Nurse Training School was a department of Jubilee Hospital in

Henderson, which opened between 1911–1912. The exact date the training school began is not certain. However, the school's documentation states that "it was discontinued when the requirement for standardization became so exacting that the department was not financially able to meet the qualifications." The movement for standardization in nursing education began in the late 1920s, and insufficient finances was a recurring theme for many hospitals and training schools. One of the biggest challenges was hiring qualified faculty, which was one of the most important factors in the grading classification for nursing schools.

THE BEGINNING OF LINCOLN HOSPITAL NURSE TRAINING SCHOOL

In 1901 Lincoln Hospital opened its doors to the Negro citizens of Durham, North Carolina. In the early 1900s, Durham was plagued with poor health that was primarily a function of environmental conditions. The city of Durham was experiencing rapid growth. People poured into the factories and mills, which led to unhygienic living conditions. The town had one main street sewer, but there were no provisions for garbage collection or for cleaning the mud- and manure-mired streets. Outdoor privies were common, and communicable diseases such as tuberculosis, smallpox, and typhoid fever were rampant throughout the community. These conditions formed the backdrop for the establishment of hospitals for all the citizens of Durham, both Colored and White.

In Durham, both the Negro and White leaderships were exerting parallel efforts to establish separate hospital facilities for their respective segments of the population. Although the populations were segregated by law and physically separated by railroad tracks, communicable diseases knew no boundaries—poor health conditions in one sector certainly affected the other. Due to the philanthropy of several Whites, Watts Hospital was opened in 1895, along with the Watts Hospital Training School for Nurses. But these institutions were exclusively for the White citizens of Durham.

In 1901 Lincoln Hospital was incorporated and began operating for Colored citizens in a framed building on the corner of Proctor Street and Cozart Avenue. The voices of a few key people launched Lincoln Hospital as well as Lincoln Hospital Nurse Training School, which followed in 1903. Dr. Albert G. Carr, who had championed the cause for hospitals in Durham, was behind the movement for both Lincoln and Watts Hospitals. Dr. Carr was the family physician for the Dukes, a prominent Durham family. Mr. W. H.

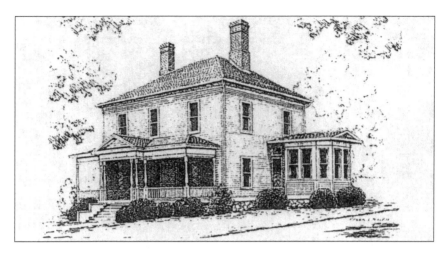

Original Lincoln hospital established in 1901. Courtesy of Durham County Hospital Corporation Archives.

Armstrong, Dr. Carr's butler, and Mrs. Addie Evans, his cook; Dr. Aaron M. Moore, Durham's first Negro physician; Mr. John Merrick, a leading Negro citizen and barber for the Dukes; and Dr. Stanford Lee Warren, an obstetrician, convinced Mr. Washington Duke that a hospital where the Negro descendants of slaves could be treated with dignity and respect would be more serviceable than a monument. Thus began Lincoln Hospital.

Dr. Moore served twenty-two years as the first superintendent of Lincoln Hospital, from its inception until his death in 1923. He was recognized for his labors as a physician, administrator, entrepreneur, and businessman as well as for his deep religious convictions.

The original charter of the board of trustees of Lincoln Hospital authorized the establishment of a training school for Colored nurses. It stated, "As such corporation they may establish, conduct and maintain a hospital in the county of Durham, for the reception and treatment of persons of the colored race, who may need medical or surgical attendance during temporary sickness or injury, and for the training of nurses under such rules and regulations as they may from time to time establish."

Lincoln Hospital Nurse Training School was founded in 1903 and incorporated into Lincoln Hospital in 1905 through the concerted efforts of Dr. Charles Shepard, one of the original pioneers and leaders of Lincoln Hospital, and Ms. Julia Latta. Ms. Latta, a registered nurse and a graduate of

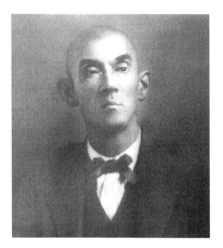

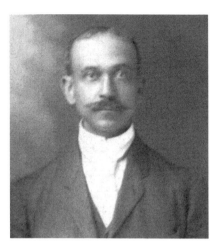

Dr. Aaron M. Moore, founder and first superintendent of Lincoln Hospital, 1901–1923. Courtesy of Andre Vann, North Carolina Central University Archives.

Dr. Stanford L. Warren, influential in the founding of Lincoln Hospital. Courtesy of Andre Vann, North Carolina Central University Archives.

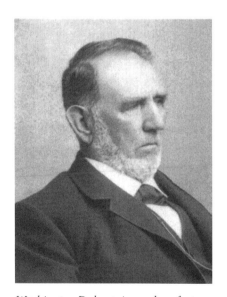

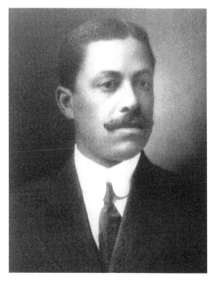

Washington Duke, primary benefactor in establishing Lincoln Hospital. Courtesy of Semans Family Papers, David M. Rubenstein Rare Book & Manuscript Library, Duke University.

John Merrick, influential in the founding of Lincoln Hospital. Courtesy of Andre Vann, North Carolina Central University Archives.

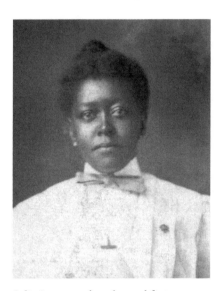 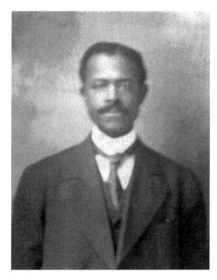

*Julia Latta, co-founder and first
superintendent of nursing service
and Lincoln Hospital Nurse Training
School.* Courtesy of Andre Vann and
Martha Donnell, North Carolina Central
University Archives.

*Dr. Charles Shepard, co-founder of
Lincoln Hospital Nurse Training School,
second superintendent of Lincoln
Hospital, 1924–1934.* Courtesy of Andre
Vann, North Carolina Central University
Archives.

St. Agnes Hospital School of Nursing in Raleigh, was the first superintendent of nursing, a position she held from 1903 to 1911.

Ms. Latta served in many roles. In addition to her administrative and educational roles, she supervised the cooking, housekeeping, and laundry for
the hospital. In 1907 the hospital employed only two paid employees: Ms.
Latta and a janitor.

The responsibilities Ms. Latta carried out were consistent with those of
other hospital nursing departments and nurse training schools at that time.
The North Carolina Board of Examiners for Trained Nurses revealed that
during the very early years of operation, most hospitals had a staff that consisted of only the superintendent and an orderly. This circumstance was
noted by the Inspector of Training Schools for Nurses, a position the board
established in 1917. The laws established by the state legislature authorized
the Board to create special positions.

Relationship Between Lincoln Hospital Nurse Training School and Lincoln Hospital

The relationship between Lincoln Hospital, its nursing service, and the training of its nursing students was a close one. Responsibility for the school was delegated to the superintendent of nursing, who performed the dual roles of supervising the nursing service as well as the nurse training school. The budget for the training school was integrated into the hospital budget; operations for the school were listed as line items in that budget. Over time the graduate nursing staff came to share the responsibility for patient care and the teaching of new students. Their salaries were apportioned between the hospital and nurse training school.

During the early years, students provided the majority of the patient care in the hospital. In addition, they also provided home care in the community. This care in private homes was a source of income for the hospital. The Board of Examiners for Nurse Training Schools in North Carolina and the Standardization Board viewed the practice of sending students into private homes as undesirable. By the 1930s the practice had been discontinued.

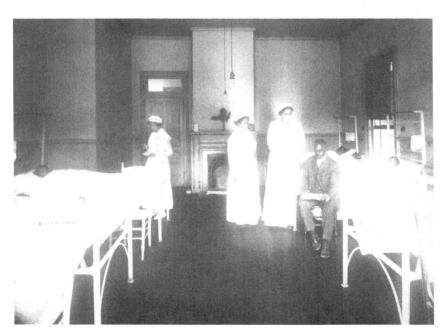

Hospital ward rounds with Dr. Joseph Napoleon Bonaparte Mills in the Pediatric Unit. Courtesy of Carolyn Evangeline Henderson.

The value of the nursing students to the operation of the hospital can be confirmed by the fact that in 1914, after thirteen years of operation, Lincoln Hospital had on its payroll only two paid employees. The rest of the patient care was carried out by thirteen nursing students. During this time the hospital averaged between fifty and seventy-five patients. It is obvious that the majority of the care was being provided by students.

BACKGROUND AND DEVELOPMENT OF NURSE TRAINING IN NORTH CAROLINA

North Carolina has the distinction of being the first state in the nation to pass a law requiring nurses to carry a professional license. The hallmark of a profession is the ability to establish and hold its members accountable to standards of practice. These standards relate to the preparation for nursing, admission criteria, the curriculum and requirements for registration, and professional practice.

In 1903, a bill entitled "An Act to Provide for State Registration for Trained Nurses in North Carolina" was passed. The bill established a minimum standard against which all graduate nurses would be evaluated for licensure as well as the composition of the Board of Examiners for Nurse Training Schools of North Carolina.

Since 1903, all nurse training schools, including Lincoln Hospital Nurse Training School, have been regulated by this board. In addition to establishing the Board of Examiners, the bill authorized the members of the board to determine the number of examinations to be given, the subject areas to be examined, and the qualifications to be required of applicants. These qualifications consisted of being of good moral character and being at least twenty-one years of age. Subjects on the examinations included Elements of Anatomy and Physiology; Medical, Surgical, Obstetrical and Practical Nursing; Invalid Cookery; and Household Hygiene. The members of the Board of Examiners consisted of both doctors and nurses. These individuals developed the examinations and determined which ones they would individually administer. A 70-percent passing rate on the examination was required. The examiners attempted to ground the examination in the realities of nursing practice. Most of the questions related to current health issues. Each examination area had between ten and fourteen questions and candidates were to choose between seven and ten questions to answer, as specified in the directions.

MEDICAL NURSING

Maria P. Allen, R. N.

EXAMINER

Greensboro, N. C., Nov. 18, 19, 20, 1919

1. State difference in general treatment between acute and chronic nephritis.

2. How long should a thermometer stay in the mouth? rectum? axilla? and what is the difference in degrees between the first two? The usual "one-minute" thermometer being considered.

3. Describe the pulse in severe hemorrhage; in the early part of typhoid fever; and in a case of apoplexy.

4. Describe the treatment of inflammatory rheumatism and nursing care.

5. What are rales and in what diseases are they found?

6. Name 4 parts of the body that may be attacked by tuberculosis.

7. Give treatment of pellagra.

8. What medical treatment is used to relieve an attack of angina pectoris?

9. Name a condition for which each of the following treatments is given: Tepid bath; Brand bath; cold pack; salt rub; hot pack.

10. Give names of two self-limited diseases and two functional diseases.

11. Describe briefly all the methods you know that may be used to stop persistent vomiting.

12. Describe the various appearances of blood in stools and the cause in each case.

13. How does the tongue appear in typhoid fever in the beginning? and during the course of the disease?

14. (a) What is sordes? (b) What is the treatment of it and the danger from it in typhoid fever?

North Carolina Board of Examiners Examination Questions on medical nursing in 1919. Courtesy of North Carolina State Archives.

The board granted a license, which authorized use of the professional title "registered nurse" (RN), upon satisfactory completion of the licensure examination. Nurses who were already practicing prior to the enactment of the bill could also be granted a license by the board. While they did not have to take the examination, they did have to demonstrate evidence of competency or achieve a rating satisfactory to the board. They also had to register their license with the clerk of the superior court and pay the specified licensing fee of fifty cents.

Practicing nurses from other states were allowed to register in North Carolina without examination. The requirements for such registration included the following: a diploma from a reputable training school connected with a general hospital in which medical, surgical, and obstetrical cases were treated; documentation of a minimum of two years work experience at one of the three state hospitals in North Carolina for the insane; or presentation of a certificate signed by three registered physicians stating that the applicant had pursued nursing for at least two years and was in their opinion competent to practice. All nurses who met any one of above requirements were to be registered by the clerk of the court.

The Board of Examiners was constantly revising the rules in order to upgrade nurse training and nursing practice. Of particular interest was the revision in 1917, which stipulated after June 1 no one could practice as a trained, graduate, licensed, or registered nurse in North Carolina without first obtaining a license through the Nurses Examining Board. Nurses already practicing could register without examination because of the passage of the Act-Waiver of February 2, 1917, which was extended to cover the June 1, 1917, revision. The law also specified that the Board would be renamed the Board of Examiners of Trained Nurses of North Carolina. Additionally, the law provided for the inspection of training schools. While the eligibility requirements for registration were essentially unchanged, the subject areas for examination were expanded to include Nursing of Children, Contagious Diseases, and Ethics of Nursing.

Two years later, in 1919, the law was amended to encourage better-educated women to enter the profession, perhaps on the assumption that doing so would increase the pool of qualified applicants for nurse training. To enhance the recruitment of better-prepared women, the amendment provided: "Training schools for nurses may give such credit for college work, on the three year course as they may deem wise, such credit not to total more than one year for any one person." The amendment was also aimed at increasing the production of nurses in order to meet post–World War I health-care needs.

(continues on page 19)

Minnie Canarah Lyon, RN '29
(1886–1991)

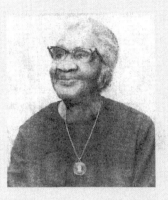

Minnie Canarah Lyon, the second of four children born to Luster and Della Hester Lyon, began her life in Granville County, North Carolina, about two miles from Oxford, in 1886. Her established birth date is December 25.

She attended Person County public schools and later Mary Potter Academy, a high school from which she graduated in 1915. Following graduation, Minnie taught for one term at the Northside School, near Oxford. She then moved to Durham, where she did domestic work because teaching afforded her little income.

In the fall of 1916 Minnie attended the Woman's Convention of North Carolina meeting in annual session at the White Rock Baptist Church, in Durham, pastored by Dr. Benjamin Brawley. It was here that she offered herself as a missionary to the foreign field. Dr. A. M. Moore, a local physician, was in the audience and volunteered to sponsor Sister Lyon's education at the Religious Training School at Chatauqua (now North Carolina Central University, founded by Dr. James E. Shepard). Minnie completed her degree at Chatauqua and continued her education in preparation for greater services to God by doing post-graduate work at Spellman Seminary in Atlanta, Georgia. Dr. Moore financed this part of her education as well. After a semester at Spellman, Minnie returned to Durham, North Carolina, and took nurse's training at Lincoln Hospital. However, she was able to finish only half the requirements for graduation.

In 1921, Minnie accompanied Dr. and Mrs. William H. Thomas to Brewerville, Liberia, in West Africa, where she served as an instructor and nurse in the mission station erected and maintained by the Lott Carey Foreign Mission Convention of the United States. Dr. and Mrs. Thomas were pioneers in the development of the Lott Carey Program in Liberia. Minnie worked conscientiously alongside them to answer the call of service to these people who lived in what was then a dark continent of the world.

Feeling that she needed more training to minister to the ills of those she served, as well as to carry to them the message of the Gospel, Minnie returned to Durham and completed the requirements for a professional nursing degree, thereby becoming a registered nurse (RN).

Continuing to answer the call to advance her training, Minnie took post-graduate work in public health at Harlem School of Nursing in New

York City. She returned to Africa a year after graduation and worked there until 1937. Somehow she was not satisfied with the support the mission was getting from her Christian friends in the States, so, in the spring of 1937, she returned to North Carolina. Under the auspices of the Lott Carey Convention, Minnie traveled throughout North Carolina and other states recruiting for the foreign fields and trying to interest more Baptists in supporting the foreign missionary program.

In the fall of 1937, Minnie returned to Africa and continued her outstanding work with the people she had learned to love so much. It was during this time that she met a little girl whom she called Hawa and took with her to the mission station to be taught the rudiments of the mission school. Minnie worked there until 1946, when she returned to the United States. She stayed in North Carolina and traveled for the Lott Carey Convention as a returned missionary. Two years later, she returned to Africa. She continued her work in the mission school until 1951. She then returned to North Carolina, where she retired from the foreign field and made her home in Durham. In 1961, she was instrumental in getting the Women's Baptist Home and Foreign Missionary Convention of North Carolina to bring Hawa to the United States. Hawa entered Shaw University, in Raleigh, North Carolina, to train for service as a teacher and missionary to her people in Africa. After completing the requirements for the bachelor's degree, Hawa returned to Africa and began working just as she had wanted so much to do, helping her African friends and trying to point them toward a better life. Thus, for Minnie, another dream had become a reality, and Hawa was certainly another star in her crown. Hawa was one of a number of African students from the mission school at Brewerville who had crossed the mighty ocean to train in an American school and then return to their native land to help others.

One would think that after such a full life of service to others Minnie would take to the familiar rocking chair of the retired and rest and rock for the duration of her life. But not Minnie. After returning to North Carolina, she continued to travel innumerable miles to carry the "light of the Gospel" to young people and encourage them to give their lives to the foreign fields and to seek financial support for the Lord's work. She did not miss a single annual session of the Woman's Baptist Home and Foreign Mission Convention until her health began to decline. Although her vision was very poor and she was nearly blind, her face lit up with a child-like radiance when she was asked to speak or to bring greetings to some church or conference. She believed that the Master had commanded her to serve to the end of her days and that only He could command her to lay down her sword and shield and come on home to rest forevermore.

(Ms. Lyon's story was compiled from her obituary published by Fisher Funeral Parlor, Inc., Durham, North Carolina.)

Based on an interview with Ms. Minnie Canarah Lyon, who entered LHSN in 1918, it seems the earliest admission standards for the school included good health, stamina, and a good recommendation. Ms. Lyon stated that LHSN's admission requirements were, first, a high-school education and, second, a good recommendation. A high-school education at this time was the equivalent of one year. Although Ms. Lyon entered in 1918, she did not complete the program of training at that time and instead traveled to Africa to begin teaching and providing care in the Lott Carey Mission as a missionary, caregiver, and educator. The ills and conditions confronting her there convinced her of the need for more nursing education and training. She returned to LHSN and graduated in 1929.

Documentation of the early years of Lincoln Hospital Nurse Training School is very sketchy. It is possible that additional information exists, but it was not found during this search. Information such as where the early students came from and how they spent their time was not available. The early students probably hailed from North Carolina and throughout the Northeast because only two schools existed in North Carolina at that time, St. Agnes and Lincoln. It is also probably safe to say that they spent their time working, working, working. Ms. Lyon could remember only working day after day, all day long, and attending demonstrations by the doctors and the superintendent. There was also time for prayer and meditation, which was a source of comfort and strength for enduring the rigors of training and patient care.

During the first eight years of the nurse training school, 1903–1911, and under the leadership of Ms. Latta, seventeen nurses graduated. However, records were not available to quantify the number of students enrolled throughout her tenure as superintendent of nursing. A 1923 Report records that the first students graduated in 1907. Given that the school was incorporated into the hospital in 1905 and it opened as a two-year program, it is plausible that the first graduates could have been in 1907. The first years of the nurse training school were likely consumed with taking care of the few patients at the hospital, along with organizing and establishing procedures and regulations for the training school. Finding the names of the earliest graduates was exciting, and consequently I have included them here:

1907   Elizabeth Spruell
Marie Antonette Gray
Elizabeth Dwane
Theda Elenor Williams
Cora L. Harris
Kate E. Creasman

1908 Pearl R. Moore
      Addie Ernestine Largin

1909 Willie F. Jones
      Mattie M. Graves
      Neil S. McKenzie
      Nannie P. Watkins

1910 Clara Lockhart
      Bettie A. Coles

1911 Emma Richardson
      Mary E. Jeffreys
      Pearl Henderson (In 1911, Ms. Henderson became a public health
      nurse with the Durham County Health Department, providing care
      to the Negro citizens of Durham.)

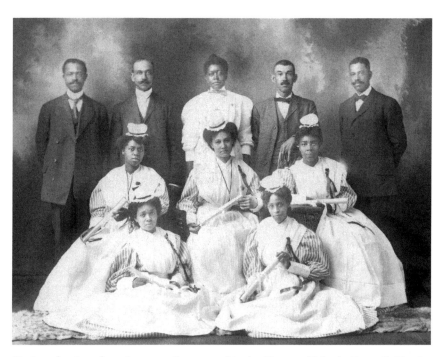

First graduation class circa 1907. Courtesy of Andre Vann and Martha Donnell, North
Carolina Central University Archives.

The earliest photograph of Lincoln Hospital Nurse Training School graduates is believed to date to 1907 and shows five graduates as well as Ms. Latta,
Dr. Aaron M. Moore, Dr. Charles Shepard, Dr. Stanford L. Warren, and Dr.
John Merrick (the photograph itself is undated). The 1907 graduate class lists
six graduates, but as the school's practice was to admit students whenever
there was a vacancy, their graduation dates varied. Also, there are other instances when the list of graduates and those in graduation photos do not
match. Perhaps some students missed the photo opportunity. The next graduation class pictured is that of 1914 along with the commencement exercise
and diploma.

Upon Ms. Latta's departure in 1911, Ms. Patricia "Pattie" H. Carter became
the superintendent of nurses, supervising, like her predecessor, both nursing services and the nurse training school. She served in this dual role for
twenty-five years. She was the daughter of Hawkins W. Carter, a representative and state senator from Warren County during the Reconstruction period. Her early education was in the Warren County schools. Later she went
to Shaw University, St. Agnes Hospital
in Raleigh, and Lincoln Hospital School
of Nursing in New York City. The organization of graduate nurses from Lincoln
Hospital School of Nursing in New York
City was later named the Pattie H. Carter
Nurses Club in her honor.

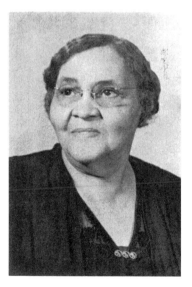

Ms. Carter received a license in North
Carolina by waiver in 1918. In 1935 she became assistant superintendent of Lincoln
Hospital. After her retirement in 1947, she
purchased a house on the corner of Merritt Street and Massey Avenue and lived
there until her death in 1950. Ms. Carter
was fondly called "Ma Carter" by many
of the nursing students. Lois Clements
Brown Thorpe, a 1948 graduate, characterized her as a stern disciplinarian, but
kind. Ms. Carter assured that the standards for competent nursing practice
were followed.

*Patricia "Pattie" Hawkins Carter,
superintendent of nursing services
and Nurse Training School,
1911–1935. Reprinted from The
Scalpel, 1948.*

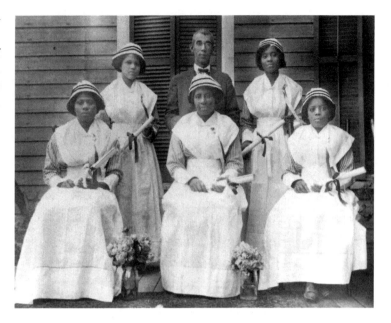

Graduating class of 1914. Courtesy of North Carolina Department of Cultural Resources.

Commencement Exercise of 1914. Courtesy of North Carolina Department of Cultural Resources.

COMMENCEMENT EXERCISES

....OF....

Lincoln Hospital Nurse Training School

MONDAY EVENING, MAY 18, 1914

Motto: "Give to the world the best you have and the best will come back to you"

Program

Music	
Invocation	Rev. Lewis
Music	
Annual Address	Dr. C. D. Hill
Music	
Presentation of Diplomas	Dr. J. O. Plummer
Music	
Presentation Prizes	Dr. W. C. Strudwick
Music	
Presentation Nurse Pins	Mrs. Ada M. Thornton
Music	
Remarks and Collection	Dr. A. M. Moore and Mr. J. M Avery
The Merrick Prize	Miss Anna E. Hill
The C. C. Spaulding Prize	Miss Clarissa E. Dukes
The J. E. Weaver Prize	Miss Gertrude L. Patterson
The Dr. A. M. Moore Prize	Miss Gertrude L. Patterson
The Dr. S. L. Warren Prize	Miss Anna E. Hill
The Dr. J. N. Mills Prize	Miss Margie D. Alston
The Dr. W. C. Strudwick Prize	Misses Alston and Hill
The Miss Carter Prize	Miss Cornelia E. Lewis

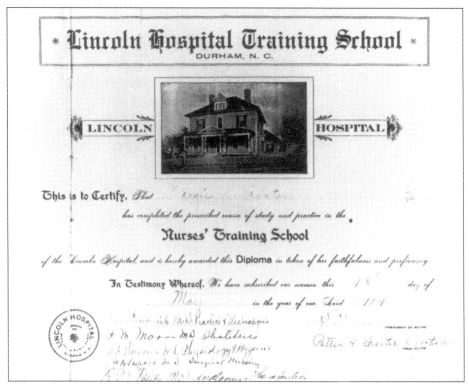

Diploma of a 1914 graduate. Courtesy of North Carolina Department of Cultural Resources.

STANDARDS FOR LINCOLN HOSPITAL
NURSE TRAINING SCHOOL

Admissions

Because the health-care conditions in the community were so poor, it was obvious that student recruits should be in good physical condition and have a desire to serve others. It was important that the students be strong and fit to endure the rigors of training and the work of caring for patients. The requirements for recruiting and training nursing students were described by the Board of Examiners in a North Carolina Nurse Training Schools document entitled "What the Board Understands as Training Given Nurses in a Training School Connected with a General Hospital." These requirements are as follows: not less than twenty years of age; program, three years in length; a high school diploma; a probationary period of not less than two months; a class term of at least eight months; written reviews every quarter, including examinations at the end of each term or completion of any subject; content to be taught by lecture, including illustrations, demonstrations, and theoretical work; passing creditable examinations; and having read one good reference textbook for nurses on the following subjects: Nursing, Anatomy and Physiology, Materia Medica, Hygiene and Sanitation, Surgical-Medical, Obstetrical Nursing, Nursing Ethics, Dietetics, and Practical Experience. Each pupil should have the care of not less than eight cases of typhoid fever, five cases of pneumonia, and other medical cases in due proportion. The required experience and classroom content reflected the health-care problems common at the time; both tuberculosis and typhoid fever were widespread in the community.

Standards and Curriculum

Lincoln Hospital Nurse Training School was especially interested in recruiting students who genuinely desired to be a nurse and were committed to serving humanity. As documented in some of the early Board of Trustee Reports (specifically those issued in 1914 and 1916), it appears that Lincoln Hospital Nurse Training School, owing to its outstanding leadership, worked vigorously to achieve compliance with the early board standards. The earliest documented admissions requirement uncovered in the course of research for this book appears in a 1923 financial report for Lincoln Hospital. The requirements are described in the following paragraph.

The superintendent of nursing was also mindful of the board requirements, as reflected in the application for entry into Lincoln Hospital Nurse Training School, entitled "Nurse Training School With A Standard Three-Year Course, Lincoln Hospital, Durham, N. C., Application for Admission." Applicants were required to write a one-hundred-word essay on the subject of "Why I Want To Become A Nurse." This essay was to demonstrate the applicant's potential commitment to nursing as well as her level of proficiency in the English language. The possession of a good moral character and physical health were key. These attributes were to be confirmed by two letters about the student's moral character and a physician's certificate of good health, respectively. The responsibility and intimacy inherent in providing care to patients required that students be emotionally mature; therefore, an age requirement of between twenty and forty years was established.

Lincoln Hospital Nurse Training School began with a two-year training program, and classes were admitted twice per year. If there was a vacancy because someone left the program, it was filled as soon as possible. It is not

LINCOLN HOSPITAL

NURSES TRAINING SHOOL

APPLICATION BLANK

What is your age?............................Weight?...............Height?...............

What is your present and former occupation?..........................

....

Are you in robust health?.................When were you last confined to bed

by illness? ....

Give disease, date and duration ....

Have you lost mother, father, sister or brother with consumption.............

Have you ever attended a nurses' training school? If so, give name,

....

Are you married, single or widowed?...

Where were you educated and to what extent?.....................................

Give name of parent or guardian..

Have you ever had scrofula or blood disease?.......................................

Are you subject to nervousness?...

Do you suffer with severe menstrual pains?...

Do you pledge to remain in training for three years?.............................

Signed...
                                                              (Applicant)

Address..

C. H. SHEPARD, Supt.
DURHAM, N. C.

Do not come until notified of your acceptance.

1923 application to Lincoln Hospital Nurse Training School. Courtesy of Durham
County Hospital Archives.

known whether the initial two-year training program required students to sign a contract, but when the program was extended to three years in 1915, students were required to sign a contract to complete the full three years. The student could, however, be dismissed for misconduct or inefficiency. If the candidate met all the requirements, they were accepted on probation for six months for what was later called the preclinical period. This period lengthened throughout the program of study from two to nine months. Successful completion of the preclinical period resulted in official admission to the program.

According to the instructions to applicants, students initially had to supply their own uniforms, which consisted of two dark-blue-wash dresses, four aprons, low rubber-heeled, easy-fitting shoes, and an adequate number of undergarments. Once students had successfully completed the preclinical period and were fully accepted into the program, they received uniforms to be worn while on duty consisting of dresses with long sleeves, detachable cuffs, and detachable aprons that extended from the neck to the hem of the dress and crisscrossed in the back at the waist.

The students' health care was the responsibility of the hospital and School of Nursing. If students became ill, they were treated free of cost for a reasonable period of time, but time lost had to be made up before graduation. This rule persisted through the duration of the school. Many students, myself included, had to make up time after graduation.

FUNDING THE COST OF ATTENDING LINCOLN

Although this book spans several time periods, this topic is addressed for the school's total years of operation because of the limited amount of information available. The first class of students in the nurse training school paid no fees; they received lodging, board, and laundry. Later, when the program was expanded to three years, students were compensated $3 per month for all three years. The monthly stipend paid each student varied over the years from $2 to $4.

In the 1920s and 1930s the cost of attending Lincoln was $25. Josephine Demmons McBride, who entered the school in 1933, stated she paid $25 dollars upon entry. Clara Josephine Miller Harris, another alumnus, reported that in the 1940s the tuition was about $90 per year. The cost continued to increase, and by the 1960s the three-year program cost approximately $900, or $300 per year. The last class of students entered Lincoln in 1968. The cost of the three-year program was by then $1,080. Although these rates were

```
                        LINCOLN HOSPITAL
                      1301 Fayetteville Street
                       Durham, North Carolina

               LINCOLN HOSPITAL SCHOOL OF NURSING

                        FEES & EXPENSES

                           FIRST YEAR
                          First Semester

Tuition - Lincoln Hospital------------------------------- $  100.00
Tuition - North Carolina College------------------------     106.25
Books --------------------------------------------------      40.00
Uniforms (Lab Coat, 6 Uniforms, 1 Cape, Buttons, &
        Name Tapes)-------------------------------------      85.00
Health Fee ---------------------------------------------      10.00
Student Nurses Assoc. Fee ------------------------------       5.50
Achievement Test ---------------------------------------       3.00
TOTAL --------------------------------------------------------$  349.75
        TO BE PAID UPON RECEIPT OF YOUR
        ACCEPTANCE LETTER------------------------------     100.00
        TO BE PAID ON ADMISSION-------------------------     249.75


                         Second Semester

Tuition - North Carolina College------------------------      77.50
        (TO BE PAID ON OR BEFORE JANUARY 1st)
Achievement Test ---------------------------------------       7.50
Books --------------------------------------------------      30.00
TOTAL --------------------------------------------------------$  115.00

                          SECOND YEAR

Tuition - Lincoln Hospital ----------------------------- $  100.00
Books --------------------------------------------------      40.00
Health Fee ---------------------------------------------      12.00
Achievement Test ---------------------------------------       6.00
Breakage Fee -------------------------------------------      10.00
Field Trips --------------------------------------------       5.00
Uniforms (set of six (6) -------------------------------      85.00
TOTAL --------------------------------------------------------$  258.00

                          THIRD YEAR

Tuition - Lincoln Hospital ----------------------------- $   50.00
Books --------------------------------------------------      25.00
Field Trips --------------------------------------------       8.00
Achievement Test ---------------------------------------       5.00
School Pin ---------------------------------------------      10.00
Diploma ------------------------------------------------       5.00
*AFFILIATIONS
        Pediatric - $130.00
        Psychiatric- 125.00 ----------------------------.     255.00

TOTAL --------------------------------------------------------$   358.00

TOTAL THREE YEAR PROGRAM                                  $1,080.75

* Travel Expense not included

THE ABOVE FEES MAY VARY ACCORDING TO CURRENT COST
```

Cost of attendance from the late 1960s through the 1970s. Courtesy of Annie Lee Phillips.

not exorbitant, many students and families had a hard time paying the fees. Over the years scholarship funds and loans became available through the Medical Care Commission, churches, and other agencies. Students also had the opportunity to work extra hours outside of scheduled tours of duty and thereby earn some extra money. The practice of students working additional hours for pay continued through the 1960s. Students were proud to have been able to earn money with which to purchase needed supplies and clothing. As a senior nursing student, I bought my first piece of clothing with the money I earned from working extra shifts. Many other students shared my experience.

EDUCATION AND TRAINING

Clinical Experience

Because the program was extended from two to three years in 1915, there were no graduates in 1917. Early school records document that the students were taught by practical demonstration and hands-on experience. The emphasis was on practical and theoretical instruction in medical, surgical, and obstetrical nursing, the care and feeding of infants and children, and the cooking and serving of meals for the sick. The superintendent of the nurse training school was assisted with classroom instruction by both White and Negro attending physicians. The nurse training schools relied on the physicians' availability and willingness to provide instruction, which was secondary to their medical practice. They taught classes related to their specialty areas. Ms. Lyon, who entered nursing school in 1918, remembers being taught by Dr. Joseph Napoleon Bonaparte Mills, who joined Lincoln Hospital in 1908 and continued to serve in numerous capacities until his retirement in 1958. At the end of each course, students sat for oral and written examinations, and those who passed were able to sit for board exams. This was the practice in hospitals throughout North Carolina, as confirmed in the records kept by the training school inspector, who surveyed hospital-based nurse training schools. The state legislature authorized the Board to establish the position of training school inspector in 1917 to improve the curriculum of training schools by establishing consistency in requirements, courses of study, and admission standards.

From the beginning of the school through the 1960s, the hours were long and the work was hard. Student nurses were treated as laborers. For example, senior students, with supervision, were placed in charge of an entire ward. Prior to graduation, students were on duty six days a week, usually for

(continues on page 30)

Marian (Smith) Smith, RN '57, BSN

My name is Marian (Smith) Smith and my story describes a trip through Lincoln Hospital School of Nursing (LHSN). There were incidents that were joyful and some that were traumatic. I enjoyed most of my training, but I especially enjoyed obstetrics, emergency nursing, and the operating rooms. It was under the steady and firm hand of Mrs. L. B. Thompson, operating room supervisor, and my advisors, Margaret Goodwin and Frances Williams, that I blossomed as a nurse and made health care my career.

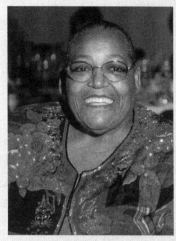

Under the direction of Mrs. Thompson, I was allowed to work in the operating room. I assumed the on-call duties and was paid a salary. This was after I had completed my classes in my senior year.

Courtesy of Marian (Smith) Smith.

I graduated in September 1957 and received the award for "Most Pleasing Personality" as well as the J. W. V. Cordice award for "Operating Room Technique." My first employment was with Old Emergency Hospital, in Washington, D.C. Within two weeks I was alternating head nurse. The hospital later combined with two others and became what is now the Washington Hospital Center.

In June 1958, I married Leslie D. Smith and from this union we were blessed with five beautiful children. I moved from the Washington Hospital Center to the operating room at Children's Hospital and remained there until my first child was born. I spent my next thirteen years doing private-duty nursing at all the major hospitals in Washington, D.C. I cared for physicians, priests, and many entrepreneurs. Most notable among the people I cared for was the mother of U.S. Attorney Harold Titus and the Honorable Senator Eugene McCarthy.

Once my children were all in school, I sought employment with the D.C. Department of Corrections. After eight years I moved to the John Howard Pavilion at St. Elizabeth's Hospital, where I held positions in forensic psychiatry. While working at John Howard Pavilion, I received my bachelor of science degree in nursing from Marymount University in Arlington, Virginia. I retired from the Department of Corrections on March 31, 1995. On May 8, 1995, I was recognized and honored by the Sigma Theta Tau International Honor Society of Nursing as one of "100 Extraordinary Nurses."

At present, I am active with my church as chairperson for the "Seasoned Saints" Ministry. We have bible study and exercise in an attempt to help us stay mobile and healthy. In addition to my five children, I now have thirteen grandchildren and seventeen great grandchildren.

twelve hours a day. This was routine at nurse training schools in the early years. My conversations with alumni who graduated during the 1930s, 1940s, and 1950s reveal long hours spent in work and study. The Board's position on hours of duty per day and week is telling:

> No medical or surgical institution nor agent or employee of the same in this state shall require, or cause to be required, any student to remain on duty for more than eighty hours in any week, or to remain on duty for a longer period than twelve hours in any day of twenty four hours, except in special and emergency cases. In such cases any student may be required to remain on duty for a period of sixteen hours in twenty-four provided that sleeping facilities are furnished in the room in which special duty is required, and that an opportunity is given the student to sleep for at least half the period on a special day.

EARLY STUDENT HOUSING

The early trend in nurse training schools was for students to live in hospital quarters, which typically were housed either in the basement or on the top floor under the roof. In the case of Lincoln Hospital, however, this seems not to have been the case. Two references give us some notion of the Lincoln nursing students' early living quarters. The caption to an image of the original hospital presented by the Endangered Durham Series reports that in 1910 an addition was made for the purpose of accommodating "nurses quarters." A 1916 hospital report also provides some information about the living arrangement of the nursing students: "The addition of a nurses home fills a long felt need and gives increased and much needed space for private patients. All Lincoln Nursing Students were required to live in the nurses' home, a frame house near the hospital." This report was signed by Ms. Pattie H. Carter, matron and head nurse; John Merrick, president of the Board of Trustees; and A. M. Moore, superintendent. So perhaps there was another building that no longer exists.

Wherever the students lived, they spent most of their waking hours in training and providing care for the patients. The rigors of training, caring for patients, cleaning, cooking, and doing whatever else was necessary allowed little time for recreation or social activity. Students looked inward for strength, resilience, and faith. It is likely that the training schools' first twenty-plus years of operation consisted of long hours of hospital and class work with little time for play.

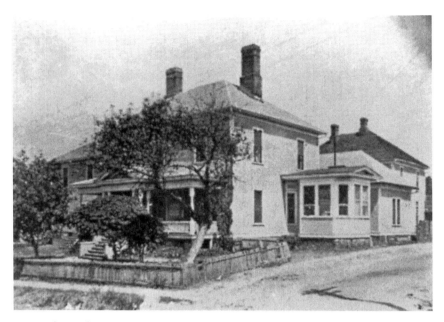

Original Lincoln Hospital with addition circa 1910–1912, located at the corner of Proctor and Cozart Streets. Endangered Durham Series. Courtesy of Andre Vann, North Carolina Central University Archives.

SUMMARY

The conditions in Durham and the lack of health care for Negro citizens were the driving forces for the establishment of Lincoln Hospital and its nurse training school. Over time, as Lincoln Hospital developed, a number of noteworthy events occurred that placed it in high regard as a Negro community hospital. In 1925, Lincoln Hospital was approved by the American Medical Association for the training of interns and residents. Lincoln Hospital essentially became a training school for Negro doctors.

By 1923 the nurse training school had been in operation for twenty years and its foundation had been laid. Rules and regulations had been established. The school was working toward complying with board standards. Due to a limited nursing staff (comprising only the superintendent and one orderly), the students were providing the majority of patient care while at the same time completing their training and becoming licensed to practice. The hospital was in higher demand and it needed more space to operate owing to post–World War I casualties and a fire in 1922 that had destroyed part of the building. Land for a new hospital was bought in 1917 on Fayetteville Street and donated by John Sprunt Hill. The Stokes Home on the old Stokesdale property was also donated. This house served as the student residence for the preclinical period as well as the residence for graduate nurses employed at Lincoln Hospital. Thus began the planning for the new hospital, nurses' residence, and school. Dr. Moore, founder and superintendent of Lincoln Hospital, died in 1923 before the new hospital and nurses' training school were complete. His death was a tremendous loss for Lincoln Hospital, the Nurse Training School, and the whole Negro community.

REFERENCES

A Tradition of Excellence: Pictorial History of Watts School of Nursing. Durham, N.C.: Watts School of Nursing, 2006.

Boyd, W. K. *Chapter XI Health Philanthropy and Relief: The Real Story of Durham, City of the New South.* Durham, N.C.: Duke University Press, 1927.

Carol, Edith, and Edna Scott. "Jubilee Hospital Department of Nursing." Henderson, N.C.: Henderson Institute Historical Museum, June 2012.

Certification of Amendment to the Charter of Trustees of Lincoln Hospital. 1901. Durham Regional Hospital Archives, Durham, N.C.

Certification of Incorporation of the Trustees of Lincoln Hospital. 1901. Durham Regional Hospital Archives, Durham, N.C.

Laws of 1907. 1907. North Carolina Board of Nurse Examiners. North Carolina State Archives, Raleigh, N.C.

Laws of North Carolina Board of Nurse Examiners. 1907. North Carolina State Archives, Raleigh, N.C. Legislation in North Carolina Brief Summary of the Nursing Laws Including Amendments and Revisions Public Laws of North Carolina, 1903. 1903. Section 1-10, Chapter 359, pp. 586–88. North Carolina State Archives, Raleigh, N.C.

Lincoln Hospital Annual Report of Hospital Operations, January 1–December 31, 1916. 1916. Durham Regional Hospital Archives, Durham, N.C.

Lincoln Hospital Report of Operations to the Durham City Alderman, 1914. 1914. Durham City Records and Archives, Durham, N.C.

Lincoln Hospital, Durham, North Carolina, Report of Hospital Operations: Financial Report, January 1 to December 31, 1923. 1923. Durham Regional Hospital Archives, Durham, N.C.

"Lincoln Hospital." Endangered Durham. http://endangereddurham.blogspot.com/2008/12/original-lincoln-hospital.html.

"Mary Seacole Biography." http://www.biography.com/people/mary-seacole-39430

McCall, Michael. "Lincoln Hospital School of Nursing Graduates: The Last Class." *Durham (N.C.) Morning Herald*, August 22, 1971.

Medical Examination Questions. 1919. North Carolina Board of Nurse Examiners. North Carolina State Archives, Raleigh, N.C.

"Medical History." *Journal of National Medical Association* 57, no. 2 (1965).

Minnie Caranah Lyons. Interview with the authors. March 1971.

Nurses Licensed in North Carolina by Waiver. 1919. North Carolina State Archives, Raleigh, N.C.

Patricia Jones. Interview with the author. May 12, 2012.

Resolution of Board of Trustees of Lincoln Hospital. 1901. Private Laws of North Carolina, Session 1901, Chapter 133. Durham Regional Hospital Archives, Durham, N.C.

Some Laws Controlling Hospitals in North Carolina in 1917. 1917. North Carolina Board of Medical Examiners. North Carolina State Archives, Raleigh, N.C.

Some Laws Controlling Hospitals in North Carolina in 1919. 1919. North Carolina Board of Nurse Examiners. North Carolina State Archives, Raleigh, N.C.

They Caught the Torch. Milwaukee: Will Ross, Inc., 1939.

Wyche, M. L. *Early North Carolina Hospitals: History of Nursing in North Carolina*. Chapel Hill, N.C.: University of North Carolina Press, 1938.

Wyche, M. L. *The Establishment of Negro Hospitals and the Progress of the Negro Nurses: History of Nursing in North Carolina*. Chapel Hill, N.C.: University of North Carolina Press, 1938.

Chapter Two

Period of Growth and Development, 1924–1944

M ANY LINCOLN GRADUATES fondly describe their school experience as an adventure. Others just speak about the good times and the blur of the bad, while still others characterize the experience as a journey. I am amazed by the creativity, talent, and recall of three outstanding graduates from 1924–1944. The musings of Ms. Josephine Demmons McBride, both poetic and spiritual, begin this part of the story.

The Class of 1936 started our journey on July 1, 1933. One hot July day, a heavily laden pilgrim marched up to the gates of Lincoln Hospital seeking admission to the Kingdom of Knowledge. This young woman was none other than Miss Mary Adams of Lynchburg, Virginia. This young lady worked diligently to prepare the way for other pilgrims who joined her later.

On August 15, 1933, four other pilgrims joined her. These were Misses Pearl Winbush of Bluefield, West Virginia, Dympha I. Brown of Boston, Massachusetts, Terri B. Isler of Kinston, North Carolina, and Jimmie Trammell of Lineville, Alabama. These students were greeted by Miss Adams and told of the many wonderful things Lincoln offered.

On September 1, 1933, three other very enthusiastic young women entered the gate, hoping to lighten the burden of those previously mentioned. They were Misses Elizabeth Ethengane of Scotland Neck, North Carolina, Willie Mae Wilkins of Roper, North Carolina, and Mary Ida Davis of Oxford, North Carolina.

On September 15, another group of pilgrims heard of the wayward travelers and decided to join them. They were Misses McLaurin of Elizabeth City, North Carolina, Evelyn H. Jeffreys of Burlington, North Carolina, Ethel Reid of Belmont, North Carolina, and Josephine Demmons of Greenville, South Carolina.

On September 19, as we were about to go forth on our journey, we heard a voice calling and, behold, it was Miss Gertrude Bullock from Bahama, North Carolina. We all greeted her and continued our journey as a band of thirteen. When we entered the gate, we found Miss P. H. Carter awaiting us. She was our beloved superintendent. She was very kind, loving, and motherly. Thus we were inspired to continue our three-year journey.

On September 20, 1933, thirteen of us entered the little room where we were to begin our class work. We spent the first week getting acquainted with our new subjects and hoping we would pass the preliminary period.

The class was organized with Miss Gertrude Bullock as president, Miss Ethengane as secretary, and Miss Winbush as treasurer. We toiled hard day by day, hoping the golden chain would not be broken. But one day Miss McLaurin decided that the farm was calling her and she must go and milk the cows. Miss Wilkins followed shortly.

Finally, the big day arrived when we were given our uniforms and caps. This meant that we had passed the preliminary period. We crashed out on the neighboring community of Lincoln Hospital as "The Nurses of 1936."

In March of 1934, Miss Bullock was selected as the "Miss Lincoln" contestant from our class. At the end of the contest Miss Bullock was crowned "Miss Lincoln," and she held that honor for three years.

The months continued to go by and again we found ourselves facing the second semester's exams. The report from the examination brought us joy because we had passed with creditable grades and without difficulty.

June 1934 brought sadness to our class. Another one of our classmates, Miss Ethengane, whom we dearly loved, departed. This left ten of us to continue the journey.

Vacation time was short, and we returned to our class to start our work for the 1934–1935 school session. New instructors greeted us and promised to help us on our journey. The months passed swiftly and at last we were ready to take our final exams. Again we conquered what we thought couldn't be done.

On September 29, 1935, one of our classmates decided that she preferred matrimony over nursing. This left nine lonely travelers. But as we were about to start on our last mile, we met four other strange travelers looking for a school where they could complete their training. So we asked them to join us at Lincoln Hospital, the Affiliating School for Nurses from the North Carolina Sanatorium. These nurses were Misses Mary McNeill, Polly Scott, Nola Harrington, and Phloy Frieson.

After each nurse had gotten acquainted with the new regime, another interesting person entered our travel. The aim of this person was to make us better fitted to overcome the many obstacles of nursing. This person was Miss Henrietta Forrest, our new superintendent of nurses. She has inspired us greatly and made our dark days seem brighter.

The second twenty-year period of the School of Nursing began with new facilities. A new hospital and a new nurses' residence and training school were completed in 1924. These new facilities represented tremendous growth and development for both the hospital and the school.

The new hospital facility increased the hospital's bed capacity by 44 percent, which in turn increased the number of nursing students needed to support the additional patient volume. The *Bulletin* of 1924 states, "Besides the head nurse at least two other graduate nurses will be needed immediately as we go to the new facility this first year, at least 20 student nurses will be required for the new hospital."

It is difficult to quantify this increase in student enrollment, but it could have represented as much as a 50-percent increase in the number of nursing students. During the early 1930s the School of Nursing graduated between seven and thirteen students each year.

NEW PHYSICAL FACILITIES

The new Lincoln Hospital, located at 1301 Fayetteville Street, in Durham, North Carolina, was completed in November 1924 and occupied the following January. The new hospital facility addressed the community's need for more inpatient beds. This need was driven by the increasing number of World-War-I casualties and by a fire that had partially destroyed the building in 1922. In addition to the eighty-seven new inpatient beds, the new hospital had an outpatient clinic area, a dietetic lab for nurse training, space for an autopsy room, and space for clinical labs and X-ray facilities. The new hospital was built at a cost of $75,000. As was the case with the original hospital, the new hospital benefited from the philanthropy of the Duke family. Messrs. J. B. Duke and B. N. Duke, sons of Mr. Washington Duke, offered to donate $75,000 for a new hospital, provided the community of Durham raised a similar amount. The city and county governments and the citizens of Durham, both Negro and White, rose to the occasion.

The new nurses' residence and training school on Linwood Avenue was a modern, well-appointed brick building. It was a gift from Mr. Benjamin N. Duke in memory of his son, Angier B. Duke. As a result the structure was

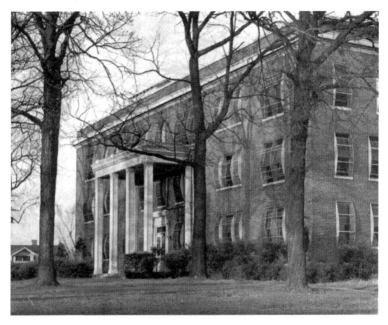

Exterior view of Lincoln Hospital in 1924. Reprinted from *The Scalpel*, 1946. Courtesy of Lois Smith Morris.

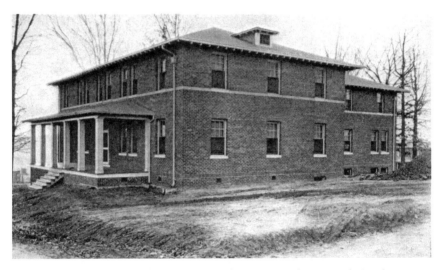

Angier B. Duke Nurses Home, Linwood Avenue, Durham, North Carolina.

named the Angier B. Duke Nurses Home. It was erected at a cost of $25,000. The home contained twenty-five bedrooms, general reception rooms, classrooms, a recreation room, a meditation room, a laundry, a library, and a science laboratory. The nurses' residence also consisted of live-in quarters for the superintendent, instructors, and housemothers.

From 1924 to 1944, the nursing students lived in either Stokes Nurses Home or Angier B. (A. B.) Duke Nurses Home. Stokes Nurses Home, located on Massey Avenue, was probably once one of the main houses on the Stokesdale property, which John Sprunt Hill had given to the Board of Trustees of Lincoln Hospital in 1917.

The new nurses' facility provided needed space for the students, faculty, and housemothers. The North Carolina Board of Examiners of Training Schools for Nurses required that students be monitored in their residence by the faculty of their nurse training school. Therefore, throughout the school's history students lived in one of the nurses' homes with the superintendent, instructors, and later the housemother. Ms. Josephine Demmons McBride, a

(continues on page 41)

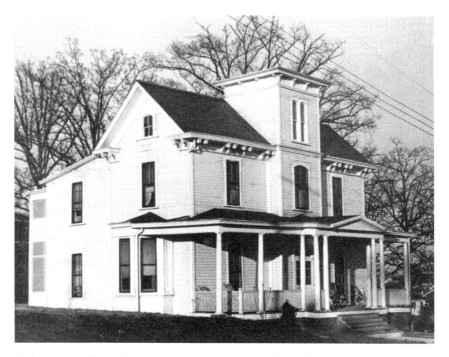

Stokes Nurses Home, Massey Avenue, Durham, North Carolina.

Life as a Beginning Student Nurse
Lincoln Hospital, Durham, North Carolina

Peggy Christine Jones Butts, RN '55
January 22, 2011

As beginning students, we were required to
undergo a full day of testing that included
physical, psychological, and course items.
Later, after about a month's time, you were
notified of whether you were accepted or
denied. A list describing supplies, suitcases,
foot lockers, prices, and so on were sent to
you.

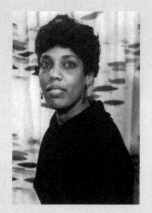

   A trial date of six months was allotted to
indicate whether you were a good candidate
and had passed all the coursework. They
were very strict with regard to attitude and
whether you were able to assimilate well.

   I was assigned to student quarters at Stokes
Nurses Home, a two-story, white frame
house with a large front porch on the hospital
grounds.

Courtesy of Peggy Christine
Jones Butts.

   I was one of four to share an upstairs bedroom with four bunk beds, two
desks, each one shared by two people, and a small closet shared by four
people.

   Lights out was between 10:00 and 11:00 p.m. and wake up time 6:00 a.m.
Then it was downstairs to the living room for morning Vespers or a
uniform check by housemother (Mama Bea).

   Once we passed the pre-clinical period, we went on to studying and
ward training with an instructor. We also took courses at North Carolina
College. And always there was church on Sunday.

   We started serious ward work or our clinicals in our junior year and
shift work in our senior year. We also were sent out of state for our pediatric and psychiatric clinicals in our senior year. This was in the early 1950s
(i.e., the era of segregation).

   As far as social activities went, you were definitely required to sign in
and out when you left campus (the school was very strict on this).

   In all, looking back, it was a very rewarding experience.

1936 graduate, stated, "I lived in A. B. Duke Nursing Home with Ms. Carter." Other alumni recalled living as preclinical students in Stokes on the second floor. Although the board permitted no more than two students to a room, Peggy Butts and Marion Miles recall sleeping in bunk beds with four to a room in Stokes. Marion was glad to sleep on the lower bunk.

Graduate nurses employed at the hospital lived on the first floor of Stokes. Students, upon completion of the preclinical period, which ranged from four to nine months, moved to Angier B. Duke Nurses Home. Be it Stokes or Angier B. Duke, this was a home away from home for the students. They had support and supervision throughout their entire training period, and the school leadership was an important part of that supervision.

LEADERSHIP

Ms. Patricia "Pattie" Carter, affectionately known as "Ma Carter," served as the second superintendent during a period of rapid growth for the hospital and its services and of increased demands on the School of Nursing from the North Carolina Board of Nursing Examiners. She led both the nursing staff and the school for twenty-three years, from 1912 to 1935. She was an organized leader and role model who exemplified total commitment and dedication as evidenced by her work ethic and her ability to manage all aspects of the hospital's operation and the students' training.

Ms. Carter was well respected by both students and hospital personnel. Her value to the hospital was so great that Dr. Charles Shepard, superintendent of the hospital, in 1924 recommended to the board of trustees that her salary be increased to $100 per month or $1,200 per year. The recommendation read, "Miss Carter has served us faithfully, doing the work of two or three women. She has been for years the head nurse, the anesthetist, bookkeeper, steward and practically everything. She has given to the hospital the best years of her life and out of our appreciation for her services (for which she has been underpaid) I ask that the board pay her twelve hundred dollars a year." According to the same report the board in 1922 had voluntarily raised her annual salary from $900 to $1,000, but she had never accepted the increase because in her opinion the hospital was not adequately financed to support that raise. By 1933 she was receiving a salary of $110 per month. She was the second-highest-paid employee following Dr. Shepard, who was superintendent of the hospital.

BOARD OF NURSING INFLUENCE

Nurse training programs continuously faced changing standards for nurse education and practice as implemented by the Board of Examiners for Nurse Training Schools in North Carolina. Two significant nursing law revisions occurred to the Nursing Law in 1925: first, the title of the board changed from the Board of Examiners of Nurse Training Schools for North Carolina to the Board of Nursing Examiners of North Carolina and, second, a standardization board was created to raise the eligibility requirements of applicants for licensure. The standardization board was charged with developing uniformity in the curriculum and in the rules and regulations governing nurse training schools. As a result of this change in the law, the Board of Nursing Examiners and the Standardization Board established a committee on the grading of nursing schools.

Following the establishment of the grading committee, a study was conducted to look at the supply and production of nurses, the average length of nurses' professional lives, and the conditions under which they worked. The training of nurses included the curriculum, the requirements for admission, and the educational requirements of instructors. The committee was composed of White men and women who were nominated either by the National Hospital Association or the Medical Association and by Nursing and Public Health organizations. In addition to medical personnel, people on the committee came from professional education organizations and the general public. Even though there were Negro doctor and Negro nurse organizations and associations, there was no representation of Negro doctors or nurses on this committee.

Some of the questions posed in the survey addressed whether there were too few or too many nursing schools; whether entrance requirements should be lowered to get more lower quality students or raised to get fewer, but higher quality, students; and whether hospitals would go out of business if they stopped functioning as educational institutions. Other questions focused on the motives behind hospitals' hosting of nurse training schools: was it to provide graduates for local needs, to maintain a stable hospital nursing service, or to save money? This study occurred over a period of three years. Nursing schools throughout the nation were surveyed in this study. A classification system was generated for rating all accredited Schools of Nursing throughout the United States. The rating was based on twenty factors including whether the nursing school had a separate Charter from the hospital, whether a high-school diploma was a requirement for admission, hospital size, daily census, and the availability of prepared instructors for the hospital-based schools of nursing.

According to the classification system of the North Carolina Grading Committee, the hospital-based nurse training schools had to employ instructors and supervisory staff specifically for the students. These staff included a night supervisor, a day supervisor, and a surgical nurse. This perhaps marked the beginning of nursing specialization. The surgical nurse, in addition to managing the affairs of the operating room, would be responsible for teaching the student nurses the details of patient preparation and operating-room techniques. Interestingly, at Lincoln Hospital the day nursing supervisor was responsible for the administration of anesthesia in the operating room. When no surgical nurse was available, these duties became the responsibility of the assistant superintendent of the hospital. Soon after the classification requirements for grading schools were established, Lincoln Hospital began to expand its nursing staff to meet the changing Board standards for nurse training.

Additionally, the report expressed concerns that an average daily census of twenty patients was the lowest census from which a student nurse could obtain proper clinical experience. Regarding high-school graduation, in 1925 only four schools in North Carolina required a high-school diploma and five schools had no educational requirements at all. By 1928 fifty-six schools in North Carolina required their students to be high-school graduates. The ratings based on the criteria for schools of nursing ranged from A to D. In 1928 LHSN was fully accredited and had an A rating. Lincoln met the requirements for admission, staffing, faculty, daily census, and patient admission. The requirement that nurse training schools have a separate charter from the hospital was being considered, according to the 1927 Lincoln Hospital annual report.

The addition of nurse instructors was an important part of LHSN's ability to meet the grading requirements for nurse training schools. In 1927, during Ms. Carter's tenure, the instructors for the school were as follows: Mrs. B. E. Jackson, RN, day supervisor; Miss E. E. Brown, RN, operating room supervisor and dietician; and Mrs. L. Hicks, house matron (housemother) for the students and laundry supervisor. Dr. Charles H. Shepard, MD, was superintendent and an instructor. The physicians, hospital attendings, and visiting staff continued to provide a major portion of the instruction for the nurse training school. The curriculum for the three years and the instructors for each course are presented in the 1927 Lincoln Hospital annual report.

The leadership role of the superintendent was extremely demanding and

36   ANNUAL REPORT OF LINCOLN HOSPITAL

SCHEDULE FOR CLASSES
SENIORS

Materia Medica .... Dr. J. N. Mills
History of Nursing .... Miss E. E. Brown
Obstetrics .... Dr. S. L. Warren
Communicable Diseases .... Dr. W. C. Strudwick
Anatomy .... Dr. J. S. Thompson
Principles and Practice of Nursing .... Miss B. E. Jackson
Urinalysis and Elements of Pathology .... Dr. L. L. Hall
Infant Feeding .... Dr. B. U. Brooks
Eye, Ear, Nose and Throat .... Dr. S. D. McPherson

FIRST AND SECOND YEARS

Dietetics .... Miss E. E. Brown
Bacteriology .... Dr. J. M. Hubbard
Materia Medica .... Dr. I. E. Turner
Gynecology .... Dr. J. W. V. Cordice
Obstetrics .... Dr. S. L. Warren
Ethics .... Miss P. H. Carter
Communicable Diseases .... Dr. W. C. Strudwick
Anatomy .... Dr. L. Bruce
Nursing Technique .... Miss B. E. Jackson
Hygiene .... Dr. R. H. Greene
Seniors—Social Service Lecture Each Month .... Rev. S. L. McDowell

Schedule of junior and senior student nurse classes and instructors, 1927. Courtesy of
Gloria Taylor Cheek King and Lillian Gray.

possibly contributed to the eventual establishment of a Nurse Training
School Committee. This committee became a valuable asset to the gover-
nance structure of the hospital-based nurse training school. In 1927 a physician, Dr. I. E. Turner, who taught courses on medical diseases and laboratory
technology, became the first chairman of this committee. Later a nurse became chairman.

RULES GOVERNING STUDENT TRAINING

The interdependence between the hospital and the training school was evident in the hospital rules. These rules governed hospital employees, nurses,
and students in nurse training. The document "Lincoln Hospital Rules and
Regulations of 1925" spelled out the responsibilities for the superintendent

of nursing and for all the hospital departments. A publication titled "The Training Schools for Nurses" was extracted from those rules in 1925 and adapted specifically for the nursing students in the training school. A few examples of these rules are as follows:

- Nurses will not be allowed to receive telephone calls and visitors while on duty.
- Nurses must rise and remain standing when physicians, superintendent, superintendent of nurses, head nurse, supervisors, instructors or visitors approach them or enter a room or ward.
- When out of the Hospital, nurses must be quiet and well behaved and maintain the dignity of the institution.
- Hours of duty are from 7:00 A.M. to 7:00 P.M. for day nurses and 7:00 P.M. to 7:00 A.M. for night nurses, during which adequate time will be allowed off duty for recreation and study when service permits.
- Nurses must address each other as Miss _____ when on duty or speaking of each other.

Ask any Lincoln graduate and she will confirm that these and many other regulations were rigidly enforced. These rules focused mostly on the moral and ethical values of the student nurses. They emphasized respect for authority, position, and age. Students always addressed each other, as well as all adults and patients, by last name. Graduates even now address each other by last name. These rules and regulations have had a lifelong effect on the graduates.

The rules at Lincoln were very specific. Students were expected to comply with these rules without fail. Between 1925 and 1931 the age requirement for admission was lowered from between twenty and forty years of age to between eighteen and thirty-five years, the passing mark was 70 in all subjects, and an entrance fee was established. The probation period lasted four months and the compensation structure was changed from $3 for each of the three years to $2 the first year, $3 the second year, and $4 the third year. The first official Lincoln brochure to use the language "School of Nursing" rather than "Nurse Training School" was published in 1931. I found no declaration of this transition in the course of my research, but the bulletin provides evidence that the change occurred.

The early efforts of the Board of Examiners and the Standardization Committee to make the completion of high school (now defined as four years) an admission requirement enabled schools of nursing to recruit better students.

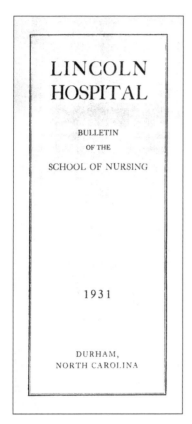

LINCOLN
HOSPITAL

BULLETIN

OF THE

SCHOOL OF NURSING

1931

DURHAM,
NORTH CAROLINA

Bulletin of the School of Nursing, 1931, reflecting the first evidence of the school's name change from the Nurse Training School. Courtesy of UNC Chapel Hill Library.

In *The Training School for Nurses Manual*, a Board of Nursing document, these efforts were clearly aimed at increasing the educational standards of the schools and preparing better future nurses. There was little concern that the high-school requirement would have a negative effect on the recruitment of students.

Ms. Mamie B. Maddox, a 1932 graduate, laughingly but seriously described her experience with the high-school requirement this way: "When I completed nursing school I could not take the board examination because I had completed two years of high school. I had to return to high school and complete the four required years. I did this and then took the State Board and became an R.N." Further discussion about recruitment stimulated the idea of allowing students to earn college credit for taking some of their nursing courses at a college. In 1930, students at LHSN began taking courses at North Carolina College (now North Carolina Central University, NCCU). Courses in sociology, psychology, chemistry, nutrition, and biology provided students with a broader foundation and enabled graduates to seek advanced educational credentials. This tradition continued throughout the life of the school. The 1931–32 *Bulletin* reflected this change in course structure. Nursing students, striking in appearance in their white-and-blue-striped uniforms and navy blue capes, walked from the hospital to the college campus. Some dreaded the walk—especially on cold, rainy days—and sought rides with the locals. This practice was strictly forbidden by the school, but nonetheless it was a part of the student experience.

During the twenty-three years that Ms. Carter served as superintendent (1912–1935), 146 students graduated from the School of Nursing. In 1935, after her departure from nursing school leadership, Ms. Carter stayed on as the assistant superintendent of the hospital, and the school entered a period of frequent turnover in the nursing leadership. From 1935 to 1945 a total of four superintendents of nursing served in the dual role of hospital and nursing leadership. These leaders were Ms. Henrietta Forrest, Ms. Mary Gray, Ms. Edith Steele, and Ms. Beulah Porter Jackson.

Between 1935 and 1936, Ms. Henrietta Forrest served as the third superintendent of the School of Nursing. According to Ms. Josephine Demmons McBride, who entered the School of Nursing in 1933, Ms. Foster began as an instructor. Under her administration as superintendent, approximately nine students graduated.

From 1936 to 1937, according to Ms. Della Mae Davison Sullins (RN '37), Ms. Mary Gray served in the superintendent's role; there were three graduates during her tenure. This is the first information we have from a creditable source about the fourth superintendent. Ms. Sullins shared this information in a conversation with Dorothy Esta Dennis Segars in June 2012.

Between 1938 and 1943, Ms. Edith Steele was the superintendent of the School of Nursing. In 1938 Ms. Steele also functioned as the chairperson of the Nursing School Training Committee, which was involved in providing administrative oversight of the school. The committee eventually expanded to include representatives from the hospital, the nursing staff, and the community. The members of the Nursing School Training Committee came from the Negro and White communities as well as various social, religious, and educational arenas. Members included: Ruth Rush, Secretary; the Reverend Miles Mark Fisher, Pastor, White Rock Baptist Church; Robert P. Randolph, MD, Lincoln physician; Harry E. Nycum; Betsy Mills; Cora Stephens, RN, Lincoln nurse; Dr. James Shepard, Founder, North Carolina College; Bessie Burgess, RN, St. Agnes Hospital School of Nursing; Joseph A. Speed, MD; Stanford Lee Warren, MD; and William Rich, Hospital Superintendent. Mr. Rich served after the departure of Dr. Charles Shepard as Superintendent of Lincoln Hospital in 1934. This committee participated in the selection of students for admission as well as the dismissal of students for due cause. Management of the School of Nursing, which had been the sole responsibility of the nursing superintendent, was now collaborative and collegial. Under the leadership of Miss Steele (1938–1943) sixty-one students graduated.

Between 1944 and 1945, Ms. Beulah Porter Jackson served as the superintendent. Ms. Jackson had a long tenure at Lincoln and the School of Nursing. Prior to becoming superintendent, she was one of the first instructors the school employed, in 1927. The hospital had also employed her as a day and night supervisor. She was involved with the State Colored Nurses Association and served as treasurer around 1940–1941, according to the minutes of the organization. During her administration thirteen students graduated. School of Nursing records and interviews with graduates confirmed the tenures of these superintendents. Ms. Clara Miller Harris remarked that Ms. Steele was superintendent when she entered the School of Nursing in 1942. Ms. Ethel McCullum and Ms. Lois Smith Morris confirmed that Beulah Jackson was superintendent when they entered the school in 1944.

There were continuous efforts to increase the size of the instructional staff in the School of Nursing. By 1938 a total of seven nurses had been employed to assist with teaching in the school: Mary Gray, RN, instructor of nurses and former superintendent (1936–1937); Beulah Jackson, RN, night supervisor; Freeland Bailey Price, RN, admitting officer; Emma Lee Randolph, RN, operating supervisor; Viola Brown, RN, and Helen S. Peach, RN, floor supervisors; and Pearl Parks, RN, night supervisor. These individuals were active in the teaching and training aspects of the school.

CLINICAL EXPERIENCE

The clinical experience, with its duties and responsibilities, marks the beginning of the application of nursing knowledge. Lincoln nursing students had at this stage in their education to translate didactic information into practice, and Lincoln nurses were steeped in clinical practice. The first level of clinical experience taught students the value of touch and of the human spirit as well as the fundamentals of interpersonal skills, communicating and establishing rapport with patients, and providing basic comfort measures. Early nursing students learned about the nutritional needs of patients with diabetes by preparing meals for them in the kitchen. They learned how to clean thermometers, sterilize instruments, and perform back rubs, which served to soothe a wrinkled brow, as did reading from the Gideon Bible when patients requested it.

Clinical experience was part of the basic foundation of hospital-based schools of nursing. As students progressed, the clinical experience taught them to function in various roles; as leader, as nurse in charge of shifts, and as caregiver on the health-care team. The daily clinical-care routines taught students how to prioritize and organize patient care. Students learned how to calculate and administer medication from a multi-dose vial, prepare normal saline and other solutions for wound irrigations and compresses,

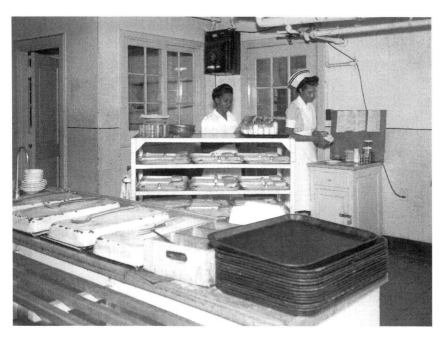

Nursing student Helen Neal Webb Jones preparing a meal for patients in the hospital kitchen.

recognize disease sequela, initiate treatment actions, and monitor patients' progress. These routines formed the foundation on which graduates could practice and in time become excellent nurses.

Many students expressed anxiety about the preclinical phrase, which culminated in the students' passage to the next level. Students were frequently eliminated at this juncture. From this point on the pace of the program accelerated. Students then had to step up their pace and apply what they had been taught, maybe in isolation, developing on that basis a care plan for the patients they were assigned. This involved integrating the clinical diagnosis into their delivery of care. Students were required to justify their nursing actions to their clinical instructors. Additionally, their documentation of these actions was gone over with a fine-tooth comb and graded. Graduates still in practice years later appreciate this attention to the details of clinical practice. Students entered their second year at this juncture, and junior students began assuming more responsibility for patient care. By their third and senior year, students had developed the leadership skills necessary to manage entire wards, albeit under the direction of the floor supervisor. Staffing

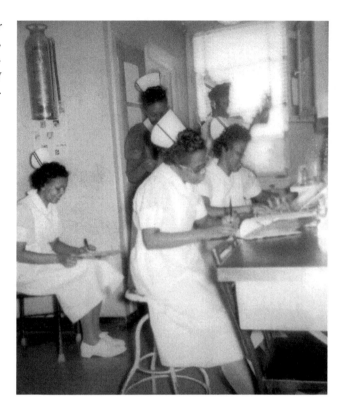

Second floor nursing station, old unit 210-212. Courtesy of Ruby Jewel Bell Borden.

consisted of a registered nurse supervisor/floor nurse, two or three students, and a licensed practical nurse or aide. The wards on the old unit consisted of eight to ten beds, male and female, and several single-bed units for private patients and those requiring isolation. In 1953, a new unit was constructed to supplement the old unit. It contained four-bed rooms, semi-private rooms, and one or two single rooms, which continued to be used for isolation patients as well as the social elite. The pediatric ward remained located on the old unit.

Reminiscing about her routines as a student nurse, Mrs. Clara Josephine Miller Harris (RN '45) recounted a typical day:

Students went on duty at 7:00 in the morning and worked until 7:00 p.m. There was a lunch break, and that was the only break allowed during the workday. Students provided a.m. care such as washing the patients' hands and faces, taking their temperatures, and preparing them for breakfast prior to going to NCC for 8:00 a.m. class. Students were usually

Nursing ward routine, night shift. Originally documented in red.

on campus for two or three hours and then returned to the hospital to resume patient-care duties. The supervising nurse told the students what to do and when they could leave. Studying was done at night following the completion of the day shift. Following the completion of a night shift, students had to attend class and perform the same as students who had slept all night.

This routine continued as Mrs. Clara Josephine Miller Harris described until the mid-1960s. The Class of 1968 recalled their hours of work as being from 7:00 a.m. to 3:00 p.m., 3:00 p.m. to 11:00 p.m., or 11:00 p.m. to 7:00 a.m. Students were allowed to leave the clinical area only when they had completed their patient assignments or there was a low patient census. Following their tour of duty they could go to the dorm to study. At times students had surprise visits from the instructors, and if they were found not to be studying they had to report back to duty (and probably got a written reprimand in their student record). One student vividly remembered studying and waiting for the instructor to visit. She had just laid down with a book and was about to drop off to sleep when she noticed the dorm door being silently opened. She glanced up over her open book and spoke to the instructor and so avoided having to return to work. Others in the class were not as lucky and several had to report back on duty. The students later surmised that this was a ploy to help staff the shifts such that the nurse/patient ratio required for safe practice was achieved. One could question the adequacy of safe practice performed by sleep-deprived students.

Affiliations

A key factor that influences the effectiveness of clinical training in a hospital is the patient census. The key areas of learning—pediatrics, psychiatry, medicine, surgery, and obstetrics—required an adequate nurse-to-patient ratio.

Students at LHSN were able to get adequate training in all the areas of practice except pediatrics and psychiatry. Lincoln Hospital had a limited pediatric service and no psychiatry service, although a psychiatry course, taught by Dr. Plummer, had been added to the curriculum in 1931. According to the 1931 *Bulletin* the pediatric service was under the supervision of a local pediatrician on staff, Dr. James Cleland, who taught pediatrics and was assisted by the nursing staff for the nursing implications. However the pediatric service had a low census and lacked diversity in diagnostic categories.

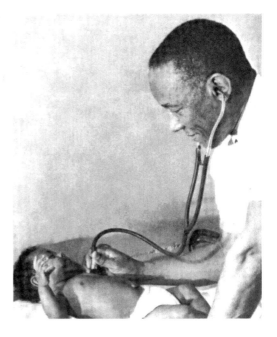

Dr. James Cleland attending a baby in the Pediatric Ward. Reprinted from *The Scalpel*, 1963. Courtesy of Bernice King.

The low pediatric census and the lack of psychiatric services in the hospital caused the Board of Nursing Examiners to be greatly concerned about the adequacy of the students' learning experiences in these areas. These concerns culminated in a new requirement; beginning in the early 1940s, the hospital was required to establish affiliation agreements with other institutions. The cost associated with the affiliations was the responsibility of the hospital. In the 1940s, as changes occurred in admission policies and students began to pay fees, a portion of these fees was applied to the cost of affiliations.

Initially Lincoln Hospital's affiliation choices were limited to other teaching hospitals that cared for Colored patients. This limitation often meant that students had to travel long distances to get their training. Students remained on these affiliations for two to three months. Affiliations continued throughout the school's existence. However, as integration opened the doors to more opportunities, pediatric clinical training became available in the local Durham area, though students continued to travel out of state to psychiatric affiliations through 1968. The last psychiatry affiliation began in the 1960s with racial integration at Eastern State Hospital in Lexington, Kentucky. The Class of 1968 was the last to participate in this affiliation. The head nurse there was a 1965 Lincoln graduate named Jimmie Ruth Gore (Persley), and she held the class to strict standards for theory and practice. The summer before graduating, the Class of 1968 completed a pediatric rotation at The Children's Hospital of South Philadelphia. The instructors marveled that completing the psychiatry affiliation before pediatrics did not hamper the students, and the Class of 1968 excelled in pediatric theory. (According to the curriculum, psychiatry was to be the last rotation before graduation, but circumstances dictated that the class take its psychiatry courses out of sequence. This pattern of taking clinical experience "out of sequence" later proved detrimental to the nursing program.) The class was introduced to pediatric growth and development while on its psychiatric affiliation. Dorothy Esta Dennis Segars, a member of that class, believes that perhaps it was the repetition and writing component that helped students retain and synthesize the growth and development information. Many of the students to this day remembered the many notebooks of theory they had to write. They were told these lectures would help them retain the necessary knowledge if they were not able to acquire clinical pediatric experience. This proved to be the case.

The Value of LHSN for Students

Students were the heart and soul of the School of Nursing, but who were these students? Where did they come from, and why did they choose Lincoln? Many students came from humble beginnings. Their parents were farmers, domestic workers, and skilled laborers; technical workers; and teachers, health-care professionals, and members of the ministry.

Students arrived at Lincoln from places near and far and up and down the eastern corridor, including small towns, cities, and rural areas in North Carolina, Alabama, Florida, Louisiana, Georgia, Michigan, New York, New Jersey, Pennsylvania, South Carolina, Virginia, Texas, and the District of Columbia. Students also came from places outside of the United States, such as various countries in Africa and territories including Bermuda and the U.S. Virgin Islands.

Students came to Lincoln for many reasons: the social history of the country, which fostered segregated schools and towns; limited economic status; family networks; association with the medical community; and the limited career choices available to women. Some chose Lincoln because an education in a three-year hospital-based program cost less than a four-year-college degree program. However, many families struggled to afford even the cost of Lincoln along with their other financial responsibilities. Some chose Lincoln for its excellent reputation and on the recommendations of high-school teachers and counselors. Lastly, many chose Lincoln for its proximity to home. Some students learned about Lincoln through their association with members of the medical community. Such was the case with Elaine Richardson Smith. She had worked with Dr. Daniel Lauray, who had previously completed his Obstetrics and Gynecology residency at Lincoln Hospital.

(continues on page 58)

Elaine Richardson Smith, RN '63, BA, BS, MA

It was an early January morning in 1961, and I awoke to see snow covering everything like a blanket. I'd never seen snow before and was amazed that so much snow could fall without me hearing it. My roommate laughed and said, "It doesn't make noise."

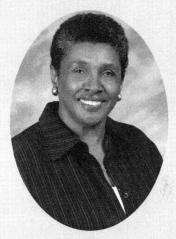

Courtesy of Elaine Richardson Smith.

My name is Elaine Richardson Smith and before I entered nursing school I had spent my entire life in Jacksonville, Florida, with a few trips to visit my mother's family in Georgia.

My mother and father were from Georgia and Alabama. My mother, Mary Edna Griffin, married my father, Crawford C. Richardson, in Atlanta, Georgia, in 1929, and they had immediately moved to Jacksonville where they would live for the rest of their lives. My mother was completing her freshman year at Spelman College, the oldest historically Black college for women, when she eloped with my father. She was nineteen and my father was twenty-five.

My father says that he only completed up to the third grade, but that's hard to believe when you consider his interests and abilities. He loved poetry and would recite poems to us, for example, "If" by Rudyard Kipling. He loved to debate any subject, could solve complex math problems, and had a determination that his children would all have a "good" education. My mother was equally as gifted. She was very creative. All of my sisters' and my clothes were made by my mother. My first store-bought dress was for class night at my high-school graduation. She possessed a quiet dignity that was subtle yet, at the same time, obvious.

They would have five children. Only four survived to adulthood. My mother worked as a domestic and later as a kindergarten teacher; my father was an entrepreneur. He first owned and operated a gas station, then a "juke joint" called The Rainbow Inn. He later owned a sawmill. He worked from the 1940s until his death in 1974 as the owner and operator of a pulpwood business. He cut and transported pine trees to the large paper mills in northeast Florida and southeast Georgia.

My sisters, brother, and I all attended and graduated from Stanton High School. It was a great school with outstanding teachers. The Great James Weldon Johnson was its first principal and, as you can imagine, we all knew every word of every verse of "Lift Every Voice and Sing." He was held up as a role model because of his local, national, and international achievements. Despite the lack of adequate books and equipment, our teachers taught well and expected us to learn and even to excel. Failure was not an option.

Despite the demeaning and cruel system of segregation, we were protected and nurtured by our family and our community.

Many national events had an effect on our lives; the death of President Franklin Roosevelt; World War II; The Korean Conflict; The Civil Rights Movement; and the ever-present threat of devastating hurricanes. The Richardson Family, guided by our mother and father, continued to move forward.

My siblings all went on to have professional careers. My oldest sister Edith became a registered professional nurse.

My brother, Crawford Jr., retired after serving twenty-six years in the U.S. Air Force with the rank of Chief Master Sergeant. He held the prestigious position of Senior Enlisted Advisor to the Commander of the U.S. Air Force, Europe, during his military career.

My youngest sister, Barbara, completed her PhD and became the chair of the History Department at Florida A&M University and later the assistant dean of The College of Arts and Sciences.

As for me, my interest in nursing started with my uncles. My mother, one of sixteen children, had two brothers who became doctors. My uncle, Joseph H. Griffin of Bainbridge, Georgia (Uncle Joe as we called him), and my uncle, David J. Griffin of Brunswick, Georgia, built a fifty-bed hospital and clinic in Bainbridge in the early 1950s. I worked various jobs in the hospital during summer vacation—from serving meals to patients to performing housekeeping tasks. I was allowed to observe in the emergency room and in surgery. I also sat in on in-service training for the nursing staff. In the interim, my sister had become a registered professional nurse. Becoming a nurse just was natural, given my experiences.

The first I heard of Lincoln Hospital was from Dr. Daniel L. Lauray. Dr. Lauray was the first Black board-certified physician in town, having completed his residency in OB/GYN at Lincoln Hospital in Durham, North Carolina. I worked for him cleaning his office and just helping out. It was the summer of 1960 and Dr. Lauray knew of my interest in nursing. He thought highly of Lincoln Hospital and its School of Nursing and wrote a recommendation to the Admissions Office. I took the Entrance Examination, passed, and was admitted in September 1960.

Lincoln was a new world. I learned so much more than the Arts and Sciences of Nursing. I learned about myself. Although I was told at home by my parents to believe in myself, Lincoln put me to the test. I came out strong and with the ability to persevere. I graduated with the Class of 1963 with the highest scholastic average. I won many awards, among them a scholarship to Duke University School of Anesthesia. I attended for a few months but left school to marry, as did my mother before me.

My husband, a medical technologist, had left Lincoln for a job in Wilmington, Delaware. It was in Wilmington that I had my first job as an RN. I worked on a surgical floor as a general-duty staff nurse. Later, I was recommended to join a dialysis team testing the clinical effectiveness of the parallel-plate dialysis machine.

In 1964, I became pregnant with my first child and resigned my position, not to work again until 1967. I returned to work on a part-time basis and almost immediately discovered that I was expecting my second child. My husband was transferred to Jacksonville, Florida, as the Director of Hematology at NAS Jacksonville Regional Medical Center. My second child was born in Jacksonville in 1968. I worked for a time with Planned Parenthood as a clinical nurse. Jacksonville was in the middle of the Civil Rights struggle and seemed to lag behind the rest of the nation.

I enrolled at the University of North Florida and completed a bachelor's degree in psychology and a bachelor of science degree in education. I later completed a master's degree in counseling psychology. After completing my MA, I worked for Family Consultation Services of Jacksonville as a psychological counselor for a year.

I was encouraged by the Urban League of Jacksonville to apply for a position at Florida Community College at Jacksonville (FCCJ). This position was a management position in the college's Women's Center. This position began my long and successful tenure at FCCJ. I was project coordinator of a program called Challenge, which provided counseling and training for women to enter or reenter employment or return to school to pursue careers. My nurses training provided me with insight into how health issues affected the success or failure of program participants. The unparalleled success of this program led to the establishment of a new department: the Department of Employment and Training. As the program operations officer and the primary grant writer, my involvement resulted in millions of dollars in program funds and indirect cost monies that provided for new programs as well as new staff positions. Most importantly, hundreds of individuals were trained and placed in full-time high-wage jobs.

In 1980 I was promoted to the position of director of resource development in the Department of Institutional Advancement. As one of five directors, I continued to write and develop grants that provided job training to special student populations. I was also assigned to develop grants that would bring new business to the city by providing incentives that would assist companies with specialized training for new personnel.

In 1985 I was diagnosed with multiple sclerosis. This diagnosis would lead to a gradual decline in certain cognitive functions that prohibited me from continuing in resource development. My last five years at the college were spent first as a member of teaching faculty and finally in Student Affairs as a counselor.

I served on many boards and received some awards. I consider my greatest accomplishment to be my children: My oldest daughter, Alice, is the director of diversity at Emory University in Atlanta, Georgia; my youngest daughter, Robin, is a vice president of E-Business with Sun Trust Bank at their corporate headquarters in Atlanta. I have five grandsons and one granddaughter, and I enjoy watching them grow, explore, and strive to find their rightful places in the world.

Well, it's been forty-seven years since I watched my first snowfall out of my dorm window at A. B. Duke Hall. It's now 2010 on a hot August day in Jacksonville. How ironic it is that I'm watching the path of Hurricane Earl as the currents steer it away from the costal United States and thanking God for that and for Lincoln Hospital School of Nursing. Without Lincoln I know my life would not have been as rich or as successful.

Student Attire and Ceremonies

The nursing uniform is symbolic. It makes a statement about a school's identity, pride, and values. The first uniform at LHSN had an apron that extended from the neck to the waist (and probably crisscrossed in the back), detachable cuffs over a blue or white dress, white shoes and stockings in summer, black shoes and stockings in winter, and a blue cape. As students were admitted, they were measured and fitted for uniforms. Through the years the style of the uniform remained fairly consistent.

The school's first uniform was one inch from the floor. By the mid-1920s according to school standards, which can be found in the 1927 Bulletin, the length of the uniform had been raised to between twelve and fourteen inches from the floor. This length remained the uniform standard throughout the operation of the school. Although in pictures of the uniform, the length appears shorter, by the end of the program the uniform length resembled that of street wear, basically, knee length or slightly above.

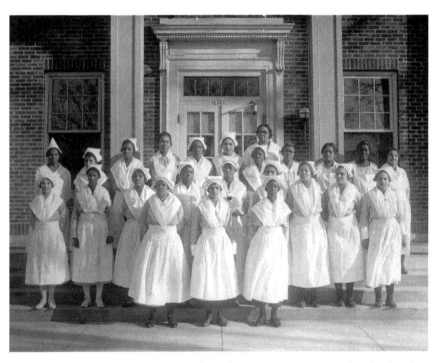

Class of 1928 wearing student uniform from the 1920s to 1930s. Notice length, detachable apron, and detachable cuff on the dress sleeves. Courtesy of Carolyn Evangeline Henderson.

It is believed that the uniform changed from a dress and detachable apron without pockets to a one-piece dress with the appearance of an apron around the late 1940s to early 1950s. The back buttons on the dress band was a place to keep one's scissors as the dress had no pockets according to Lois Clement Thorpe in a discussion about the uniform in October 2010. In the late 1950s the one-piece uniform had gained pockets for carrying scissors, pens, and the small Gideon Bible. See the changing length of uniforms as shown in the 1936, 1948, 1965, and 1968 graduate class photos.

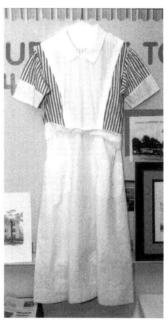

Replica of student one-piece uniform with pockets from the 1950s to 1970s. Courtesy of Gloria Johnson Fulton. Jerry Head, photographer.

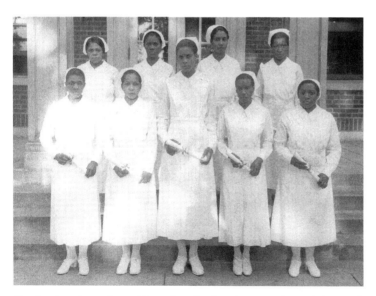

Graduating class of 1936. Notice length of uniform. Back row left to right: *Pearl Winbush, Terri B. Isler, Jimmie D. Trammell, Evelyn Jeffreys.* Front row left to right: *Josephine Demmons McBride, Ruth F. Reed, Gertrude Bullock Henry, Dympha Brown, Mary Adams.* Courtesy of Carolyn Evangeline Henderson.

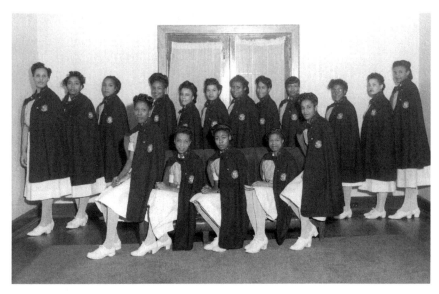

Class of 1948 wearing striking blue capes. Seated left to right: *Mary Lois Clements Brown Thorpe, Elizabeth Williams Thorpe, Corona McClary Umstead, Muriel Harris Daniels, Zella Perry Thompson.* Back row left to right standing: *Dorothy Farley, Thereasea Clark Elder, Margaret Davis, Georgia Major, Rosebud Roderick Beverly, Fannie Choates, Othello Cave Williams, Catherine Carter, Helen Black, Alice Williams, Lillian Brown and Annie Coley.* Courtesy of Carolyn Evangeline Henderson.

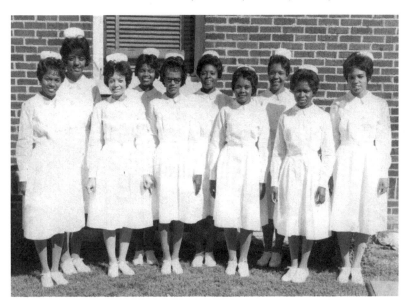

Graduating class of 1965. Front row left to right: *Carrie Stone Reavis, Christine Henderson Groover, Geneva Vann Dees, JoAnn Moore, Penny L. Davis, Patricia Martin Blue.* Back row left to right: *Shirley Ann Oliver Scott, Betty Evelyn Dalton Brown, Jimmie Ruth Gore Persley, Jeronica Williams Hardison.* Courtesy of Patricia Martin Blue.

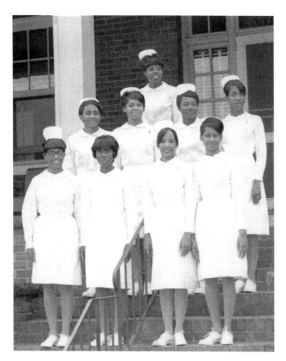

Graduating class of 1968. Notice the length of the uniform is more like street wear. First row left to right: Myrna Watson Hughes, Dorothy Esta Dennis Segars, Carolyn Beatrice Martin, Theresa Fields Andrews. Second row left to right: Linda Floyd Hill, Mary Ellen Price Britton, Alice Harrell Young Tharrington, Brenda Howell Shephard. Third row: Yetta Hardy Clark. Courtesy of Dorothy Esta Dennis Segars.

Students strictly adhered to the uniform length requirement. Mrs. Ethel Brown McCullum (RN '47) described the daily ritual of measuring the length of her uniform before going on duty. If the uniform did not meet the inspection of the housemother or superintendent, then one had to make changes until the correct measurement was achieved. Alumni who were students in the 1960s report the same ritual.

The cape was an essential part of the student uniform. It was navy blue with a red interior and a button closure. LH and SN were embroidered on the right and left sides of the neck collar, respectively. It featured the school emblem on the upper left side. The student nurses wore the uniform and cape with much pride. The uniform, the dress, shoes, stockings, the cap, the pin, and the cape made a statement about the character and pride of the student and the school. Collectively, they were the image of professionalism.

The 1931 School of Nursing *Bulletin* stated, "While on duty nurses are required to wear the school uniform, length of skirt being not more than 12 inches from the floor. They are not allowed to wear the school uniform on the streets and in public places without the consent of the Superintendent of Nurses. No jewelry except a watch with second hand, training school pin or badge or ring was to be worn while on duty. In the early years student nurses could wear black oxfords and black stockings while on duty in winter and white shoes or oxfords and white stockings while on duty in summer." Later the practice was changed to white stockings and shoes in summer and winter. Additionally, the uniform was used as a disciplinary tool for student indiscretions. Can you imagine being stripped of your uniform? Mrs. Elizabeth Thorpe (RN '48), a longtime obstetrics supervisor (now deceased), admitted that she hardly knew what a complete uniform looked like, she was so often on disciplinary action or campused. Mrs. Thorpe probably was not the only one to have that experience. Students were permitted to keep their uniforms upon graduation. Many shared them with other students. However, if nurses severed their connection with the school before graduation they were not permitted to take any part of the uniform with them. The late 1960s witnessed changes in dress styles. Between 1967 and 1971 shorter uniforms and pants as street wear became the norm.

By 1968 graduates were being asked to leave the uniform with the school upon graduation; the finances to purchase new uniforms for incoming students were limited even though the cost of uniforms and supplies was supposedly included in the tuition.

Professions are characterized by standards, codes of ethics, distinct cultures, responsibilities, and accountability for their practice. Inherent in the culture of a profession are ceremonies that mark milestones along the way. For students at Lincoln, these ceremonies were capping, pinning, and graduation. These were the rites of passage that marked one's progress toward becoming a professional nurse.

The Cap

Students were taught to wear "the cap" with dignity and to treat it with the utmost respect. Students received their caps at the end of the preclinical period, and the cap marked the student's clinical and theoretical achievements as they progressed through the nursing program. The following description of the cap worn between 1907 and 1936 is based on photographs alone. The cap worn in the graduation picture taken circa 1907 was cuplike with ruching along a horizontal stripe and perched atop the head. The 1914 picture shows a bowl-like cap with two horizontal stripes; it probably was a senior cap worn at graduation. The bowl-like shape of the cap changed to one reminiscent of fly-away wings between the 1920s and 1940s. In the 1950s it returned to a smaller cup-like shape, which remained through the school's closure in 1971. Regardless of the shape of the cap, the stripes it bore denoted a student's status as either a junior or a senior. The students' first cap was plain without a stripe. Lula Cowan McNair, RN '53, recalls the following:

At the end of the first year, which ended our preclinical period, caps were received. I was not too excited about receiving my cap because this meant full-time on the floor, with a full-time patient load and a cap that I could never keep straight on my head! Theory was no problem for me, but at this point, I thought I should know everything about all I had studied. I was a little uncomfortable about all the hard work before me. The second year was the year of hands-on practice in medical nursing, surgical nursing, obstetrics and gynecology, and the operating room.

(continues on page 65)

Lula Cowan McNair, RN '53, BSN, MS

My name is Lula Cowan McNair. I was born in Henderson, North Carolina, on June 12, 1932. I had one sibling, a brother who was four-and-a-half years older. I graduated in 1950 from Henderson Institute, a local high school. I was an average student, graduating in the upper one-fourth of my class.

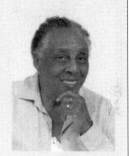

I chose nursing as a career because there were not a lot of choices for Black women and I had a desire to learn how to help sick people after learning how to administer insulin and check urine sugars at the age of twelve.

Courtesy of Lula Cowan McNair.

There were no counselors at my high school; therefore, I used the library, talked with the nurse at our local hospital across the street from my high school, and requested information from different schools. I applied to the Lincoln Hospital School of Nursing (LHSN), was accepted, and entered the Class of 1953 in the fall of 1950. There were twenty-two students in this class; ten of those twenty-two entrants graduated in 1953. The attrition rate was high due to the failure of several of my classmates to meet academic requirements and to other circumstances.

On admission there were four students in each room of the dormitory and a housemother who was like a real "mom." Our spiritual needs were supported by early morning prayer at the start of the day, led by our housemothers. We also attended Vespers on Wednesday evening led by a local minister in addition to another Vespers at North Carolina College (now North Carolina Central University) on Sunday evenings. This service was monitored and required. Seats were assigned and grade points were lost if you did not attend. Students were also expected to attend a church of choice on Sunday mornings. We were part-time students at North Carolina College.

Our social life was monitored closely. We had a late leave on Friday nights until 11:00 p.m. and could never see the ending of 9:00 p.m. movies. We could not go out of the city limits or walk through the business area of Hayti and Pettigrew Streets.

Professional Ethics was one of the first courses offered. This was the only course taught by the director of nurses, who was a good example of professionalism. We were taught to respect each other as well as patients and anyone else with whom we had contact. We were taught to dress properly, including clean shoes and laces. When a director entered a room or a doctor approached a nurses' station, we stood and remained standing until we were given permission to sit. Our director of nursing had the foresight and interest in our future education to instill these things in us. We attended North Carolina College for most of our preclinical classes, which gave us college credit. This was an advantage to those who continued their education. Students were also taught the importance of involvement in professional organizations such as the National and State Nurses Association. At the end of the first year, which ended our preclinical period, caps were received. I was not too excited about receiving my cap, because this meant full-time on the floor, with a full-time patient load and a cap that I could never keep straight on my head! Theory was no problem for me, but at this point, I thought I should know everything about all I had studied. I was a little uncomfortable about all the hard work before me. The second year was the year of hands-on practice in medical nursing, surgical nursing, OB/GYN, and the operating room.

We affiliated at Crownsville, Maryland, for psychiatric nursing and during our senior year at Meharry School of Nursing for Pediatrics in Nashville, Tennessee. I took the North Carolina State Boards in the fall of 1953. Only one student failed, and by only one subject. She later passed with flying colors. Lincoln Hospital School of Nursing had a long history of excellent State Board Examination results.

I retired in 1992 after working eleven years in general hospitals and twenty-eight years in staff nursing education and staff development. I was also a nursing instructor for staff and nursing students affiliating in psychiatric nursing.

I graduated from LHSN in 1953. Upon completion of a further course of study I received a bachelor of science degree in nursing in 1963 and a master of science degree in education in 1975 from North Carolina Central University.

Lincoln Hospital School of Nursing provided me with a strong foundation of knowledge and skills as well as a desire to improve my current situation. I am very proud of LHSN and of its graduates before and after my own graduation.

In the second year of training (the junior year) students received two black stripes, which were vertical or horizontal depending on the year. In the third year of training (the senior year) students received two more black stripes, again either horizontal or vertical. They wore those stripes until graduation. Upon graduation the cap reflected a single horizontal stripe.

Based on the photographic evidence, students wore their black stripes horizontally on the cap through the 1940s. In the 1950s the stripes were placed vertically on the cap, and the size of the cap decreased to approximately half that of the original cap. Notice the differences in the shapes and sizes of the caps through the years.

Circa 1907 student nurse cap. Courtesy of Andre Vann and Martha Donnell, North Carolina Central University Archives.

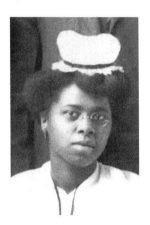

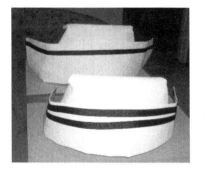

right: *Replica of student nurse caps from 1914* (top) *and 1920s to 1940s* (bottom). Courtesy of Gloria Johnson Fulton. Photographed by Mary Richardson Baldwin.

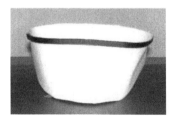

left: *Replica of graduate nurse cap from the 1950s to the 1970s.* Courtesy of Gloria Johnson Fulton. Photographed by Mary Richardson Baldwin.

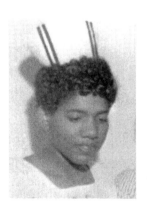

left: *Student nurse cap from the 1950s to the 1970s.* Reprinted from *The Nightingale*, 1959. Courtesy of Marion Glen Miles.

Capping: A Sacred Ritual

The capping ceremony was a sacred ritual. On this spirit-filled, serious, and sober occasion, each student came forward to receive their professional dignity. At first, students struggled with the initial adjustment to school life, including the long hours of study and the academic demands. In time, the intensity of the academic demands, coupled with the long hours of clinical work, imbued the cap with symbolic significance, and the capping ceremony became the pinnacle of the student experience. The ceremonies were held at different churches in the Negro/Black community, namely, White Rock Baptist, Saint Mark AME Zion, Mount Vernon Baptist, St. Joseph AME, the Covenant Presbyterian, and the Seventh Day Adventist.

The capping poem captures the heart, soul, and spiritual commitment of the student nurse's journey.

As part of the capping ceremony the students received the Nightingale Lamp. The candle in the first lamp was lit by a nurse advisor, after which the light was passed from student to student and each student lit her neighbor's lamp, symbolizing their professional bonding and illuminating the nurse's student path.

Student nurse capping ceremony. Lucille Zimmerman Williams capping student Jimmie Ruth Gore Persley. Reprinted from The Scalpel, 1962. Courtesy of Patricia Martin Blue.

The Capping

He wore a crown of thorns that I
Might wear a crown of light,
And so in deep humility
I'll wear this cap of white.
I'll walk in quiet confidence,
Befitting one who knows
The path He trod once long ago,
The way a Christian goes.

And as I minister to those
Who need His healing touch,
I'll serve them in the name of Him,
Who gave for me—so much.

And somehow may His light shine forth
Through me from day to day,
That those entrusted to my care
Will find the living Way.

For Him who wore a crown of thorns
I'll wear this cap of white,
That when He calls I'll worthy be
To wear a crown of light.

Alice Hansche Mortenson

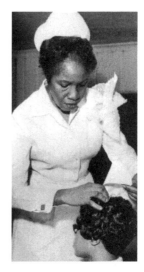

Nightingale Lamp Poem

I
Shine on dear lamp, we love you very truly.
Tho you may grow older with age each day,
You've placed a beam in our hearts so dearly,
And we'll hold on, and never from it part.

Chorus:
You are the best lamp anyone desires.
You've helped a many hearts to grow each day.
Dear Lincoln, how will we ever thank you?
Your bright glow, we pray, will shine forever more.

II
You've led the way for many hearts before us,
And we're assured that our career is best.
For you have rendered us the best of service,
And may your light forever beam that way.

Tune: Londonderry Air
Words by: Nora M. Kendall

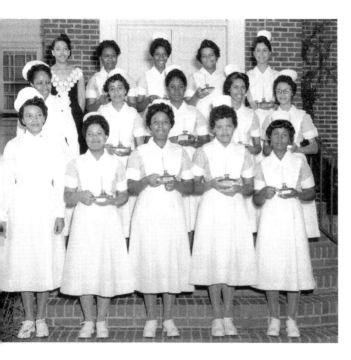

Class of 1961 student nurse capping ceremony. First row left to right: Mary K. Wilkerson (Instructor), Marion Patricia Godley Wilson, Eva Johnson Geer, Roberta Elliott, Gloria Atkinson Armstrong. Second row left to right: Lucille Zimmerman Williams, Betty Jean Talford Fisher, Ola Ruth Putman Davis, Norcy McDaniel (left early), Margaret Elda Parker. Third row left to right: Unidentified, Ernestine Smith Thomas, Christine Coleman Calhoun, Shirley Jean Long Bethel, Evangeline Boone Harrell Rickman. Courtesy of Carolyn Evangeline Henderson.

Graduation Ceremony

The graduation ceremony was filled with pomp and circumstance. The procession into the church with graduates dressed in all white professional uniforms, white cap, white stockings and shoes was a beautiful sight to behold. The ceremony included the address by a guest speaker, presentation of the class, and awarding the diplomas and the school pin. Frequently the presiders of the ceremonies were members of the Lincoln Hospital Board of Trustees, senior attending physicians, and community personalities. A final highlight of the ceremony was the presentation of special awards recognizing professional behaviors and excellent performance of the students throughout their tenure in the school. Throughout the history of the school, dating back at least to the 1914 graduating class, physicians awarded "prizes" (as they were called) to members of the graduating classes. Awards were also presented by the hospital graduate nurse staff and the Alumni Association. Names of some of the awards changed through the years but the awards to the 1971 class were as follows: The J. W. V. Cordice Prize to the student excelling in Theory and Practice in Operating Room Technique, Carolyn Evangeline Henderson; The Leo G. Bruce Award to the student maintaining the highest scholastic average for three years, Janie Lee Canty-Mitchell; the R. P. Randolph Prize to the student who had been most courteous for three years, Ruth Foy; The Dr. and Mrs. Clyde Donnell Individual Prize to all members of the graduating class; the Graduate Nurses' Staff Nurse Prize to the student who had been the most technically competent nurse for three years, Barbara Davis Porter; The Lincoln Hospital School of Nursing Alumnae Prize to the student who had been the neatest for three years, Dorothy Terry Justice; and the C. C. Spaulding Prize to the student who had been the most courteous to patients for three years, Mary Carmichael.

The Nursing Pin

Each graduate received a school pin that identified them as graduates of LHSN prepared to serve the health needs of society. Mary Richardson Baldwin describes the Lincoln pin as a four-pronged gold pin with a red cross in the center. The left prong bears the letter L for Lincoln. Directly across on the right prong is the letter H for Hospital. On the top prong is the letter S for School and on the bottom prong is the letter N for Nursing. In the center of the pin is a cross, a religious symbol of Christianity. No records revealed who designed the Lincoln pin. (See pin image on front cover.)

The uniform, cap, and nursing pin are all sources of meaningful memories of the graduation ceremony. Many nurses recalled the setting, the place,

---

Florence Nightingale Pledge

I solemnly pledge myself before God and in the presence of this assembly to pass my life in purity and to practice my profession faithfully. I will abstain from whatever is deleterious and mischievous and will not take or knowingly administer any harmful drug. I will do all in my power to maintain and elevate the standard of my profession and will hold in confidence all personal matters committed to my keeping and all family affairs coming to my knowledge in the practice of my calling. With loyalty I will endeavor to aid the physician in his work and devote myself to the welfare of those committed to my care.

---

and the family members who witnessed the event. During the ceremony, the graduates took the Nightingale Pledge with reverence and with a deep spiritual commitment to caring for humanity. Lincoln nurses were required to memorize and recite the Nightingale Pledge. It remained a source of pride at graduation.

The students' deep honor, respect, and sense of accomplishment is reflected in graduate testimonies on their nursing attire. Carrie Stone Reavis (RN '65) expressed the following:

The uniform was worn as a source of accomplishment and pride. It, and especially the cap, was to be treated with respect and almost reverence. I wore my Lincoln Cap proudly with the black band across the top, my starched white nurse's uniform, blue cape, white nurse's shoes, and white stockings. This was the professional RN nurses' attire back-in-the-day; and there were no identity clashes with other medical personnel. RNs practiced an unspoken language of respect for physicians, devoted care and concerns for patients, and dignity for our profession. We were called Angels of Mercy dressed in white uniforms. The RN professional dress code changed with the new millennium to casual and colorful scrubs. I think RNs lost their professional identity and sense of respect when they started wearing scrubs. What will prevail for RNs tomorrow?

(continues on page 72)

Carrie Stone Reavis, RN '65

"Say It Loud Now . . . Black and Proud": A Voice of Pride and Principles

This phrase from a well-known Black singer, James Brown, was a major hit and indeed most appropriate in describing my point of view as a student nurse back-in-the-day at Lincoln Hospital School of Nursing in Durham, North Carolina. Women of African descent had been a part of nursing history since the days of Harriet Tubman and Mary Mahoney in the 1800s. Now it was time for me to take a stand to help make a better life for my people and myself.

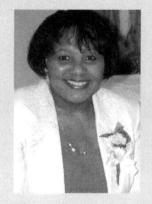

Courtesy of Carrie Stone Reavis.

Discrimination and segregation in the 1950s and 1960s were societal norms and existing thorns in our lives. In search of comfort, harmony, and meaning in the harshness of life, we listened to rock & roll music, now called doo-wop, and motivational speeches for racial equality from our civil rights leader and the internationally known advocate Martin Luther King Jr. Choosing a financially affordable profession was a priority and another challenge during the difficult times of the 1960s. My nonprofessional, hard-working mother's opinion that Negros could not succeed in life without a higher education, as she knew it, supported my ideas and hopes toward advancing my education. My guidance counselor at high school helped us locate a suitable school . . . Lincoln!

Proud, young, and inexperienced, I left Richmond, Virginia, in August 1962 to attend Lincoln Hospital School of Nursing. With perseverance and determination in my blood, I prayed to do my best so Mom would be pleased having me as the only professional nurse in our family. Life at Lincoln was not fancy but it was meaning-ful, and most students were full of purpose and educationally inspired; supported and impressed by voices from the administrative faculty and hospital staff; ener-gized and refreshed by participating in community events; spiritually strengthened by weekly reverent requirements; mentored and nurtured by inherited big sisters; restrained, approved, and questioned by a forceful but caring housemother; and taught by others the art of frying and dying hair the Lincoln way. We learned win-ner's luck at being a card-playing ace, and I embraced this sisterhood of education, friendship, networking, trust, and respect at Lincoln to become empowered to be the "Best of the Best" in professional nursing.

I moved through life at Lincoln on my mother's wisdom, love, and optimism, striving for a better future than what was handed to her as a company seamstress. She said, "Be a professional nurse. You will always have a job and people will look up to you as someone special." Graduating from Lincoln Hospital School of Nursing (RN '65) provided me with a bigger purpose in life, a sense of security, and a feeling of readiness. I had no identity crisis or inabilities as a young nurse, but instead the competency "to learn wisely from today . . . to do better tomorrow."

Sure enough in 1965 I was a proud graduate nurse and later "RN" after passing the state boards. I returned home to Richmond to seek work. I was hired immediately by the Medical College of Virginia, our largest Hospital, as a charge nurse in a med-surg ward for the indigent—a sector called St. Phillips Division. I felt strong and ready for the challenge. In 1968 my mother influenced me to change jobs and seek employment with the federal government at McGuire Veterans Hospital in Richmond. She said, "Government benefits, salary, and retirement plans are the best," and she was right! My experience at Lincoln touched many areas of training and gave me the confidence needed to accept the job offer as a VA recovery room nurse, now called a PACU nurse.

In 1972, I capitalized on a window of opportunity to graduate from MCV School of Nurse Anesthesiology, Allied Health Division as the first Black student to complete the program. It was a tough and unexpectedly challenging experience to go through alongside being married with a young son. Racial issues and discrimination confronted my every move in student training; each day I felt like Sidney Poitier, the Black actor, in the movie "Guess Who's Coming to Dinner." Agonizing harassments came from White patients as well as physicians. The song "Tears On My Pillow and Pains In My Heart Because of You," by the Black singer Little Anthony, clearly captured my feelings during this miserable time in my life. Coping with this madness was almost unbearable. Mom said, "Stick with it . . . time goes by faster than you think," and she was right; it worked! I became chief nurse anesthetist at the VA Hospital and retired after thirty years in June 2000. I experienced salary discrimination on many jobs, and it was difficult to correct in many instances.

The closing of Lincoln Hospital was also difficult to comprehend, but changing times can produce necessary evils. Our voices as professional nurses from Lincoln are still being heard throughout these United States of America: in communities, associations, sororities, affiliations, and on jobs here and abroad. Through the services our hands and hearts provide, we continue to make a difference in peoples' lives. I am proud of my "life-line" in the Lincoln legacy and will remain a conscientious supporter of alumni events.

I'm not a trailblazer in this profession but I left a small mark as the only registered nurse in my family; as a member of the American Nurses Association; as an officer of NER, Chi Eta Phi Sorority, Inc., and Zeta chapter; as a Saint Paul Baptist Church usher; as a community association participant; and as a dedicated and caring worker.

The nursing profession has been rewarding to my family and me (I have a husband of forty-six years; two children; four grandchildren; and my parents, who are deceased). My faith and trust in God has sustained me. I have no regrets, only R-E-S-P-E-C-T taken from soul singer Aretha Franklin's popular song. I credit my accomplishments to my Mom and all the wonderful people who gave me advice along the way. I'm saying it loud, yes . . . "I'm Black and Proud" and very thankful for all the lessons taught and learned at Lincoln that prepared me for my job as a devoted and passionate professional nurse, a journey that started forty-five years ago.

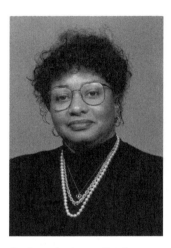

Barbara Anderson Leathers.
Courtesy of Barbara Anderson
Leathers.

Barbara Ann Leathers (RN '69) seems to agree. Although she doesn't wear her old uniform, she still wears one. She explains thusly:

I pride myself on being one of the few nurses (if not the only nurse) who still wears a lab coat, white skirt, and white support hose. I don't dare go to work without wearing my nursing pins from LHSN and North Carolina Central University. Very frequently patients and others stop to compliment me for still "looking like a real nurse." They find it comforting.

Dorm Life

Dormitory life was an adjustment for most nursing students. It meant having to share a bathroom, shower, and other spaces with someone other than a family member. But, in time, the dorm became a home away from home.

The North Carolina Board of Nursing Examiners and the standardization committee were concerned about the well-being of student nurses in training and in particular about their living quarters. They issued a regulation that required the superintendent of nurses and/or instructors to live in residence with the students. Interviews with graduates confirmed these living arrangements. Ms. McBride (RN '36), Mrs. Armstrong (RN '38), Mrs. Thorpe (RN '48), and Mrs. McCullum (RN '45) confirmed that the superintendents lived in residence with them.

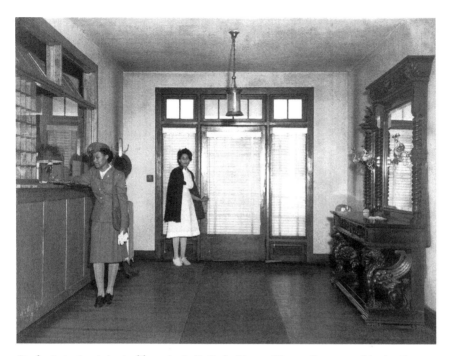

Student signing in/out of foyer in A. B. Duke Nurses Home. Courtesy of Andre Vann, North Carolina Central University Archives.

The Board also felt that a comfortable and clean environment with adequate space and furniture was necessary for the students' well-being. When A. B. Duke Nurses Home was completed in 1925, part of the financial contributions from the Duke Family and Dr. Aaron Moore's estate provided for adequate furnishings for the residence.

The A. B. Duke Nurses Home was a stately building with a long porch that stretched across the entire front of the building and had wide front steps and tiered stoops on either side. The front porch was lined with rocking chairs, which provided a great source of pleasure for many of the nurses.

A. B. Duke Nurses Home had a beautiful entry foyer with an elaborate breakfront.

The living space on the first floor of A. B. Duke comprised a small kitchen, a Seniors Room, and a parlor with a piano. The Seniors Room was a small private room where seniors could receive guests. However, the door had to remain open. Students were oriented to the protocol for using the room. There was the oft-repeated cry: "That's the Seniors Room!" Junior students did get invited out of the Seniors Room; seniors were accorded that level of

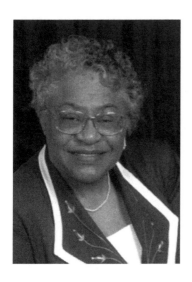

Emily Carrington.
Courtesy of Emily Carrington.

respect. The parlor could be used by all for receiving guests and dates, and for other social events, especially Sunday afternoon tea.

The kitchen in the nurses' residence was a valuable asset. Many of the students had few discretionary funds with which to purchase snacks at Page's Store on Fayetteville Street across from the hospital. Some students developed friendships with the hospital kitchen staff and were able to obtain food to cook in the nurses' home kitchen. Thus, the small kitchen in the nurses' home was used for storing food and preparing simple meals. Can you imagine cooking cakes, steaks, chicken feet and rice? All were delicacies of the 1966 Class. A frequently heard comment was, "Someone used my mayonnaise for their sardines!" Some students didn't even have money for sardines. Many of the students received care packages from home that contained all sorts of nonperishable food stuffs. When care packages arrived, many hungry friends arrived as well. Betty Evelyn Dalton Brown's (RN '65) parents always delivered great care packages containing fried chicken and homemade cakes, and Patricia Martin Blue (RN '65) vividly remembers always being there when they arrived. Other students organized grocery-shopping expeditions, pooling their few coins. Such was the case with Emily Carrington, Thenia Craig, and Louise Adams. Thenia Craig was my big sister in the Big Sister Program, which is described later. She became a licensed practical nurse, and we still share the sisterhood bond.

It is unclear when housemothers were first hired, but students who were enrolled in the mid-1940s talked about these ladies. The term "housemother" became popular as these women were hired specifically to monitor the students along with performing other duties, at times, in the hospital. From the mid-1940s through the closing of the school five women served in this role. The housemothers included Ms. Albertine Mason, Ms. Beatrice Moore, Ms. Beatrice White "Mama Bea," and Ms. Ricks, who also served as the housekeeping supervisor in the hospital.

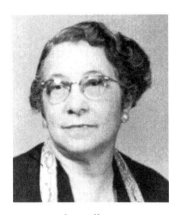

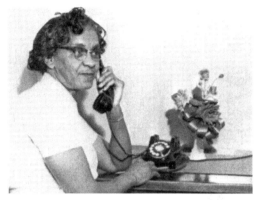

*Housemother, Albertine
Mason. Reprinted from The
Scalpel, 1956.*

*Housemother and hospital housekeeping super-
visor, Beatrice Moore. Reprinted from The Scalpel,
1962. Courtesy of Patricia Martin Blue.*

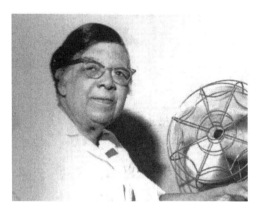

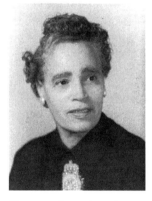

*Housemother and housekeeping supervisor,
Ms. Ricks. Reprinted from The Scalpel, 1963.
Courtesy of Bernice King.*

*Housemother, Ms. White,
"Mama Bea." Reprinted
from The Scalpel, 1956.*

Students shared that being monitored by a housemother sometimes felt like being checked by the police; however, their orders came from the nursing administration. There were rules for everything: sign in, sign out, clean your rooms, lights out by 10:00 p.m., no loud music, check your uniform when you leave the dorm, are you wearing a girdle as part of the foundation, is your uniform fourteen inches from the floor, are there runs in your stockings. The housemothers' voices were memorable: "Ms. Andrews, you have a caller." "Man on the hall!" "That's the Senior Room!" "Young lady, you didn't sign in." Some students signed neither out nor in. They were adept at exiting

LINCOLN HOSPITAL
DEPARTMENT of ADMINISTRATION *For your General
information & files*

Job description for the House Directress and Relief in the Nurse's Home.

Hours on duty:

3 P.M. to 7 A.M.
4 " " "
Each person is to be relieved by Mrs. Speed or Mrs. Duffin at 7 O'clock every morning.

Specific duties

1. answer the door bell
2. check all windows for closure each night before going to bed. In the event that
   it is necessary to close windows before night, please recheck the same windows
   for closure.
3. Blinds and or shades are lowered at a reasonable hour in the classroom. You may use
   some judgement as to when the blinds are to be closed in the lobby, office room
   etc.

Lights

The front porch, Kitchen(outside) light and the fire escape are to be turned on
immediately before dark and off each morning before leaving off duty. This is
the responsibility of the house directress or the relief person.

Inside----Leave lights on in the front hallway near the door, the stairways leading
to the upper floor and to the basement. Turn lights off in the long hallways
kitchen, the two lounges and classrooms. Be sure to check for same within the
basement where the library is located.

Doors

All door are to be checked nightly. These will include the front door, base-
side doors and windows(especially the library) the basement door and windows
of the Nursing Arts Room, and hair parlor.

Kitchen

Check the stove to see if the burners are left on through mistake.
" for cleanliness in general especialt following a party or if a group have
used the kitchen.

Parties

Following each party given the students are responsible for placing of chair
back into the room from which they were taken, taking down decoration,
sweeping the floor and moping the kitchen floor if unduly dirty. Also, the
emptying of excess waste and trash. Any thing borrowed from the hospital kitchen
must not be left in the home but to be returned to the lender.

Morning Duties

Unlock the front and basement doors (especially the door which leads to the
laundry room and library. In unlocking the front door ,see that the catch is taken off.
Raise the blinds in the hallways, office room, classroom, kitchen and lounges before
leaving off duty.
Turn lights off (the outside lights and the porch lights). Leave the one on
in the office room ower the signing out desk.
Students room are to be checked every morning. Beds must be neatly made,
floors swept, wastebaskets emptyed, shoes or uniforms in proper place, bottles
not left in the rooms. See that the blinds are raised. The above applies to those
students going on duty. If the rooms does not pass inspection the same should be
reported. (You may leave a note in case the Educational Director is not available
before your leaving off duty)

Mail

It is a must that the house directress or the relief person pick up the mail
daily from the secretary office. On Saturdays check with the switchboard operartor
for the mail to find out if it is im and it is your respobsibility to go to the
office and check for the students mail.

cc L.A.Crockett

and entering through both the fire escape and a basement door on the side of the nursing residence. The most frightening part of the basement door was the sleeping dog that belonged to Mr. Scott, the hospital administrator at the time. One wonders just how many students he didn't report! The fire-escape door was locked on the side of the nurses' residence adjacent to the hospital (across from the emergency room). One could not linger on the fire-escape stairs without risking being seen and reported.

The duties and responsibilities of the housemothers reflected their role as monitors of the student body. Can you imagine assisting an unstable class-mate or roommate up the stairs to the second floor without being discovered by the housemother whose living quarters was just beyond the stairs? Or, being campused with your roommate for not divulging her misadventures or mischievous activities? Or, not divulging the location of "spirits" stored in a bucket hanging outside from the student's bedroom window? Or, dressing hair in the room rather than the designated area in the basement? These were some examples of the bonding of the sisterhood.

Locking down and opening up the dorms was quite a ritual and was completed on time every day. The housemothers took the welfare, wellbeing, and success of the students to heart. Some were motherly. Others were motherly to the point of being almost smothering.

Social Life and Religion

Although there was plenty of work to do, students did have some time for rest and relaxation. The students in the 1930s and 1940s had more time for social activities than their predecessors did. Dances such as the Miss Lincoln Ball started in the 1930s. Ms. McBride talked about the queen selected from her class to be Miss Lincoln. In 1934 Ms. Gertrude Bullock was selected as Miss Lincoln. The primary social activities revolved around the dormitory and interactions with people in the community. Many students established relationships with people in the community based on their family networks, which in many cases had influenced their decision to come to Lincoln in the first place.

Religion and an abiding faith in God have always been important parts of Negro life. Many of the students talked about their religious upbringing and going to church on Sunday—some walking several miles to get there. The students were introduced to the churches in the surrounding area because their feet were their only means of transportation. They had to be able to return to campus in time to get lunch and collect their sandwich and fruit for

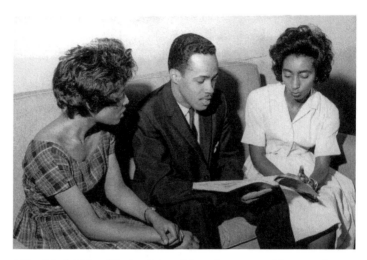

Miles Mark Fisher III, chaplain, with student nurses Miron Andrews Wilkerson and Yvonne Goolsby Spencer. Reprinted from *The Scalpel,* 1962. Courtesy of Patricia Martin Blue.

dinner on Sundays. According to Dorothy Esta Dennis Segars (RN '68), when her class entered they received hot meals on Sundays.

When the students began attending North Carolina College, they gained access to the Vesper services held on Sunday evenings. In later years Vesper services were conducted in the dormitory. Beginning in the 1940s, local ministers coordinated the Vesper services. A Baptist minister, Miles Mark Fisher III, from White Rock Baptist Church was a member of the School of Nursing staff and served as chaplain, counselor, advisor, and recreational coordinator in the 1960s. Student participation in local churches continued until the school closed and many graduates continue as members of those fellowships today.

Political Events Affecting Students

Students at LHSN, though fairly isolated from the world, were nevertheless affected by the larger social and political events. For example, LHSN students had lived through World War I. When the Japanese attacked Pearl Harbor on December 7, 1941, the United States was again at war, and LHSN students lived through World War II. This war imbued the country with a sense of panic. There was concern about whether the supply of nurses could meet the demand for civilian and military services at home and abroad.

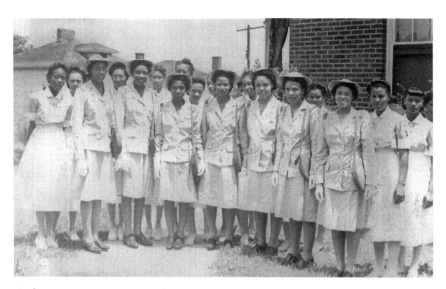

Cadet nurses, 1947. Courtesy of Carolyn Evangeline Henderson.

Congress enacted the Nurse Training Act of 1943, which authorized the U.S. Public Health Service to create the United States Cadet Nurse Corps. The main purpose of the Cadet Nurse Corps was to increase the enrollment of students in schools of nursing. The Cadet Nurse Corps offered students free education, attractive uniforms, and stipends for thirty months. It offered participating institutions maintenance fees for students for a period of nine months, tuition reimbursement, and assistance in securing funds for expansion of residential and educational facilities. Between 1943 and 1945 many Lincoln student nurses joined the segregated Cadet Nurse Corps, among them Ms. Helen Neal Webb Jones, Lois Clements (Thorpe), and Beatrice Coleman. Twenty-eight students graduated from the Cadet Nurse Corps.

Several Lincoln nurses received recognition and acclaim for their service in the military forces of World War II. Della Raney Jackson (RN '37) Major, U.S. Army (Retired), described her journey to becoming a military nurse this way.

When I entered nursing more than forty years ago, it was serious business with me. It was a commitment to give my life for a cause—that of caring for those who were ill. Today, though I've been a retired nurse since 1972, nursing to me remains the same.

In my school of nursing at Lincoln Hospital, Durham, North Carolina, the Nightingale pledge was administered to every student upon

(continues on page 81)

Edna Martel Jones Moore, RN '47, BSN

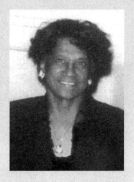

Courtesy of Edna Martel Jones Moore.

I was born in Taylorsville, North Carolina, and graduated from Happy Plains High School in 1944. I am the middle child of three girls. My mother died when I was five years old and our maternal grandparents raised us.

I always wanted to be a history teacher. However, this changed in 1942 when my grandfather had a massive stroke that paralyzed him and left him almost speechless. He had been a loving father figure to my sisters and me. We assisted our grandmother and the community volunteers in taking care of him. I enjoyed caring for him and seeing the thankful look in his eyes and the smile on his face when he was fed or given water. Caring for him helped me to make the decision to become a nurse. When I saw an advertisement about the Cadet Nurses, I applied to Lincoln Hospital School of Nursing and St. Phillip School of Nursing. I was accepted at both but chose Lincoln because it was closer to my grandmother.

Student Cadet Nurses who had completed all of their classes and affiliations were permitted to spend their last six months of training in a Veterans Administration Hospital. I met my husband during this period, got married, graduated, passed my State Boards, and went to Tuskegee, Alabama.

Louis J. Moore and I will be married for sixty-three years in August 2010. We had three children, two daughters and a son (we lost our son in 2006), three grandchildren, and four great grandchildren. I was a nurse at the Veterans Administration Hospital in Tuskegee, Alabama, and at the Veterans Administration Hospital in the Bronx, New York, for a total of thirty-seven years of service. I worked as a staff nurse, assistant head nurse, head nurse, and trained as an evening supervisor but declined further promotion because I enjoyed working with patients. I earned a bachelor of science degree in nursing from Tuskegee Institute (now Tuskegee University). I retired in 1985 following many rewarding years of service. From 1985 until today, I have been a volunteer in the community.

I am a member of Greater St. Mark Missionary Baptist Church and an active member of both the Tuskegee University Alumni Association and the Tuskegee University Nurses Alumni Association. I am active with the Cancer Research Foundation, the National Active and Retired Federal

Employees Association, Habitat for Humanity, the National Coalition of 100 Black Women, the Alabama State Nurses Association, the American Nurses Association, Chi Eta Phi Sorority, Inc., and am a life member of Delta Sigma Theta Sorority. I hold or have held leadership positions in most of these organizations. I am also a volunteer with the Montgomery Health Department focusing on AIDS research.

I have received several awards throughout my career. To mention a few: Chi Eta Phi, Epsilon chapter's Sisterhood and Nurse of the Year Award, Habitat for Humanity's Angel Award, and several appreciations awards from Tuskegee University. I was named an Outstanding Retired Nurse by the Alabama State Nurses Association and was inducted into the Alabama Senior Citizen Hall of Fame. I was a special guest at a Harvard University graduation exercise recognizing my inclusion in a dissertation titled "Professional Commitment and Activism in the Lives of Five Southern African-American Nurses." The dissertation appeared in book form, and an article about us, titled "Nurses Making a Difference" appeared in the *American Journal of Nursing* in February 2001.

acceptance into the program. Though I am no longer a practicing nurse, the words of this pledge are just as clear and vivid in my memory as they were forty years ago. Particularly do I relive the words, "I will do all in my power to maintain and elevate the standard of my profession." I believe that every nurse, whether retired or practicing, should constantly strive to promote nursing in every way possible wherever she is.

It was this strong desire to elevate my profession that led me to volunteer for military service in 1940 with the U.S. Army Nurse Corps. Getting accepted by the American Red Cross was difficult for graduates of Black schools of nursing in the South. But I persisted in overcoming this barrier to the point of writing to Miss Mary Beard, who at that time was director of nursing for the American Red Cross, telling her of my desire to serve my country and practice my profession. Miss Beard replied with my membership card, certificate, and pin.

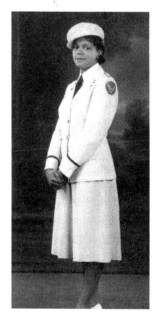

Major Della Raney Jackson, U.S. Army (Retired).
Courtesy of Janie Cooke.

After serving for six months, I was given the chief nursing examination and promoted to First Lieutenant. All of this was the result of my love for my profession and the love I had for patients, which I expressed in the care I gave to them. Without a commitment to the profession and a love for patients, one cannot be successful. This I believe about nursing.

At the time of this writing, Ms. Raney is deceased. Her accomplishments ensure she will not be forgotten. Della H. Rainey [Raney], the first African American nurse commissioned as a lieutenant in the Army Nurse Corps, was also the first nurse to become part of the famed Tuskegee Airmen. There

---

Minnie Mae Williams-Beverly, RN '53
Lieutenant Colonel, USAF (Retired)

I was born on July 3 in Grab Township, Johnston County, North Carolina, and raised on a farm where my parents worked. Later we moved to Princeton, North Carolina, and my family continued farming. I graduated from Dillard High School in 1950 and then decided to pursue nursing. The majority of my life was spent taking care of members of my family; therefore, I felt that nursing was the career for me. Immediately after high school I was accepted into Lincoln Hospital School of Nursing (LHSN) in Durham, North Carolina. Based on that education I enjoyed the following career accomplishments in my life: After graduation I went to work

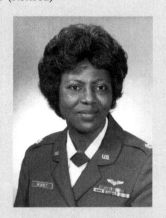
Courtesy of Minnie Mae Williams Beverly.

in Washington, D.C., at St. Elizabeth's Hospital as a registered nurse in charge of the Psychiatric Unit. I lived on the grounds in the nursing quarters and worked there from 1954 through 1957. I went on leave from St. Elizabeth's when I decided that I wanted to see the world and joined the U.S. Air Force. Because of my nursing experience, I enlisted as a First Lieutenant. My military experience started at Gunter Air Force Base (AFB), Alabama, and continued at Wright-Patterson, Ohio, Johnson Air Force Base, Japan, and Travis AFB, California. When I had completed active duty I joined the Reserves and went back to St. Elizabeth's for a year to honor my commitment.

is a Della H. Rainey Nursing Scholarship that was established by the Tuskegee Airmen Scholarship Foundation and the National Black Nurses Association for nursing students enrolled in at least their sophomore year at an accredited BSN degree program.

In later years other Lincoln nurses have been recognized for their distinguished service in the military: Minnie Mae Williams-Beverly (RN '53), Lt. Colonel, USAF (Retired); Margaret Aquilla Watkins Stanfield (RN '58), Lt. Colonel, U.S. Army (Retired); and Nora Kendall Noble (RN '57), Colonel, USAF (Retired).

(continues on page 88)

From there I went to Walter Reed Medical Center in Washington, D.C. In 1962 the Cuban crisis occurred and I was called back into active duty. I stayed on active duty from 1963 to 1966. I was stationed at Andrews AFB, Maryland, and attended flight school to become a flight nurse. I was sent to Wiesbaden, Germany, to work at the Wiesbaden United States Air Force (USAF) Hospital for three years. From 1969 to 1971 I was in Cam Rahn Bay, Vietnam, as a hospital nurse supervisor. From 1970 to 1972 I was stationed at Andrew AFB in Maryland and ran my own little dispensary in the Air Force Systems Command. I then got orders to go back to Travis AFB, California, for my second tour there. I worked from 1972 to 1973 as a flight nurse bringing home the prisoners of war (POWs) from Hanoi. Finally in 1974 I went back to work at the hospital at Travis AFB in California.

In the course of my career I received the following military awards: Bronze Star Medal; Meritorious Service Medal with one Oak Leaf Cluster; Combat Air Crew Medal; National Defense Medal; Air Force Longevity Service Award with four Oak Leaf Clusters; Vietnam Campaign Medal with four Service Stars; and Republic of Vietnam Medal with Palm Leaf.

My civilian awards include a City of Goldsboro, 2006, Human Relations Award for Notable Achievements for volunteering with the Red Cross. I went to Baton Rouge on one twenty-one-day trip and to New Orleans for twenty-one days on another trip with the Red Cross during the aftermath of Hurricane Katrina. I received a Certificate of Appreciation from the local American Red Cross chapter. I have been an AARP member since 1985. I have been a member of the founders of the local Tuskegee Airmen Member chapter since 1998. I am a long-standing member of the Dillard/ Goldsboro alumni association, which provides numerous community services to youths. I served on the Wayne County Nursing Homes Advisory Board for several years and was an adamant advocate for improving the quality of care for patients in county nursing homes.

Margaret Aquilla Watkins Stanfield, RN '58, Lt. Colonel, USAF (Retired)

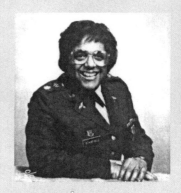

I, Margaret Aquilla Watkins, was born on June 13, 1932, in Milton, North Carolina, to Sterling and Maggie Watkins. I attended elementary school in Blanch, North Carolina, and Milton High School in Yanceyville, North Carolina. Reared on my parents' farm I had only two jobs in my life: the first was on my daddy's farm and the other was nursing. Daddy always said, "No working until you finish school and then you can hire yourself out." I was one of eleven children—five girls and six boys and one that my mother and dad adopted at the age of five when his mother passed away.

Courtesy of Margaret Aquilla Watkins Stanfield.

My mother passed away when I was fifteen years old and my oldest sister Wynolia stepped in and took the lead. Wynolia taught sixth grade eighteen miles from home in Roxboro, North Carolina. She came home every weekend to check our schoolwork and clothes and prepare us for church on Sundays where I was a member of the choir and taught the Youth class. My father, along with Wynolia, made sure I completed post-secondary school along with seven of my siblings, all of whom graduated from professional/academic institutions. My siblings are entrepreneurs, teachers, principals, and a railroad engineer.

I made the honor roll each month in the eleventh grade. I received two Cs, both in Home Economics. When asked why, I replied, "I never could cook or sew." I played the clarinet in the marching band in my senior year. My grades were so high that I did not have to take the final exam. I attended the Duke Practical Nursing Program from May 1951 to May 1952 and earned an LPN diploma. Following the completion of the LPN program, I worked at Duke Hospital for about eighteen months and then decided to further my career in nursing and was accepted at Lincoln Hospital School of Nursing (LHSN) on September 8, 1955. It was tough, but thank God I made it!

On Christmas Day in 1956 I became engaged to the love of my life, Melvin Stanfield. Because there were no married students allowed at Lincoln, I had to receive permission to marry in order to remain in school. Permission was granted and we were married on June 30, 1957. I was the first married student to attend LHSN. In September 1957 I went to Crownsville State Hospital, Crownsville, Maryland, for a three-month internship in psychiatry. It was very special because I was able to spend my weekends in Washington, D.C., with my husband. I then interned at Meharry School of Nursing in Nashville, Tennessee, for training in the area of pediatrics. I graduated on September 8, 1958, from LHSN. For the next sixteen months I worked at North Carolina Mutual Insurance Company as a company nurse and then returned to Lincoln Hospital and worked on the maternity ward. I enjoyed working hard on the 3:00–11:00 p.m. shift as well as taking vacations, going to the beach on weekends, and shopping. I was never too busy to get up and go to St. Joseph A.M.E. Methodist Church on Sunday mornings. I joined St. Joseph Methodist Church in April 1959 where I worked faithfully in the church and was the president of the Mary C. Evans Missionary. In October 1960 my life changed drastically when I passed the State Board and became a registered nurse. Thank God!

In September 1965 I obtained employment at the Veterans Administration Hospital in Fort Howard, Maryland. In June 1966 I transferred to Walter Reed Army Medical Center and in June 1969 I was commissioned First Lieutenant. I became busy with classes: basic training at Kirkland AFB in Albuquerque, New Mexico, Army Medical Advance course at Fort Sam in Houston, Texas, and Army Medical General Staff College at the Academy of Health Sciences, United States Air Force Base, also at Fort Sam. In 1973 I worked with the Public Health Nursing District Government. I spent every summer in school and made my rank right on time.

As for my decorations on my uniform, I received Army Service ribbons, National and Defense Service medals, Army Achievement medals, and two oak-leaf-cluster Armed Forces medals. My tours of duty included: Walter Reed Army Center, Head Nurse; Fort George Meade, Head Nurse; Indiantown Gap, Pennsylvania, Retention Officer,; Fort Dix, New Jersey, Area Coordinator; Fort Drum, New York, Area Coordinator; and last but not least, Walter Reed Army Medical Center, Desert Storm, Assistant Chief Nurse of the 2290 U.S. Reserved Hospital. After Desert Storm and twenty-three years of service, I retired.

I had opportunities to do extensive travel including to Germany, France (Paris), and other countries. Currently, I stay busy with my church and conferences. I am a member of Ward Memorial A.M.E. Church where I am a member of the Steward and Missionary groups, as well as of nurse and church clubs. Additionally, I became a member of Chi Eta Phi Sorority. I give credit for my accomplishments to God first, and then to my elementary school teacher Mrs. Ophelia White Stephens as well as my principal and other teachers. I particularly give credit to the Lincoln Hospital director of nursing Mrs. L. Z. Williams (a great lady), the nurses and instructors, Mrs. Geraldine Butler, Mrs. Elizabeth Thorpe, Mrs. Lelia Miller, Mrs. Mary L. Thicklin Jones, and all the others who lent their support during my stay at LHSN. Finally, I also give credit to the housemothers, "Mama Bea" White and Mrs. Albertine Mason. Lincoln Hospital School of Nursing was a great school and I will always be grateful to it.

I maintain close contact with Dot Collins Rhodes, Lucille Thomas Lawrence, Marion G. Miles, the late Sharon D. Winston, Margaret Goodwin, Frances Williams, and Jessie Lyons, who kept her nurse's cap pretty and white. The sisterhood we shared while at Lincoln continues.

I retired a GS 12 from the District of Columbia government after thirty-one years of service and twenty-three years in the military. Thank God I made it!

Nora Kendall Noble, RN '57, Lt. Colonel, USAF (Retired)

I am the youngest of two daughters born to Rev.
Joseph Kendall and Dr. Aggie Nora Kendall-Simpson
in Maxton, North Carolina, on August 5, 1936.
At the age of fifteen years I was baptized by the
late Reverend Wertz at her home church of Shiloh
Missionary Baptist Church in Maxton. My fondest
childhood memories include my church girls' leader,
Mrs. Etta McLaughlin. She took us on Vacation Bible
School day trips to Jones Lake in North Carolina.
At the age of sixteen I was inspired by God to seek a
career in the military.

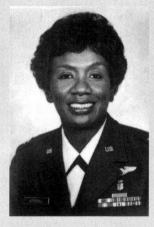

Courtesy of Nora Kendall Noble.

On December 31, 1960, I joined the United States
Air Force as a First Lieutenant at Dyess AFB in
Abilene, Texas. Eventually I became a staff nurse and
was later promoted to Captain and stationed between
Wiesbaden, Germany, and the Bangor, Maine, AFB.
I attended flight nursing school in San Antonio,
Texas, and became a flight nurse at Rhein-Main Air Base near Frankfurt, Germany.
Eventually I was promoted to Standardization Evaluation Flight Nurse, which made
me responsible for administering flight-nurse qualification exams in the Air Force.
I had an early promotion to Major and in 1968 I volunteered as a flight nurse in
Vietnam. Following a one-and-a-half-year tour in Vietnam, I went to McGuire AFB
in New Jersey and then to Andrews AFB in Maryland where I was again promoted,
this time to charge nurse supervisor of the Outpatient Clinic. In 1976 I received the
bachelor of science degree from the Air Force Institute of Technology via Catholic
University of America in Washington, D.C. Later I became a primary nurse practi-
tioner and eventually was promoted to the military position of Lieutenant Colonel.
Following this promotion I was sent to Denver, Colorado, as the Chief Nurse of the
Air Force Reserve Nurses.

In Denver I was blessed with my most precious gift from God, the birth of my
daughter, Celia Kendall, in 1981. Eventually I was promoted to full Colonel and was
deployed to Elmendorf AFB in Anchorage, Alaska. In Alaska I was dual-hatted as the
Alaskan Air Command Nurse and Chief Nurse of the Elmendorf Medical Center.

In June 1984 I left Alaska and was transferred to Newark, Ohio, as the first female
base commander of the Newark Air Force Station. I retired there in 1987 after completing twenty-seven years of consecutive military service.

Upon my arrival in Newark I immediately joined the Shiloh Missionary Baptist
Church. The Lord blessed me in Newark and I married the widowed Reverend Dr.
Charles W. Noble Sr., pastor of Shiloh Missionary Baptist Church on November 9,
1985. The wedding ceremony was a jubilant affair, with the sanctuary filled to capacity and the members delighted with how God has restored the church with a very

talented and capable First Lady! I am the longest-serving first lady in the history of Shiloh.

Following my military career I co-founded with my husband the Par Excellence Learning Center and accepted the full-time position as its administrator. The center opened its doors despite considerable odds on August 25, 1987. In 1988 I was able to get the new elementary school fully accredited in a year's time, which had never been done before in Ohio.

My community and civic roles have also been extensive from the time I first began public speaking in high school. I was a member of the Advisory Nursing Council of Central Ohio and a board member of the Private Industry Council. I served on the YWCA board of directors and was a member of the United Way Planning Division, a board member of the Center of the Visually Impaired, a board member of the Licking County Aging Program, a board member of the SCORE program, and a past president of the Ohio State Medical Board.

I have had the opportunity to speak on the local, state, and national levels throughout the country. I have served as a Sunday School Teacher, a Hattie Jackson Guild Girl advisor, a Shiloh Women's Prayer Breakfast Leader, a choir member, a teacher, and an orator for the Eastern Union Missionary Baptist Association and the Ohio Baptist General Convention. I have also served as past chairman of the Baptist Pastor's Minister's Wives and Widows of Columbus and Vicinity Ministry.

I have also been privileged to be the first Black female Colonel to become the Command Chief Nurse of the Air Force Reserve Nurses, the first Black Air Force nurse to become the Command Nurse of the Alaskan Air Command with a dual hat, the first female to command the Newark AFB in Newark, Ohio, the only Black female in my Aeromedical Evacuation Unit to be promoted to Major one year ahead of all of my contemporaries, the first Black Air Force Colonel to be placed in the Ohio Veterans Hall of Fame, and the first female in Ohio to establish a private fully accredited elementary school in nineteen months.

On May 11, 2003, I was awarded the Doctor of Humane Letters from Tri-County Bible College and Seminary in North Carolina. In 1990 I was inducted into the Ohio Veterans Hall of Fame. I also received the Vietnam Service Medal, the National Defense Service Medal, the Air Force Longevity Award, the Air Force Outstanding Unit Award, the Air Force Organizational Excellence Award, the Meritorious Service Medal with two oak-leaf clusters, and the Legion of Merit Award with one oak-leaf cluster. I hold a teaching certificate in grades K–8 from the state of Ohio. My husband and I were invited to the inauguration of President George H. W. Bush and were included in the President's "inner circle."

My faith has been my leading force in life. The most influential persons in my life have been my grandparents, the late Reverend Henry and Maggie McRae, and my late mother. My mother was my mentor and "my everything." My lifetime aspiration has been to motivate people to live a healthy and spiritual life. My faith has also been key in my twenty-five years as a cancer survivor. A favorite scripture for my daily living is "Cast all your cares upon Him; for He careth for you," 1 Peter 5:7.

During the Depression and President Roosevelt's New Deal, developments in infrastructure offset unemployment. Unemployed men between the ages of eighteen and twenty-five were eligible to join the work-placement camps, which provided labor for construction projects, reforestation, road building, and the like. These camps were located throughout the states and provided both employment opportunities and skilled labor training.

Lincoln Hospital provided a Civilian Conservation Corps Camp Clinic (CCCC Clinic) under the leadership of Dr. Leroy Swift, the attending obstetrician. As a student in the CCCC Clinic during the war, Mrs. Clara Harris recalled that the military brought soldiers who had contracted venereal diseases, such as syphilis and gonorrhea, to the Clinic at Lincoln:

> This clinic allowed us (nursing students) to practice our skills in the administration of medications, especially penicillin. Penicillin had been discovered and was being used in the mid-1940s. We were assigned to go to this clinic and give the soldiers injections to treat their syphilis and gonorrhea. Penicillin was distributed only at Duke Hospital, and therefore Lincoln and other hospitals had to pick up their supply of this medicine from Duke. Penicillin came in a vial and had to be activated by adding sterile water and then vigorously shaken prior to administration. This was a tremendous practice experience.

COMMUNITY AROUND LINCOLN AND EXTENDED FAMILY

Throughout its existence, the School of Nursing enjoyed good relationships with the Negro community. Individuals, churches, and formal groups provided various kinds of goods and services to the hospital and the school. The various boards that impacted hospitals and nurse training schools were made up of community leaders, wives of Lincoln physicians, and interested citizens who valued the work of Lincoln and wanted to see it succeed in meeting the needs of the Negro/Black community. One of these groups, called "The Lady Board," primarily provided services to the hospital, but students also benefited from these volunteer efforts. Later, the Women's Auxiliary, sorority sisters, Candy Stripers, and volunteers were big supporters.

Lincoln Hospital, with its grand lawn graced with large oak trees, was a friendly and welcoming place. Mrs. Julia Simpson Armstrong (RN '38) always viewed the hospital and front lawn as a spot to meet someone or wait for the bus—it was a landmark. Lincoln Hospital, the lawn, and the nurses' residences were sites of frequent hospital and community events in addition to the graduation ceremonies and activities held for the students. Lincoln Hospital worked very closely with the Durham City and County Health Department to host the Well Baby Clinic for babies born at Lincoln and elsewhere. Nursing students were able to experience caring for children while helping the public health nurses manage the clinic. Mrs. Lydia Flintal Betts (RN '36), a supervisor for the Well Baby Clinic, went on to have a long career in public health.

As we bring these twenty years to a close, we reflect on the changes that transpired at LHSN. By 1944, the title "Nurse Training School" had been changed to "School of Nursing"; the age for admission had been reduced to eighteen; the education requirement had been increased from one year of high school to four years; and the employment of graduate nurses in instruction and supervisory positions had been initiated. The hospital continued to provide a large amount of charity care and had grown in status as a training place for interns. In 1925 the American Medical Association approved Lincoln Hospital for the training of interns and residents. Student nurses developed professional relationships with the doctors and gained their respect with their nursing skills. The rotation of interns from Freedman's hospital, and later from the Philippines, proved an asset to the recruitment of nursing students. As the physician networks broadened, so did the recruitment of students from places farther away. Students also developed an appreciation for the teaching and learning experiences that doctors from the White medical community could offer them. Although there were anxious times, the respect between the students and the physicians remained mutual. Ms. Ethel McCullum (RN '47) smilingly stated, "I was always nervous with Dr. Copperidge, a urologist, and those urethral dilators. I never could get those straight."

In 1944, despite several changes in nursing leadership, LHSN once again rose to the accreditation challenges of the Board of Nursing Examiners and remained fully accredited. Students were fully engaged in the school and its activities. The social and political climate of the country was changing. The School of Nursing and its students were adapting.

Lydia Ruth Flintal Betts, RN '35
(1913–1996)

Mrs. Betts was born August 31, 1913, in Durham, North Carolina, the third of ten children. Her father worked at North Carolina Mutual Insurance Company and her mother was a housewife. At about the age of twelve, she experienced the death of her mother and a sibling. Being the eldest girl she was given the responsibility of caring for the other children. This resulted in her inability to attend school for a while. She and her siblings were assisted by family members during this period. Later, she returned to school and was a 1932 graduate of Hillside High School and a 1935 graduate of Lincoln Hospital School of Nursing. She received a bachelor of science degree in nursing from North Carolina College (now North Carolina Central University) in 1966. She also held a

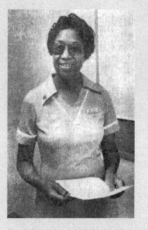

Reprinted from the *Durham Morning Herald*, August 30, 1978.

certificate in public health nursing from St. Phillips Medical College of Richmond, Virginia, and attended the Certified Public Health Nursing Supervisor Training Program at the Public Health Nursing Section of the North Carolina State Board of Health. She died in November 1996.

Mrs. Betts has been recognized as an early pioneer in public health in Durham County. She was the first African American to be appointed supervisor of the Public Health Department in Durham County in 1971.

During her interview, she said that her grandmother had been a midwife and that she had accompanied her at some birthing events. These events influenced her decision to become a nurse. She held supervisory positions at Lincoln Hospital and worked in several hospitals outside of North Carolina. Before joining the Durham County Public Health Department in 1944, she was a public health nurse at the Wayne County Health Department, Goldsboro, North Carolina, and at the Pearson County Health Department, in Roxboro, North Carolina.

Mrs. Betts was very active in both community and professional orga-
nizations. Her professional involvements included: President, Lincoln
Hospital School of Nursing Alumni Association; member, North Carolina
Central University Alumni Association; member, American Nurses
Association and District 11; board member and chairperson of the Bylaws
Committee of the District 11, North Carolina Nurses Association; chair-
person, Nominating Committee, North Carolina Conference of Public
Health Supervisors, Directors and Consultants; member, Legislative
Committee, North Carolina Conference of Public Health Supervisors,
Directors and Consultants; and member, Governing Council of the North
Carolina Public Health Association, where she earned a life membership.

Mrs. Betts loved the Chi Eta Phi Sorority, Inc., of which she was a
life member. She was the chapter's first Anti-Basileus, and she served
as Tamias for more than twelve years, as Tamiochus, as chair of the
Nominating and Finance Committee, and as treasurer of the southeast
region.

She was also a life member of the NAACP, a member of the National
Council of Negro Women, Inc., a member of the Coordinating Council for
Senior Citizens and AARP, a member of the YWCA and Women-in-Action
for the Prevention of Violence and its causes, and a board member and
Secretary of the American Cancer Society, Durham Unit. Mrs. Betts provided voluntary transportation for cancer patients and was appointed to
the Patient Advocacy Committee of the Durham County Nursing Homes,
for which she served as secretary.

A deeply religious person, she was a life-long member of White Rock
Baptist Church, in Durham, North Carolina; a member of the Senior and
Sanctuary Choirs, for which she served as Financial Secretary and Chair
of the Bylaws and Policy Committee; a leader, and for several years the
secretary, of the church's College View District; a member of the Susie
V. Norfleet Sunday School Class; and a member of the Rosewood Street
Community Club.

Mrs. Betts listed her grandmother; Mrs. Helen Miller, the chairman
of the Department of Nursing at NCCU; Dr. Warren; and Mrs. Shirley
Callahan, the director of nursing at Durham County Department of
Health, as persons who were influential in her life choices and who
supported her throughout her career.

REFERENCES

Annual Report Lincoln Hospital and Nurse Training School. 1924. Durham Regional Hospital Archives, Durham, N.C.

Annual Report of Lincoln Hospital. 1927. Durham, North Carolina. Lillian Green Gray (RN '28) and Cornelia Jackson Hardie (RN '43) Collection. Information compiled by Gloria King, April 2004.

Harris, Clara J. M. Interview with the author. August 1998.

Lincoln Hospital Annual Financial Statement. 1933. Durham Regional Hospital Archives, Durham, N.C.

Maddox, Mamie B. Interview with the authors. October 1972.

McBride, Josephine D. Interview with the author. August 2010.

McCullum, Ethel B. Interview with the author. August 25, 2011.

McCullum, Ethel B. Interview with the author. March 25, 2012.

Miller, H. S., and E. D. Mason. *Contemporary Minority Leaders in Nursing: Afro-American, Hispanic, Native American Perspectives.* New York: American Nurses Association, 1983.

Morris, Lois S. Interview with the author. August 25, 2011.

Morris, Lois S. Interview with the author. March 25, 2012.

Public Law 74: The Bolton Act Highlights in Nursing in North Carolina, 1935–1976. March 1977. A 75th Anniversary Project of North Carolina Nurses Association.

The Grading of Nurse Training Schools in North Carolina. 1928. North Carolina State Archives, Raleigh, N.C.

The Scalpel. 1963. Lincoln Hospital School of Nursing yearbook. Lincoln Hospital School of Nursing Archives, Durham, N.C.

Thirty-Eighth Annual Report Lincoln Hospital. 1938. Stanford L. Warren Library, Durham, N.C.

Thorpe, Elizabeth W. Interview with the authors. March 1971.

Chapter Three

The Changing Tide, 1945–1971

Class Poem: Class of 1948

On August twenty-fourth of forty-five,
We were so darn glad to be alive,
To enter into Nurses Training;
Glad too, that it wasn't raining.
As we ventured on into our chosen profession—
We've had many, many a session.
Some proved good, some proved sad,
And on the other hand that wasn't so bad.
Professional Adjustment, Oh! What a course,
But we dug into it with a terrific force.
Trying to gain knowledge needed,
To prevent quick packing, instructions we heeded.
Don't be fooled, that's really tough;
Nursing instructors can dig out some stuff.
Vitamins, minerals, and medicine too—
Sometimes we thought [t]hat we were really through.
Crying, studying, we worked like mad;
Each other, at times, were all we had.
Settling some nights for a game of pinochle,
Which now makes us sit down and chuckle.
That was the time set aside for study.
But, if you wanted to cut, there was always a buddy.
Don't forget Vespers on Sunday;
If you failed to go, there was a conference on Monday.
When coming in, please don't be late,
Miss Mason will show you that you really don't rate.

Campus! Campus! That word we dread
And for the least little thing that word was said.
In your room, please don't sing,
Or the faithful buzzer you would soon hear ring.
At ten-thirty, turn out every light
For all rest and sleep must be gotten at night.
That is, unless someone decided to operate;
You'll go over stat, and you won't be late.
Stat! Stat! that awful word.
While in surgery that was all you heard.
You washed the windows, you scrubbed the floor,
You turned around, and there was still much more.
In the wee hour of the morn,
There comes a wail—a new life is born.
It doesn't matter if all packs are depleted,
A Lincoln nurse will find what's needed.
So, after all is said and done,
It has been three years, but at last we've won.
Our motto we carry, and try to preserve,
"Enter to Learn—Depart to serve."

—Author unknown

THE PROGRESSIVENESS OF PROFESSIONAL NURSING

The period extending from the mid-1940s to the closing of Lincoln Hospital School of Nursing (LHSN) was perhaps the most challenging, rewarding, and disappointing in the history of the school. During this time Lincoln Hospital and LHSN experienced significant internal difficulties in maintaining adequate resources. The physical facilities were deteriorating and becoming obsolete, personnel for patient care were in short supply, and the patient population in the hospital declined and lacked the diversity needed to meet the clinical-practice requirements of nurse training.

Professional nursing at the national, state, and local levels underwent bold changes that affected the hospital and the School of Nursing. On the national front, the American Nurses Association and the National League of Nursing became the official organizations representing nursing. They faced uphill battles in establishing control of nursing practice, the educational direction of nursing programs, and economic security for nurses. At the state level, a triumvirate composed of the North Carolina League of Nursing, the Board of Nursing Examiners, and the North Carolina State Nurses Association determined the standards for nursing education and practice. Nursing in the 1950s primarily focused on readying nurses for atomic warfare, improving nursing education and practice (i.e., its functions, qualifications, and standards), expanding nursing research, informing legislative changes, and establishing economic security. The needs of the nursing profession were emphasized, as was the preparation of nurses to serve as qualified administrators, educators, and supervisors for meeting the challenges of the changing health-care landscape.

Events on the international scene (ending of World War II, the Cuban Missile Crisis, the Civil Rights Crisis of the 1960s, and the Vietnam War) challenged the nursing leadership at every level. Changes in health policy and law, with the implementation of government-sponsored health programs and insurance for the very young and elderly populations, provided many with access to health care for the first time. The Civil Rights Movement provided Negro citizens with new freedoms and access to opportunities in all areas of life.

This era also saw increased social freedoms, and nursing students began to experience some balance between school, work, and their personal lives. For students who trained at Lincoln during this period, the era became known as the "L. Z. Era." Miss Lucille Zimmerman joined LHSN as the director of nursing service and nursing education in 1945 and remained in this position through the school's closing in 1971.

The last twenty-six years of the school (1945–1971) can be metaphorically described as the "Years of the Changing Tide." Internal and external factors made the waters turbulent. The tide ebbed and flowed and then, in 1971, went out to sea to return no more. Ms. Zimmerman (later Williams) navigated those changing waters. She aimed to prepare students to adapt to a changing world, regardless of the circumstances, and to meet the challenge of the corresponding changes in nursing and in health care in general.

Ms. Zimmerman was raised in a deeply religious home. Her father was a Baptist minister and her mother was a missionary. She received her nurse training at St. Agnes Hospital in Raleigh, North Carolina; attended Morrison College in Sumter, South Carolina; and in 1958 earned a bachelor of science degree in public health from North Carolina College (now North Carolina Central University), in Durham, North Carolina. Prior to joining Lincoln she was engaged in public health practice, traveling from Maine to Florida to provide health care for migrant workers. She also worked at Community

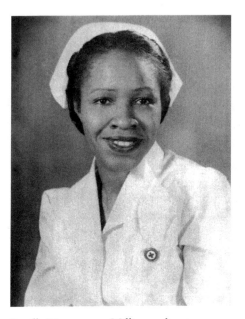

Lucille Zimmerman Williams, director of nursing service and nursing education, 1945–1971. Reprinted from The Scalpel, 1948. Courtesy of Marion Glen Miles.

Hospital, in Wilmington, North Carolina. She married in 1948 and became Mrs. Williams.

Ms. Z, as she was fondly called, was a stickler for grooming. Stately in her appearance, with her uniform immaculately starched, her cap a bright white, her handkerchief tucked neatly in her breast pocket, and her hands perfectly manicured, she portrayed a professional image and always greeted students with a smile. She cautioned students to "Keep your hands pretty; after they see your smile, they see your hands, the tools of your profession." She stressed to students that when they were in the public, even if they were not in uniform, they needed to look well put together, saying, "You girls cannot afford to be casual." This was another reminder of how important she felt image was to the nursing profession.

Ms. Z was well known in the Durham community. She was described as very friendly, outgoing, and involved in community affairs. Her personality, communication skills, and involvement in the community benefitted the school. She participated in a weekly radio broadcast on wDNC with Northley Whitted covering educational topics for the local community. Students accompanied her on these weekly broadcasts. Her involvement in the community, coupled with her communication skills and bright smile, probably accounted for a statement she made in an interview with Ruby and me: "I had been able to gain support to get whatever I needed for the students from the people in the community."

Ms. Z was a commonsensical and practical person. She had many maxims by which she lived. Many of us remember these: "If it ain't broke, don't fix it" and "Don't worry about the mule going blind." A favorite when students were somewhat rebellious was "Pack your pie box and go home." Many of us took that seriously. A longtime family friend and caretaker remembers her saying, "Whatever will happen, will happen on Thursday."

Mrs. Elizabeth Williams Thorpe (RN '48), a longtime supervisor and instructor in obstetrics, spoke of Ms. Z this way:

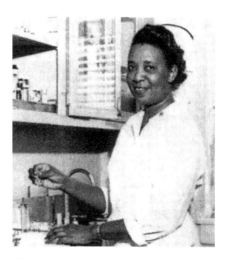

She knew every student; she knew where they were coming from. She could read you like a book. She was thinking before you started. You tried to fool her but underneath, psychologically, she was one of the greatest. She could fool you to death, like she was going to murder you and scare the daylights out of you—but it was all for the student's benefit . . . the students were her uppermost concern. She said, "You must be a

Elizabeth Williams Thorpe. Reprinted from *The Scalpel*, 1963. Courtesy of Marion Glen Miles.

good student, you must perform. You are going to minister to patients and you must prepare yourself spiritually before you go to the patient's bedside." Before we went to minister to a patient, we had to go to the library and we had a short service. She would read a scripture from her book and a short prayer. This was important to me. As I entered Lincoln in 1960, this devotional ritual was not routine but the importance of spiritual devotion was continuously emphasized.

She had an especially strong interest in the professional growth and development of individual students, and she set high standards for scholarship and practice. In fact, the first class admitted under her administration in 1945 was a class with distinction—in 1948 everyone passed the State Board Examination on the first writing. Below are the members of this class.

Rosebud Roderick Beverly
Lillian Brown
Annie B. Coley Boyd
Helen J. Black
Muriel Harris Daniels
Thereasea D. Clark Elder
Dorothy A. Farley

Zella Perry Thompson
Elizabeth Williams Thorpe
Lois Clements Brown Thorpe
Margaret Davis Reeder
Corona McCoy Umstead
Alice Williams
Othello Cave Williams
Mary B. Worley

(continues on page 99)

Laura Hart Harrison, RN '58

I am a 1955 graduate of Everglades Vocational High School, in Belle Glade, Florida, Palm Beach County. It was the only high school in the area for "Negroes" and was always seven to ten years behind in terms of textbooks and other educational equipment. But, thanks be to God, our Black principals and teachers were masters at improvising and taught us how to compete in the academic world. The first time that I sat in a classroom with White students was when I wrote my college entrance exam, which was required by Lincoln Hospital School of Nursing (LHSN) for acceptance.

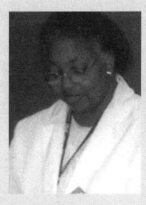

Courtesy of Laura Hart Harrison.

My parents lived in a village called Azuca, Florida, where people worked in the sugarcane industry. I was born the forth of eight children. My mother did domestic work to add to the family's meager income. One day when I was eleven years old, I came home from school and found my mother, who was eight or nine months pregnant with her eighth child, unconscious and breathing funny. I knew that a lady named Nurse Porter worked in the emergency clinic for the village, so I ran to get her. She came and assessed mother's condition and arranged for her to be admitted to a hospital some miles away. As I observed Nurse Porter caring for my mother, the desire to help other people was born in me. I wanted to be a nurse. Nurse Porter became my friend and told me about Lincoln Hospital in Durham, North Carolina, where she had worked. She told me that my parents could afford to send me there, even on their small income. Once I went to high school, my dream of being a nurse continued, and my family was so proud when I was accepted to LHSN.

Lincoln Hospital School of Nursing was personified by our nursing director, Mrs. Lucille Zimmerman Williams, RN, who emphasized professional ethics, social graces, humanity, and spiritual nourishment. She also emphasized other qualities that were needed to relate with the individuals and communities that we serve and the healthcare teams with whom we work. The expertise of our nursing arts instructor, Geraldine Butler, RN, enabled us to develop excellent nursing skills. Our performance was outstanding while on affiliations for the study of pediatric and psychiatric nursing.

My nursing career has led me down many paths over many years including head nurse, Surgical Unit, North Shore University Hospital, Manhasset, N.Y.; head nurse, Recovery Room, Jamaica Hospital, Jamaica, N.Y.; nurse consultant, Division of Day Care Department of Health (DOH), N.Y.; and nurse supervisor and clinical manager, Fed Cap Home Care Agency, New York, N.Y. The most rewarding service of my career was with the Fed Cap Rehabilitation Service, Inc., New York, under whose auspices a Joint Partnership Training Act (JPTA) Program for training home health aides was begun. I was responsible for planning, developing, and submitting the curriculum to the New York State DOH for certification. The program passed on the first submission. I trained and certified over three thousand home health aides. Many of the trainees were welfare recipients and were so grateful to finally be members of the job force of New York City.

Fed Cap nominated me to the New York State Legislature's 1993 Nurse of Distinction Award Program. All the nominees were honored at the National League for Nursing in New York City. We were also rewarded with a two-day conference held in Albany, N.Y., under the direction of Michael J. Tully Jr., state senator. I was cited at Fed Cap for twenty years of service. As clinical manager of Fed Cap Home Care, I was instrumental in the Home Care Department receiving its Joint Commission on the Accreditation of Health Care Organizations.

This class was well guided by Gertrude Bullock, nursing arts instructor and class advisor. She was a 1936 Lincoln graduate. She presented the following message to the graduating Class of 1948:

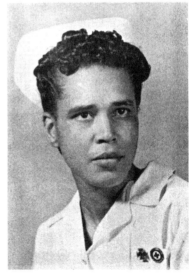

Many have been the days when you sailed along smoothly, depending mostly on others to steer your course. Now you have reached the crossroads where you must say goodbye to the familiar scenes and associates and launch out for the great beyond. The ocean lies before you—take advantage of the sailing. The waters will be deep and you know it, at times the sailing tough, and you know it, but when the waves begin to toss you about speak to the King of Kings and ask for the abating of the waters. Have faith, then the sailing will be smooth to the end.

Gertrude Bullock, nursing arts instructor and class advisor. Reprinted from The Scalpel, 1948.

(continues on page 101)

Glenda Howard Harris, RN '70
"Building A Dream"

Having a dream is what makes our lives worth living and it keeps hope alive. My story is probably just ordinary to some, but my dreams of someday achieving the one thing that I could do for a lifetime and still love even when I was older started when I was in high school. Nursing is that one thing in my life that was born of a dream and became a reality after I was accepted to Lincoln Hospital School of Nursing (LHSN). I was born in 1948 to a wonderful family. My dad was a self-made Chemist, who had pride in himself and felt that he could do anything that anyone else could do. My mom was a meek, wonderful woman who was a domestic worker. I was the eldest of six children and, naturally, the task of being an example and taking care of everyone fell on my shoulders. We were very poor, but were rich in love and good things. I always wanted to take care of everyone and everything, for everybody. It was not hard to choose nursing as a career because it just seemed like the right thing to do, and I felt that God "called" me to do so. I attended an all-Black high school, York Road High School, in Charlotte, North Carolina, in the early 1960s when things were tough and money was tight. At that time, Black women could choose only teaching or nursing, and of course I didn't want to teach or so I thought. I was awarded a scholarship to attend LHSN, which in itself was a miracle because there was very little money for education at that time.

It was so hard being at Lincoln that first year. I had never been away from home, and I was scared and cried a lot. We were in a disciplined environment, which taught me dignity, self-respect, and respect for others. Lincoln Hospital students were charged to achieve and excel, and we had better not get less than a B in any class at North Carolina College (now North Carolina Central University). Our director of nursing, Mrs. Williams, was very strict and would send you home if she had to. For that, I will never forget her. Lincoln Hospital graduates were being prepared to come out of school and take charge right away. After graduation, many of us became charge nurses after only two or three weeks of orientation. When given an assignment as a new nurse, I for one felt that God had blessed me to rise to the top, and I was so proud of that. Additionally, we were given the opportunity to work in the hospital after classes and earn a little money to help pay our way. We learned so many things that made us strong and prepared us for twenty-first century nursing. I am so proud that I attended LHSN when I did because I was given the opportunity to give back to God what He had given to me. While at Lincoln, God favored me to be mentored by some wonderful women who were LPNs, such as Lottie Hall, Ellen Webster and Connie Brown. They took me under their wings and looked out for me, which helped me through.

It wasn't hard for me to write my story about my love for our school. It would take a lot of paper to describe every experience I had at Lincoln that shaped my life. I have been a nurse for forty years, and it seems like it was just yesterday that I graduated from nursing school. My training at Lincoln forever changed my life. Because of Lincoln I have been able to experience so many avenues in health care. I have been a surgical charge nurse, a psychiatric nurse manager, a hospice nurse, a triage nurse, a long-term care nurse, an outpatient clinic nurse, a nurse educator in a high school, and now a medical-surgical telemetry nurse with oncology experience. Some of the children who I taught in high school loved my stories about my nursing-school experiences and were inspired to seek careers as doctors and nurses. WOW, all of this because I attended one of the best schools of nursing, LHSN. Even if my story is not chosen for our book, it has been a pleasure writing it. I thank God for giving me the opportunity to serve His people and become a nurse. The steps of good men are ordered by the Lord, and God truly guided my steps to Lincoln Hospital School of Nursing.

May God keep the memory of LHSN alive.

Many changes were initiated under the administration of Ms. Z in accordance with board standards. Perhaps one of the most substantive was the change in the admissions procedure. From the early years through the late 1920s, students were admitted during the year whenever there were vacancies. Between the mid-1930s and the mid-1940s students were admitted just two times a year. Soon after her appointment in 1945, Ms. Z implemented the practice of admitting students just once a year, in the fall. Once-a-year admissions provided more consistency, uniformity, and structure for the school, administrators, instructors, and students. However, this change created new staffing challenges for the hospital.

Two other changes that occurred under her leadership were the admission of younger students (the minimum age was decreased to seventeen-and-a-half years old) and the admission of married students. Previously, married students were not allowed in nursing schools. Although the new policy was not implemented at Lincoln until 1960, in 1947 Lois Morris Smith received special permission to marry on the day of her graduation. In 1958 Margaret Aquilla Watkins Stanfield received special permission to marry while she was a student, and the marriage ceremony took place on the Lincoln campus.

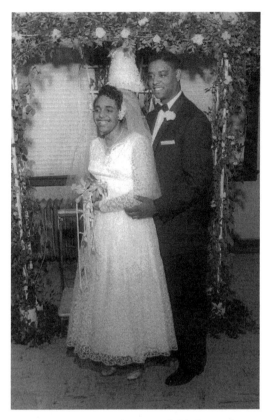

Margaret Aquilla Watkins Stanfield obtained permission to marry while attending Lincoln Hospital School of Nursing. Married June 30, 1957. Courtesy of Margaret Aquilla Watkins Stanfield.

In 1960 three married students were admitted to the program: Thelma Hayes Thornton, Gertrude Carson Meadows, and Yvonne Goolsby Spencer. These students exhibited great maturity and frequently counseled their younger, unmarried classmates. All three graduated in 1963.

FACULTY IN THE SCHOOL OF NURSING

From the mid-1940s on, the Board of Nursing became increasingly stringent in its scrutinizing of schools of nursing. The Board of Nursing Examiners and the standardization committee began to raise the standards regarding consistency and uniformity of the curriculum, admissions standards, and

Thelma Hayes Thornton, RN '63

I am the daughter of Lucious Hayes and Pearlie Bass Hayes and was born in Person County, North Carolina. I was the fifth of eight children and was educated in the Person County schools. I graduated from Person County High School in 1955. Later I entered Durham Technical School (now Durham Technical Community College) and became a Licensed Practical Nurse. I worked at Duke University Hospital, in Durham, North Carolina, for three years.

I married the love of my life, Tom Thornton Jr., in 1959. We were blessed with three daughters.

I applied to Lincoln Hospital School of Nursing (LHSN) and graduated in the Class of 1963. I was one of the first married students allowed to attend, along with my roommate Yvonne Spencer. I passed the State Board of Nursing Examination on the first attempt and continued my training in public health. I've been employed as a school nurse, in the Vance County School System and later in the Granville County School System in Oxford, North Carolina. I was also a nurse in a doctor's office and a camp nurse at Camp Oak Hill in Oxford, North Carolina.

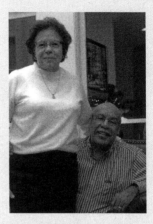

Thelma Hayes Thornton was already married on admission to Lincoln Hospital School of Nursing. Courtesy of Thelma Hayes Thornton.

I am a member of many church ministries and civic organizations, and I most recently became a member of the Trustee Board of the Granville Health System.

I am grateful for the excellent training I received from the faculty and staff of LHSN and would like to thank them, the wonderful students I met, and my husband for their unwavering support, which gave me the incentive to stay and complete nursing school.

student work hours. Additionally, the hiring of faculty devoted exclusively to the supervision and teaching of students became an imperative. The faculty's support of the students' emotional and spiritual development was as important as their advisement and academic counseling. However, securing qualified faculty was difficult due to the limited supply of trained nurses and the limited fiscal resources of the hospital. Another recurring issue was the students' difficulty in passing the board examination on first writing. Eventually they all passed, according to Ms. Z in a conversation with Ruby and me in 1971. Several instructors who taught at the school from the mid-1960s through the end had ideas about the reasons students had difficulties with the board examination. Julia Oliver, a graduate of Winston-Salem State University, North Carolina, taught in pediatrics. She described the students as hard-working, bright, and committed to patient care. Their challenges, she felt, included their backgrounds and their deficiencies in critical-thinking and problem-solving skills, which she attributed to poor preparation in elementary and secondary schooling. She felt the students would have benefited from having materials to review before taking their state boards; these materials were reportedly available at White schools. Julia Oliver later obtained her license as a Nurse Anesthetist and shared that she and her classmates had practiced on an old test before taking their boards. She too felt that this resource would have been helpful to the students at Lincoln. We will never know whether this was the case.

The School of Nursing only had one White clinical instructor, Elizabeth Robin Gordon. Ms. Gordon expressed similar opinions and felt that students at Lincoln were unfairly judged because they did not all start from the same place as their White peers in general. Some students were well prepared, while others fell short on basic skills such as reading, writing, and math. Their baseline skills were a reflection of social inequities for which the school could not make up. Another contributing factor to the low board passing was the lack of diversity among the patient census. Nevertheless, Elizabeth Robin Gordon characterized the students as motivated, caring, hardworking, high achievers despite their backgrounds and limited patient experiences. She worked as a clinical instructor alongside Joan Miller Martin Jones Mathews in the 1967–68 school year.

Lincoln Hospital and the School of Nursing worked very hard to maintain their A rating. The hospital's hiring of instructors and several graduate nurses for supervisory positions (upon their becoming registered nurses) greatly facilitated this achievement. Below is a list of most of the instructors and supervisors who worked at Lincoln in the period after the hospital's first achievement of the A rating:

A. Mildred Crisp, Operating Room Supervisor, 1940
Mary L. Thicklin Jones, Outpatient Department Supervisor, 1956–1971
Laura Walker, Pediatric Instructor, 1962
Joyce Roland, Instructor, Medicine/Surgery, 1962
Manice P. Banks, Nursing Arts Instructor, 1959–1960s
Sylvia Overton Richardson, Director of Nursing Education, Assistant
     Director of Nursing Services, Drugs and Solutions Instructor, 1959–1966

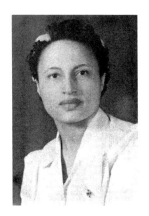 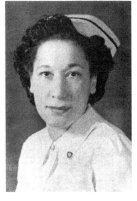

Left: *A. Mildred Crisp, operating room supervisor, 1940.* Reprinted from *The Scalpel,* 1948.

Right: *Mary L. Thicklin Jones, outpatient department supervisor, 1956–1971.* Reprinted from *The Scalpel,* 1948.

Left to right: *Joyce Roland, medicine/surgery instructor, 1962; Manice P. Banks, nursing arts instructor, 1959–1960s; Sylvia Overton Richardson, drugs and solutions instructor, 1959–1966.* Reprinted from *The Scalpel,* 1963. Courtesy of Bernice King.

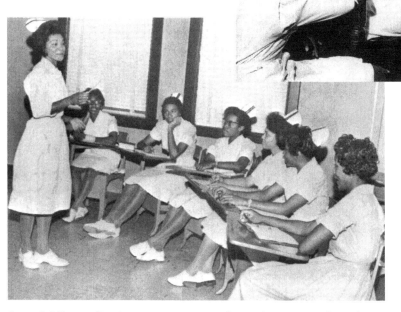

Laura Walker, pediatrics instructor, 1962. Left to right: *Attemerell Smith, Otelia Blanks Smith, Mary Bass Satterwhite, Altamease Riley Arnold, JoAnna Neal Dowling, Maggie Lee Ledbetter.* Reprinted from *The Scalpel,* 1962. Courtesy of Patricia Martin Blue.

Lelia P. Thompson, Obstetrics Supervisor, 1948
Julia Oliver, Pediatrics Instructor, 1962
Marion G. Elizabeth Sanders DeGreffread Rogers, Night Supervisor, 1948
Elizabeth Robin Gordon, Clinical Instructor, 1968 (the only White clinical
   instructor on campus)
Joan Miller Martin Jones Mathews, Clinical Instructor, 1968
M. L. Smith, Supervisor of Surgery, 1948

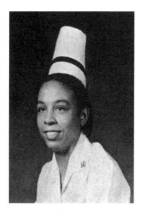 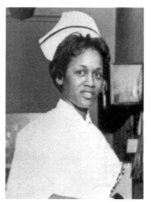 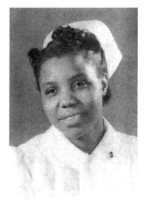

Lelia P. Thompson,   *Julia Oliver, pediatrics*   *Marion G. Elizabeth*
supervisor of obstetrics,   *instructor, 1962.* Reprinted   *Sanders DeGraffread*
1948. Reprinted from *The* from *The Scalpel,* 1962.   *Rogers, night supervisor,*
Scalpel, 1948.   Courtesy of Patricia Martin   *1948.* Reprinted from *The*
                              Blue.   *Scalpel,* 1948.

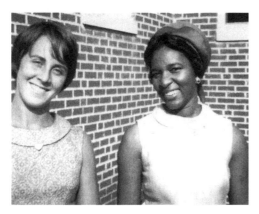 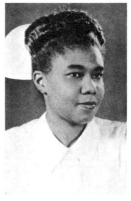

Elizabeth Robin Gordon, clinical instructor,   *M. L. Smith, supervisor of*
1968 (the only White clinical instructor on   *surgery, 1948.* Reprinted
campus); Joan Miller Martin Jones Mathews,   from *The Scalpel,* 1948.
clinical instructor, 1968. Courtesy of Elizabeth
Robin Gordon.

Ruth E. Parlor Amey, Supervisor of Obstetrics, 1947
Elizabeth Williams Thorpe, Supervisor and Instructor of Obstetrics,
    1956–1971 (see picture on page 97)
Julia Simpson Armstrong, Night Supervisor of Medicine, 1948
Lelia B. Miller Thompson, Supervisor of Operating Room, 1951–1971
Corona McClary Umstead, Supervisor of Central Supply, 1959, and Head
    Nurse of Obstetrics, 1962
Marion Glen Miles, Night Supervisor, 1959, Recovery Room, 1960s

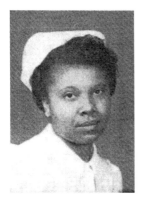 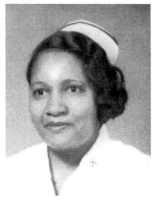 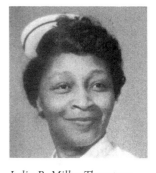

*Lelia B. Miller Thompson,
supervisor of operating room,
1951–1971. Reprinted from The
Nightingale, 1958. Courtesy of
Marion Glen Miles.*

*Ruth E. Parlor Amey,
supervisor of obstetrics,
1947.* Reprinted from *The
Scalpel,* 1947. Courtesy of
Lois Smith Morris.

*Julia Simpson Armstrong,
night supervisor of medicine,
1948.* Reprinted from *The
Nightingale,* 1958. Courtesy of
Marion Glen Miles.

*Corona McClary
Umstead, super-
visor of central
supply, 1959, and
(later, 1962) head
nurse of obstetrics.*
Reprinted from *The
Nightingale,* 1958.
Courtesy of Marion
Glen Miles.

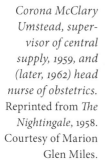 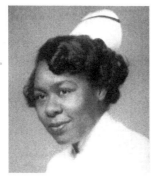 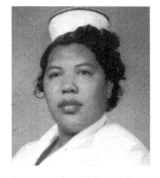

*Marion Glen Miles, night
supervisor, 1959, and supervisor of recovery room in the
1960s.* Reprinted from *The
Nightingale,* 1958. Courtesy of
Marion Glen Miles.

Lois Clements Brown Thorpe, Supervisor, Pediatrics, 1956
Laura Robinson, Supervisor of Medicine and Second Floor, late 1950s
    through the 1970s
Lula Cowan McNair, Instructor, 1963 (see picture on page 63)
Josephine Plummer, Instructor and Night Supervisor, 1962
Helen Neal Webb Jones, Supervisor of Second Floor, 1959

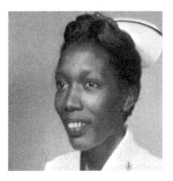

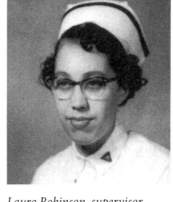

Lois Clements Brown Thorpe,
supervisor of pediatrics, 1956.
Reprinted from *The Nightingale,*
1958. Courtesy of Marion Glen
Miles.

Laura Robinson, supervisor
of medicine and second floor,
1950s–1970s. Reprinted from *The*
Nightingale, 1959. Courtesy of
Marion Glen Miles.

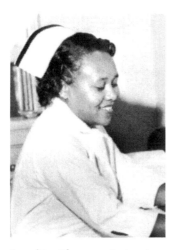

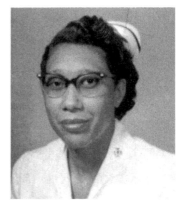

Josephine Plummer, instructor
and night supervisor, 1962.
Reprinted from *The Scalpel,* 1962.
Courtesy of Patricia Martin Blue.

Helen Neal Webb Jones,
supervisor of second floor, 1959.
Reprinted from *The Nightingale,*
1958. Courtesy of Marion Glen
Miles.

Although many of these instructors were prepared at the diploma level, they participated in continuing education to prepare them for their instructional and supervisory roles. For example, Elizabeth W. Thorpe, a supervisor and instructor in obstetrics, attended a post-graduate course at Margaret Hague Hospital, in Jersey City, New Jersey, and Lelia B. Thompson, an operating room supervisor, attended a post-graduate course at Michael Reeves, in Chicago, Illinois. Others attended workshops at institutions such as Duke University, in Durham, North Carolina.

Other instructors external to Lincoln included Mr. Stahl, Pharmacology, Watts Hospital; Ms. K. C. Darden, Pharmacology, Xavier College, New Orleans; Mr. Butts, Chemistry, NCCU; Drs. Lee and Vernon Clarke, Microbiology, NCCU; Mrs. Dejarmon, Nutrition, NCCU; Ms. Gloria K. Saunders, Diet Therapy, NCCU; Ms. S. Hopper, Nutrition, NCCU; J. Himes, James Taylor, Psychology, NCCU; Mrs. Cooke and Mr. Slappy Brown, Sociology, NCCU; and the renowned Dr. Leroy Walker, Physiology and Anatomy, NCCU.

The title "Superintendent" was changed to "Director of Nursing" in the late 1940s. This change paralleled other changes in the hospital administration. Ms. Z became known as the Director of Nursing Services and Director of the School of Nursing. Her administrative assistant was titled the Assistant Director of Nursing Services and the Director of Nursing Education. Mr. Rich became known as the Director of the Hospital and subsequent administrators bore the same title.

Throughout her tenure, Ms. Z worked with several assistant directors of nursing, whose responsibilities lay with both the hospital nursing service and the School of Nursing. Some of the nurses who occupied these roles were:

Ella Ferguson Hargrave, Assistant Director of Nursing Education, 1950s
L. H. Houston, Assistant Director of Nursing Education and Nursing Arts
   Instructor
Geraldine C. Butler, Director of Nursing Education, 1956
M. K. Wilkerson, Acting Director of Nursing Education, 1956–1957
Alice C. Kennedy, Assistant Director of Nursing Education, Assistant
   Director of Nursing Services, 1956–1957
Sylvia Overton Richardson, Director of Nursing Education, Assistant
   Director of Nursing Services, 1959–1966
Leona Crockett, Director of Nursing Education, Instructor, 1968
Margaret Wilson, Clinical Instructor, 1968

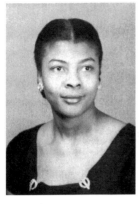

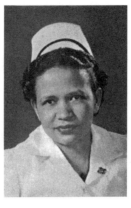

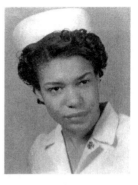

Geraldine C. Butler, director of nursing education, 1956. Reprinted from *The Scalpel*, 1957. Courtesy of Marion Glen Miles.

L. H. Houston, assistant director of nursing education and nursing arts instructor. Reprinted from *The Scalpel*, 1948.

Ella Ferguson Hargrave, assistant director of nursing education, 1950s. Reprinted from *The Scalpel*, 1956. Courtesy of Marion Glen Miles.

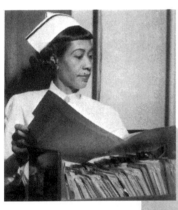

right: Leona Crockett, director of nursing education, instructor, 1968. Courtesy of Carolyn Evangeline Henderson.

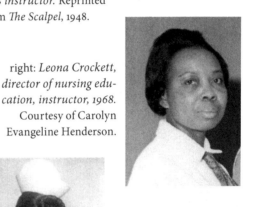

Alice C. Kennedy, assistant director of nursing education and assistant director of nursing services, 1956–1957. Reprinted from *The Nightingale*, 1958. Courtesy of Marion Glen Miles.

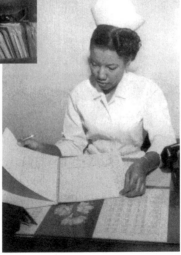

M. K. Wilkerson, acting director of nursing education, 1956–1957. Reprinted from *The Nightingale*, 1959. Courtesy of Marion Glen Miles.

Sylvia Overton Richardson, director of nursing education and assistant director of nursing services, 1959–1966. Courtesy of Sylvia Overton Richardson.

BOARD STANDARDS

The Board of Nursing Examiners for Schools of Nursing, in conjunction with the Standardization Committee, had continuously upgraded the standards for schools of nursing in order to produce better graduate nurses. The Board felt that by increasing the quality of the students, it could assure that the graduate nurses would be eligible for registration, reciprocity, and employment in federal service.

In addition to increased course requirements and a decrease in the age of admission (to seventeen-and-one-half years), changes were made to the students' work hours. The board mandated that students should be on duty only for necessary practice during the first two or three months of the pre-clinical period. The time students spent on duty was to be gradually increased during this period. Moreover, the combined number of hours spent in clinical practice and in class could not exceed forty-eight hours per week because students needed adequate time for study and recreation. Of equal concern was the hospital daily census. The hospital was required to have an average daily census of fifty patients.

On a visit to LHSN in the mid-1940s, the board emphasized the urgent need for additional graduate nurses, practical nurses, ward helpers, and orderlies so that the student nurses might be relieved of the major portion of the nursing load at Lincoln Hospital. For example, of the 335 nursing hours an average daily census of fifty patients required during a twenty-four hour period, the hospital could render only 156 hours with its present nursing staff. The Lincoln Hospital Board of Trustees immediately authorized the hiring of additional staff. The funding to support the additional salaries was achieved by increasing the daily rates of wards, semi-private, and private patients by $1 per day. This increase had a direct impact on all insurance carriers and an especially negative impact on the welfare departments throughout the state that sent patients to Lincoln Hospital. This change was effective on January 1, 1949.

In addition to the recommended staff changes, the Board of Examiners in 1948 established a general plan of the curriculum for schools of nursing in North Carolina. The plan included the required minimum clinical experience over the three-year period.

General Plan For Clinical Experience

Students in all classes entering January 1, 1948, and thereafter shall be given the following minimum clinical experience.

Minimum Experience

Pre-clinical period .... 24 weeks
Medical Nursing .... 20 weeks
Surgical Nursing (including GYN, E.E.N.&T., Ortho.) .... 20 weeks
Pediatric Nursing (including Infant Feeding) .... 12 weeks
Obstetric Nursing .... 12 weeks
Operating Room .... 8 weeks
Diet Kitchen .... 4–6 weeks
Vacations .... 8–9 weeks
Night Duty, to be included in the above and not to exceed .... 22 weeks
Psychiatry (recommended) .... 12 weeks
Community Nursing, Public Health (recommended if public
    health has been integrated with the entire curriculum) .... 1–6 weeks

It is recommended that other services such as outpatient, communicable disease, and tuberculosis nursing be included in the remaining twenty-seven to thirty-five weeks.

Pre-clinical Period: During the pre-clinical period of at least twenty-four weeks, the school shall endeavor to determine the student's fitness for the duties that will later be required of her. Her ability to understand the principles involved in the procedures taught her requires that she have time to study. Her duties on the ward during this time shall therefore be confined to practice periods under close graduate nurse supervision. The safety of the patient and the education of the nurse make it essential that these students shall not be given the responsibility of nursing care of patients during this time.

Subsequent Terms. Hours attending class and on duty after the pre-clinical period shall not exceed forty-eight hours per week for any student. The hours in class shall be considered to be time on duty, but the hours for meals shall be regarded as time off duty. The following allotment of hours is recommended:

6 to 8 hours daily in practical work.
1 to 2 hours daily in class work.
1 to 2 hours daily in study.
2 hours daily in recreation.

No student should be required to spend more than eight hours per day in practical work and should have an average of four hours for recreation and outdoor activities.

CURRICULUM

The curriculum at LHSN was planned in accordance with Board standards. It recognized the needs of the students, changes in nursing practices and skills, and the emerging social issues of the nursing profession. The curriculum consisted of didactic instruction in the classroom, clinical instruction in the lab, and clinical experience in the hospital. Successful student outcomes would be the yardstick by which the curriculum and its execution would be measured. As the school progressed, the planning of the curriculum became a collaborative effort between the director of nursing of the hospital and the School of Nursing, the educational director, the faculty, and the supervisors. The plan incorporated day, evening, and night rotations. The maximum evening and night rotations were each eighteen weeks in the course of the entire program. This strikes me as strange as it seems as if I only worked nights. I must have completed another student's night rotation in addition to my own eighteen weeks.

Although the curriculum did not originally include extracurricular activities, The Board and Lincoln leadership recognized that leisure activities were necessary for a well-integrated individual. In contrast with the students who matriculated during the first thirty years of the school, students now had many more activities and opportunities in which to participate. These activities, be they social, religious, or professional in nature, facilitated the students' growth and development. They became more confident and self-assured as they moved through Lincoln and entered the broader public stage.

Admissions

Most students who attended Lincoln found out about the school through word of mouth or a referral from a family member, a family network, a teacher, or a high-school counselor. Later, as physician networks were established and doctors began to share how outstanding Lincoln nurses were, the School of Nursing became a source of pride and a popular choice among those who wished to train as a nurse.

The recruitment of nursing students became more structured and focused in the 1950s and 1960s. Mrs. Sylvia Overton Richardson, Assistant Director of Nursing and Director of Nursing Education (1959–1966) was very involved in student advising and the recruitment process. According to Sylvia, "Mature, stable students predicted to be able to survive the rigors of training

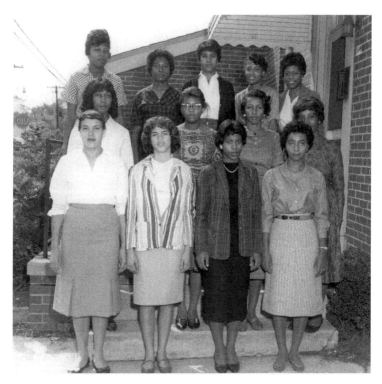

Class of 1963 as entering students. First row left to right: *Thelma Hayes Thornton, Norma Roberts Lipscomb, Gertrude Carson Meadows, Yvonne Goolsby Spencer.* Second row left to right: *Evelyn Booker Wicker, Jennie Woodard Slade, Elaine Richardson Smith, Irene Wright.* Third row left to right: *L. Thompson, Mary Davis Wright, Marion Johnson, Miron Andrews Wilkerson, Mary Lassiter Howell.* Reprinted from *The Scalpel,* 1962.

were recruited. Good grades also were important." High-school transcripts had to meet certain requirements, which are described in detail below. Sylvia viewed recruitment "as an interesting and exciting activity." She frequently attended high-school career days and college days with her colleagues from Durham Business College on Fayetteville Street and North Carolina College (now NCCU) on Fayetteville Street, in Durham. Recruitment materials included brochures and single flyers.

The transition in the admissions standards that began in the 1950s reflected the progressiveness of the board and the Standardization Committee. Nursing schools were required to pre-test applicants before accepting them. Passing (or failing as the case may be) the entry test was not the only

The

SCHOOL OF NURSING

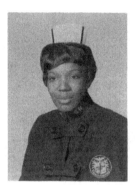

Lincoln Hospital

Durham, North Carolina

GENERAL INFORMATION

THE LINCOLN HOSPITAL SCHOOL OF NURSING offers a three-year course of study which includes instruction in all branches of nursing. The school is accredited by the North Carolina Board of Nursing. It is connected with Lincoln Hospital with a capacity of 105 beds. The Hospital has an A rating and is approved by the American College of Surgeons.

REQUIREMENTS FOR ADMISSION

AGE: 17 to 35 years of age.

MARITAL STATUS: Preferably single. Married applicants are given special consideration on individual basis.

PERSONALITY: Applicants should possess personality traits and attitudes which will make possible a satisfactory adjustment to professional nursing.

HEALTH: Must be in good health. (Dental and medical forms are included with all applications.)

EDUCATION: Graduated from an accredited high school with 16 units of credit, preferably consisting of the following:

ENGLISH	4 UNITS
MATHEMATICS (ALGEBRA, ETC.)	2 UNITS
FOREIGN LANGUAGE	2 UNITS
SOCIAL SCIENCE	2 UNITS
NATURAL SCIENCE	
(PREFERABLY CHEMISTRY	
AND BIOLOGY)	2 UNITS
ELECTIVES	4 UNITS

PRE-ENTRANCE TESTS: After all application materials have been received the applicant will be notified by letter to come for pre-entrance tests and an interview. The cost of the test battery is $10.00, payable at the time the test is given. Application to take the pre-entrance nursing examination should be made to the Director of Education, Lincoln Hospital, Durham, N. C.

DIRECTIONS FOR MAKING APPLICATION

Write to the Director of Nursing, Lincoln Hospital, Durham, N. C. and ask for applica-

The 1965 School of Nursing bulletin with admission requirements.

factor that determined whether a student was admitted to nursing school because admission was based on an overall profile. Lincoln wanted the student to be in the upper third of her high-school graduating class with an average grade of 85 percent. Most of Lincoln's students were outstanding students in their local schools, graduating as valedictorian or salutatorian. As many of the students entered Lincoln during segregation and before integration was firmly applied, their primary and secondary educational experiences were limited. Skills in test-taking, critical thinking, and reading comprehension were marginal in many of the students due to the inequality of the educational system and its allocation of resources, including facilities, equipment, supplies, and teacher training. A number of Lincoln graduates reported that they did not pass the entry test but were accepted conditionally. They went on to apply themselves and become outstanding graduates. Negro/Black families have always highly valued education and that value was instilled and drilled into Negro/Black children. A common refrain in their communities, and especially among teachers in segregated schools, was, "Get an education; that is something no one can take from you." Lincoln students had the passion, the discipline, and the motivation to achieve; they did not

Janie Lee Canty-Mitchell, RN '71, BSN, MSN, PhD

My paternal and maternal ancestors were settled in Pinewood, Wedgefield, and Sumter, South Carolina, for at least five known generations. My parents, James Ernest Canty and Janie Geter Canty, were married when twenty-one and sixteen years old, respectively; neither graduated from high school, as was the case with many in the earlier generations of my family. Six children were born to my parents' union, all within eight-and-a-half years of each other. I was the second child, sandwiched between an older sister and a younger brother. During the early years of my life, through the fifth grade, my parents were tenant farmers. The children were expected to assist the adults by planting, caring for, and gathering cotton, peanuts, soybeans, vegetables, and fruit crops, especially watermelons. There were farm animals at my paternal grandparents' home that we

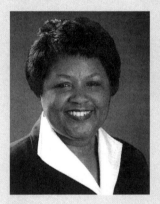

Courtesy of Janie Lee Canty-Mitchell.

were at times asked to care for, including feeding horses and milking cows. I attended segregated elementary, middle, and high schools in Sumter, often using second-hand books from the "White" schools in town. I graduated from Lincoln High School in 1968 at the age of seventeen.

Nursing had been my career interest since elementary school, sparked by a nurse who came to Green Elementary School to immunize the first graders. In my senior year of high school, my aunt Carrie Bell Canty informed me about Lincoln Hospital School of Nursing; one of her classmates was a Lincoln graduate. I applied to Lincoln and as a requirement for admission I had to travel from Sumter to Durham, North Carolina, to take a pre-nursing standardized examination. This was my first bus trip and my first ever trip out of South Carolina. Lincoln accepted me as a probationary student because my scores on the standardized test were unacceptable. From the

want to disappoint themselves or their families, who struggled in many cases to support their education. A 1971 student, Dr. Janie Canty-Mitchell, described her experiences and her achievements in her story.

During the 1960s Lincoln participated in regional testing sites throughout the southeastern states. One of the testing sites was in Birmingham, Alabama. Patricia Martin Blue, a 1965 graduate and a resident of Alabama, related that she was undecided about nursing as a career and about Lincoln as a school. By the time she settled on nursing and found out about the test-

beginning, I knew I had to succeed because failure meant going back to Sumter where few opportunities for growth existed. I excelled in classes at North Carolina College (now North Carolina Central University) and was surprised when the Lincoln Alumni Association awarded me a prize for having the highest grade point average in my second (junior) year. The culmination of my Lincoln experiences was receiving the award at graduation for achieving the highest academic average. I did not know how much the nursing program would contribute to my growth and development as a person and as a nurse.

Since leaving Lincoln in 1971, I have earned a bachelor's degree in nursing (BSN), a master's degree in nursing (MSN), and a doctor of philosophy (PhD) degree in nursing—all from schools in Florida. My nursing career includes experiences in psychiatric/mental-health nursing, public health nursing, supervision and administration, program development, project management, coalition building, teaching, and research. Between 1988 and 2007, I worked as a faculty member in higher education, teaching in schools of nursing at Florida International University, the University of Miami, Indiana University, and the University of Florida.

Since 2007, I have worked at the University of North Carolina in Wilmington in the roles of associate dean/director of research, community partnership, and sponsored programs. My research and scholarly activities have focused on children's mental health and quality of life, adolescent risky behaviors, health disparities, and environmental stressors on children's health and well-being. I have presented fifty-five podium speeches and scholarly posters at local, regional, national, and international conferences and have published twenty peer-reviewed articles or book chapters.

From 2004 to 2008, I served as a charter member and nurse consultant on the National Institute of Health, Center for Scientific Review, Children and Family Study Section. In 2009 the Robert Wood Johnson (RWJ) Foundation selected me as one of twenty fellows in the nation-wide Executive Nurse Fellows (ENF) Program. The RWJ ENF Program is an advanced leadership program for nurses in senior executive roles who aspire to lead and shape the U.S. health-care system of the future.

ing site in Birmingham, the date of the test had passed. She had to come to Durham, N.C., for testing. The hospital had begun a monthly publication, *The Dispatch*, which was a local publication shared among the Durham medical community. *The Dispatch* listed the monthly pre-nursing testing dates for candidates. It's possible that it was disseminated to guidance counselors in the various high schools in the surrounding area. I remember coming to Durham for the interview and taking my test. It was a frightening experience for a naïve, small-town, country girl. I apparently did well on the test. I was admitted without probation.

Higher Academic Standards

In addition to the testing requirement, the academic standards were exceedingly high. These standards, or the grading scale, were determined internally by the school's nursing administration. Students who could not meet these standards were dismissed. The attrition rate ranged over time from 15 percent to as high as 60 percent. Many classes started with high numbers, but far fewer completed the curriculum. The grading scale from 1945 to 1959 consistently reflected these higher standards. The academic expectations at LHSN as stated in the 1945–1946 *Bulletin*, were very clear: "A passing grade of 80% must be made in each subject. A final grade for the course within five points below passing grade will pass the student on condition; however, this does not apply to the major in Nursing. The grading in Nursing Arts was 75%. A failing grade in this course automatically eliminated the student from the school." By 1959 the Nursing Arts passing grade had been raised to 85 percent, and preferably 90 percent. By the end of the 1960s, requirements in all areas had increased and the expectation was that students would comply. A concern about the academic performance of Dorothy Esta Dennis Segars, who potentially was failing, was communicated by letter to her parents. She maintained that she had been studying very diligently despite the poor grades. Maybe what was needed was a diversion from her stress. Esta, now a successful, retired graduate, cleaned up her act, became a card expert, completed the program, and passed her Board exam on first writing. In her own words:

By the 1968 graduation, nine completed the program out of a group of twenty-one. They left for various reasons and, yes, grades were a reason for dismissal. I managed to stay one step ahead. Previously 76 and 81 were considered passing; however, not at Lincoln, these grades were failing. At one point I received two failing grades and called my mother wanting to

```
                    LINCOLN HOSPITAL SCHOOL OF NURSING
                          DURHAM, NORTH CAROLINA

                              Grade Sheet

To:  Mr. & Mrs. Purvis Dennis
     Post Office Box 213
     Holly Springs, North Carolina

Report of:  Miss Esther Dennis           Period  1st & 2nd Semester 1965-66
```

	1st Year		2nd Year		3rd Year	
Subject	1st Sem.	2nd Sem.	1st Sem.	2nd Sem.	1st Sem.	2nd Sem.
Anatomy & Physiology	92					
Chemistry	85					
Microbiology		85				
Nutrition and Cookery		89				
Nursing Arts	89	92				
Psychology		79				
Nursing History (Included in Nursing Arts)						
Sociology		79				
Professional Adjustment I (Included in Nursing Art)						
Professional Adjustment II						
Drugs & Solution		89				
Pharmacology II		83				
Introduction to Medical Science		85				
Medical & Surgical Nursing						
Diet Therapy						
Operating Room Technique						
Communicable Disease Nursing						
Eye, Ear, Nose & Throat						
Orthopedic Nursing						
Gynecology & Obstetrics						
Pediatrics						
Dermatology						
Urology						
Public Health						
Psychiatry						
Neurology						
English	93					

```
Key:  A+  99-100   C+  90-91     Comments: Borderline student in most subjects,
      A   98        C   88-89
      A-  96-97     C-  86-87     however, over-all performance has improved.
      B+  94-95     D+  84-85
      B   93        D   82-83     Strives to do well.
      B-  92        D-  80-81


Date:    June 30, 1966          Signed: L. A. Crockett, R.N.

                                Title:  Director Nursing Education
```

Grade Sheet of Dorothy Esta Dennis Segars. Courtesy of Dorothy Esta Dennis Segars.

go home. She told me to hang up the phone, go upstairs, and study; my mother's decisions were law. I went upstairs, learned to play pinochle, and played every chance I got. It was a good stress reliever. I continued to study as usual and my grades improved. I received an award at graduation for technical competency (no errors in medication administration), and I passed State Boards on first writing.

(continues on page 122)

Dorothy Esta Dennis Segars, RN '68, BSN

I am one of seven siblings, born and raised
in Wake County, North Carolina. I attended
Fuquay Consolidated High School in
Fuquay Varina, North Carolina, until the
tenth grade when I transferred to Apex
Consolidated High School, in Apex, North
Carolina. After graduation I attended
Lincoln Hospital School of Nursing, in
Durham, North Carolina. I had aspired to
be a nurse since the fourth grade when I saw
what I thought was a nurse in my geography
book taking care of a native in Africa. Later
I learned the picture was of a Catholic
nun. At that time I had not been exposed
to other religions except the usual Baptist
and Methodist faiths. Before continuing
my education, I took a one-year sabbatical
before moving on to nursing school.

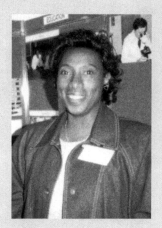

Courtesy of Dorothy Esta
Dennis Segars.

I arrived at Angier B. Duke Nurses Home late, the last in my class to
arrive. Waiting for me were two upper classmen named Davis and Flateau.
My father had driven me to school in a borrowed old red truck; we were
lucky to make it at all. We could not go the speed limit so I kept a good
lookout for Linwood Avenue. I arrived in time for the group photograph.

By my graduation in 1968, only nine of out original group of twenty-one
had completed the program. My classmates left for various reasons and,
yes, grades were a reason for dismissal. I managed to stay one step ahead.
Elsewhere 76 and 81 were considered passing grades. However, not at
Lincoln; these grades were failing grades. To make things worse, the
terminology had different meanings; for example, "sponge" was used for
cleaning at home. The first chance that I got I looked up the use for sponges
in medicine. It might have helped initially if there was a show and tell for all
the new preclinical students. We had a lot of material to digest in a matter
of months in order to be prepared to care for assigned patients. I received
an award at graduation for technical competency, no errors in medication
administration. At one point I received two failing grades and called my
mother wanting to go home. She told me to hang up the phone, go upstairs,
and study; my mother's decisions were law. I went upstairs, learned to
play pinochle and played every chance I got. It was a good stress reliever. I
continued my same study routine and my grades improved. I passed state
board on first writing.

I became a nurse because I wanted to care for people, to help them feel better, and to assist in curing their ills. I did that and much more in many areas of employment. After graduating from Lincoln Hospital School of Nursing, I was recruited to work at Baptist Hospital in Winston-Salem, North Carolina. I returned to Lincoln Hospital, paid my dues by working one year in the Emergency Room under the guidance of Mrs. T. Jones and Ms. Edwina Sellers. Then I accepted a position in the Psychiatry Department at Duke University Medical Center (DUMC), in Durham, North Carolina. Later I worked at the Veterans Administration Medical Center, also in Durham, North Carolina, in the Department of Medicine. Then I transferred to the area I love the most, the Department of Psychiatry at the Veterans Administration Medical Center. While at the Veterans Medical Center, I returned to school to earn my BSN. Due to scheduling problems, I resigned my position and went to work part-time in the Infirmary at North Carolina Central University and also did private duty nursing.

My degree allowed me to work in leadership and supervisory roles with the State of North Carolina. While working in Geropsychiatry with the state of North Carolina I established a behavioral model program that was very successful. I praised the staff for wanting to try new ways of doing patient care and the physicians for being extremely supportive. I returned to DUMC in 1981 to the psychiatry unit. Later I worked in the Duke Outpatient Surgery Program, Duke Comprehensive Sickle Cell Center and a Women's and Children's Medical Outpatient facility. I assisted the Department of Social Work as a Discharge Nurse Coordinator; served as night supervisor (later changed to Assistant Director of Nursing) of Duke South (now Duke Clinics) and Duke North; and assisted with several research programs in the Department of Oncology and Hematology. I was employed at North Carolina Central University on two occasions in my nursing career; first in 1994 as night charge nurse in Student Health and in 1998 as a tutor/counselor on a special grant in the Department of Nursing. Six years ago I worked with a community owned Health Education Company to teach non-nursing personnel to administer medications, and taught blood-borne pathogens and seizure precautions. While employed with this company I became certified in the Medicaid Personal Care Services Curriculum.

Over the years I have received awards for job performances, as well as received Civic and church recognition. I can honestly say my initial education from Lincoln Hospital School of Nursing prepared me for a variety of positions. What do I hope to leave as a legacy, besides my rite of passage? I hope that I did make a difference in all the lives I touched, for the better.

Lastly, in my leisure time I was an amateur bowler and have won several tournaments. I am also a lifetime member of the WIBC National 600 Club.

ATTRITION

Attrition was an issue at Lincoln, and the weeding-out process began in the preclinical period. This period, which was a combination of classroom, on-unit guided observations, and "hands-on" practice, provided faculty (and students) with the opportunity to assess each student's aptitude for nursing. By the time this period ended, typically after between four and nine months, the attrition had begun. The attrition rate in the 1950s ranged from 13 percent to 42 percent. See the chart below.

Attrition of Student Nurses at LHSN, 1951–1956

Entry	End of 1st Year	End of 2nd Year	End of 3rd Year	Retention	Attrition
1951: 19	15	13	13	68%	42%
1952: 16	12	12	12	75%	25%
1953: 14	12	12	12	80%	20%
1954: 29	28	25	21	72%	28%
1955: 31	28	18	18	58%	42%
1956: 16	16	14	14	87%	13%

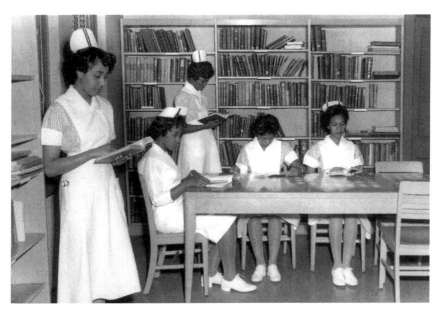

Study hall in the library. Left to right: *Betty Talford Fisher, Sylvia Overton Richardson (Instructor), Josephine Wood, unidentified, Joan Miller Martin Jones Mathews.* Reprinted from *The Scalpel,* 1963. Courtesy of Bernice King.

The attrition rate increased to 60 percent through the 1960s. For example, twenty-two students entered the Class of 1966, but by the end of the first semester only eight remained. These eight went on to graduate.

However, not all attrition was the result of poor performance or grades. Some students left because they were homesick, missed their boyfriends, chose to get married, or for some other traumatic reason, for example, the death of a family member. Believe it or not, some were asked to leave simply because they refused to conform to the dress code—specifically, uniform length! Rules at that time were not as forgiving as today.

PHILOSOPHY

What were LHSN's beliefs, values, and guiding principles, that is, its philosophy? One's philosophy guides one's actions, and in the case of nursing it provides the foundation for practice. The questions, "Why do I want to be a nurse?" or "Why did I choose nursing as a career?" have been posed, most probably, from the very beginning of nurse training schools. The first documented evidence of the question appears in the 1923 Application. Applicants in the early years of the program responded to this question. Here is one account from a student, Gloria Johnson Fulton (RN '56).

I chose Nursing as a profession because nursing is not merely an occupation, temporary and superficial in its scope, but it is a great vocation. It is so well known to be difficult that it is seldom undertaken by any woman who has not, in the depths of her consciousness, an earnest desire to serve humanity. This desire should be so great that no unpleasant or disgusting experience will overcome one's humanitarian motives. In the first place, one should be interested in all kinds of people, not merely in those who have tastes in common with one's own. The pain, misery, and distress of the dirtiest tramp should appeal as much as the suffering of a child, or the rich, and to see the sick grow strong and well under one's ministration are the activating motives of a true nurse.

The world has no room for human parasites. Each individual owes something to mankind.

A nurse may become very well-versed in the cause, treatment, and prevention of disease; she may give very good care to a great many patients; she may keep up with the newer, better methods, but she has not done her full duty unless she contributes something creative as well. The art of Nursing has still marvelous, undeveloped possibilities, especially

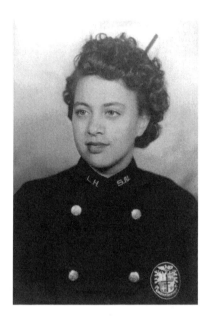

Gloria Johnson Fulton. Courtesy of
Gloria Johnson Fulton.

the more difficult and delicate art of nursing
sick minds and spirits. The science of
nursing is still in its earliest infancy, and
even our present knowledge is very imper-
fectly grasped and applied by the majority
of those who practice nursing. We have here
the great task of perfecting our art, and
building up our body of knowledge. Though
it is impossible to lay too much stress on the
aforementioned, we must never overlook
the fact that the root and spring of all good
nursing is still as ever the inborn nursing
instinct with its eager spirit of service, deep
human interest, and warm and spontaneous
sympathy.

A nurse should be one of the finest of
women. No other is worthy of being trusted
with human lives, and those things that go
to make up human happiness. She should
be pure of speech and thought. She should
be kindly, yet firm when occasion demands. She should always take good
care of her own health, yet never hesitate to give care to another who
needs her. She should never divulge the secrets of another, yet she should
be ready to listen to the troubles of her patients. She should believe in, and
obey, the Golden Rule for Nurses: "Do unto others as ye would that others
should do unto thy Mother. Angels themselves can do no more."

All this and much more, the nurse should be, and often is.

The philosophy of the School of Nursing and its objectives were first
drafted in 1954. The objectives were achieved through engaging students in
educational, clinical, social, and professional activities that would enable
them to adapt to a changing society. Though undocumented, we can assume that fundamental beliefs and values about nursing, health, and human
nature also guided the early leaders of the school. They certainly had goals
and objectives for the educational program, which may or may not have
been written down, and were keenly aware of the foundation the students
needed and the standards they had to reach if they were to play their part
in nursing and the health-care field at large. Miss Carter, in a 1931 report to
the Lincoln Hospital Board of Trustees, described that graduates, in addi-

tion to their nursing practice, should be about the uplift of the Negro race. She recognized the need for Lincoln nurses to be responsible for self and for the broader community.

The first documented philosophy and objectives of the school reads as follows:

The Philosophy of Lincoln Hospital School of Nursing

The Lincoln Hospital School of Nursing, being aware of the need for adequately prepared nurses to meet the demands of the nursing profession, believes that these needs can be best accomplished by the careful selection of students who have the intelligence and special aptitude for nursing, and show a desire for motivation.

It is our goal to provide learning experiences and other advantages by which the student may obtain scientific knowledge and develop skills and understanding that they may become reflected in the learner's personality and practice.

The curriculum is arranged to provide opportunities for the student to participate in teamwork with allied workers through planned conferences and ward-rounds with emphasis placed on the physical, mental, social, and spiritual aspects of nursing.

The health service allows for preventive and remedial care, which helps the student to apply clinical practice to her personal health needs and those with whom she serves.

The guidance program is planned to aid students in educational, professional, social, and personal problems in terms of student needs.

Objectives of Lincoln Hospital School of Nursing

- To select students who possess high personal standards, wholesome attitudes, and who will be able to maintain a satisfactory scholarship and will make satisfactory adjustments to their environment and other conditions relating to growth and development in their chosen profession.
- To provide a course by which students gain empathy and give efficient nursing care, to understand and teach sound principles of health, and to prepare themselves as useful citizens in community activities.
- To help the student to develop mental abilities and skills which will enable her to appreciate civic, cultural, and spiritual values, and thus become a well-integrated individual.

- To prepare graduates who have a knowledge of nursing principles which will enable them to care adequately for the ill, and encourage them to assume leadership in disease prevention and promotion of better public health.
- To influence and guide students in their personal and professional progress toward the highest ideals of moral virtue.

Clinical Experience

The clinical daily-care routine helped students to prioritize and organize the care to be done. Their routine formed the basic foundation on which graduates practiced and became regarded as excellent nurses. They could get the work done in a manner that respected the dignity of the patient. Former patients and physician colleagues used the phrase "real nurse" to capture the essence of a Lincoln nurse.

(continues on page 128)

Della Marie Harris Clemons, RN '46

I was born in Wendell, North Carolina, one of twelve children. My father was a farmer and my mother was a housewife.

While in nursing school I was a cadet in the Nurse Cadet Corps. I attended St. Joseph and White Rock Churches while in school. I worked a short time at Lincoln after graduating, while preparing for the licensure exam. After receiving my RN license, I took a short course in anesthesia. This course of work proved very challenging but not as satisfying as I had imagined. My work experiences included: St Agnes Hospital in Raleigh, N.C.; school nurse with a Federal Program under the Supervisor of Public Health Department in Raleigh, N.C.; supervisor in the Department of Corrections, later known as the Correctional School for Women. I was the first Black nurse and the first RN at the Corrections Department. I had applied at Dorothea Dix Hospital after I graduated, but they would accept me only as an aid. As a continuous learner I earned the bachelor's degree in nursing in 1965, and I continued to be involved with the Lincoln Hospital School of Nursing Alumni Association. I retired from the Department of Corrections after twenty years.

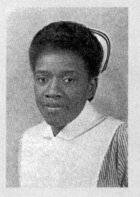

Reprinted from *The Scalpel*, 1946. Courtesy of Lois Smith Morris.

Students providing patient care.
Reprinted from *The Scalpel*, 1962. Courtesy of Patricia Martin Blue.

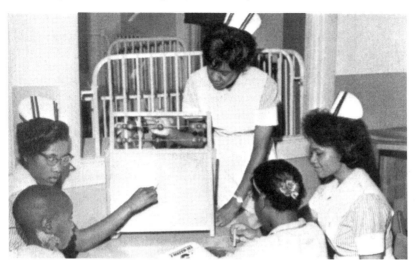

Mary Bass Satterwhite, JoAnna Neal Dowling, Altamease Riley Arnold.

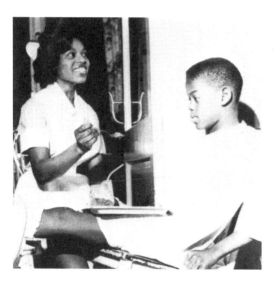

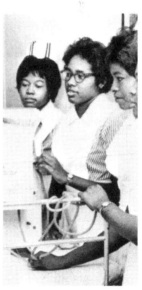

Anna Gertrude Brown Lubatkin.

Jennie Louise Adams,
Maggie Lee Ledbetter,
Geraldine Richardson.

From the beginning of the School of Nursing, the clinical experience had a twofold purpose: for the hospital it was a source of patient care and for the student it was a source of preparation for their practice as a registered nurse upon successful completion of the licensure examination. The day, evening, and night supervisors were responsible for planning, teaching, and supervising the clinical services. Through the early 1940s, all clinical experiences were onsite; the hospital census was adequate for providing the necessary clinical experiences for the students. However, for the area of psychiatry, content and case analysis were presented through lecture by visiting physicians. Amazingly during the 1940s students were able to successfully pass the psychiatry portion of the board exam without specific clinical experience in this area. The passing score for the board exam was 70 percent, and Della Marie Harris Clemons (RN '46) recalled that she had the highest scores of her class. Student rotations through medicine, surgery, pediatrics, obstetrics, and psychiatry followed a plan predicated on the acquisition and application of increasingly complex information as the student progressed and matured in her nursing education experience. Below, Ethel Brown Mc-Cullum (RN '47) reminisced about her clinical experience as a very innocent nineteen-year-old.

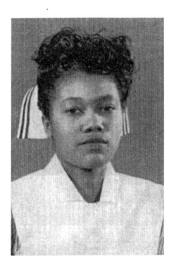

Ethel Brown McCullum.
Reprinted from *The Scalpel*,
1947. Courtesy of Lois Smith
Morris.

I was nineteen years old when I entered nursing school and never had groomed men (only my brothers). I was scared to death when I had to help them with a bath and nearly died when I had to assist Dr. [John Walter Vincent] Cordice [Jr.] with prostate dilatations. And, Dr. [Max] Schiebel! I got nervous when I heard his name! I don't care how many needles I threaded before he got started, I still couldn't keep up. And, Ms. [Mildred] Crisp, our supervisor, just walked around looking, made no comments and gave no assistance.

We were assigned five to six patients. If two or three were diabetics we had to prepare their food and take it to them and do AM care.

Back rubs, wet-to-dry dressings, saline compresses, learning how to safely turn a patient on a Stryker Frame Bed who was being treated for pressure ulcers were memorable clinical experiences. Vital signs, giving injections with dull needles, autoclaving instruments before you could use them, preparing meals in the kitchen for patients with diabetes, working in Central Supply, taking out flowers at night, and making rounds were the routines we were expected to follow daily with great care. The level of care demonstrated by our supervisors and nursing instructors made an indelible impression on students.

As the Board of Nursing raised its standards for clinical hours, the hospital census, and the diversity of patient contacts, it became obvious that to assure student success, other avenues for clinical experience had to be established. Hospital-based schools of nursing were expensive to maintain, and a number of schools began closing. In 1948 the board approved guidelines for the use of affiliations as an avenue through which small hospitals could secure the desired student clinical experiences. McCain, a two-year tuberculosis hospital in North Carolina, utilized LHSN for clinical experience. Sarah McKoy Rhynie (RN '42), initially a student at McCain Sanatorium, was admitted to Lincoln to complete her formal education. Ms. Rhynie shared an amusing incident about the State Board Exam in a conversation with Dorothy Esta Dennis Segars on June 5, 2012.

I completed my first two years of nurse training at McCain Sanatoria in North Carolina. I came circa 1940 and graduated in 1942. The nurses who attended the sanatoria were not able to complete nurse training and be eligible to sit for the licensure exam without completing the third year at a general hospital.

Before coming to Lincoln, my exposure to surgical procedures was practically nil. On the board exam, which occurred over a period of three days in Winston-Salem, I had to clean a tracheostomy tube. I had no knowledge of or familiarity with tracheostomy care. Luck would have it that the White nurse administering the examination accidentally dropped the tracheostomy tube on the floor and it came apart. It became obvious to me that the two pieces needed to be cleaned individually. I acted as if I knew exactly how to perform the procedure and passed the exam.

One of the earliest affiliation experiences for students at LHSN was in pediatrics at Freedman's Hospital in Washington, D.C., in the 1940s. Della Marie Harris Clemons (RN '46) recalled this affiliation as a good experience.

Sarah McKoy Rhynie, RN '42

I was born in Laurinburg, North Carolina, on
May 30, 1921, to Henry and Ethel McKoy, the third
of six children. I graduated from Laurinburg
Normal Industrial Institute High School. After
completing two years at McCain Sanitoria, I
went on to Lincoln Hospital School of Nursing in
Durham, North Carolina, from which I graduated
in 1942. After receiving my nursing license as a
registered nurse, I traveled north to Maryland. I
was one of the first African American registered
nurses to work in the City Hospital of Baltimore.
Later I moved to Brooklyn, New York, and worked
at the Brooklyn Jewish Hospital as a staff nurse, a
head nurse, and later as a supervisor in the Brooklyn Home for the Aged.

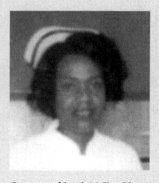

Courtesy of Sarah McKoy Rhynie.

In New York I met husband, Victor Rhynie, and we were married in August 1963.
I retired from nursing after working in many hospitals in the Brooklyn area. My
patient after retirement was my ailing husband until his death.

My church has been a source of great joy. My Christian journey began as a child,
having being baptized in a river in North Carolina. After relocating to Brooklyn,
New York, I continued my journey by joining the Greater Mt. Pleasant Baptist
Church in 1970. I have been a devoted member, having perfect attendance in Sunday
School, feeding and encouraging people in the community through the Church's
Soup Kitchen, and serving as President of the Willing Workers Club. My greatest joy
of all is to encourage others to build strong Christian values in the many children
whom I have loved and helped over the years.

I have enjoyed extensive travels to Europe, the Holy Land, and Jamaica, W.I. These
travels have given me more insight into Christianity, and I continue to impart my
Christian values and mentoring skills, sharing what I have been blessed to learn and
experience as a result of my relationship with God.

I am the proud mother of one daughter and one step daughter, and I have one
grandson and one great grandson.

She and her classmates had the privilege and opportunity to meet and make
rounds with Dr. Charles Drew, the inventor of blood plasma. She said, "Dr.
Drew asked questions as they made joint rounds with the medical students.
The medical students were often 'shamed' because the nursing students
could answer the questions better than the medical students." Affiliations
were the nursing students' last intensive clinical experience before gradu-

ation. Several students shared specific stories about their affiliation experience. Here is one from Carolyn E. Henderson.

I lost my one and only pediatric patient during my senior nursing affiliation in 1971 at Children's Hospital in Cincinnati, Ohio. I saw almost every pediatric anomaly from cancer to hermaphroditism while rotating there!

My patient, who was less than seven years old, had leukemia and had no idea how sick she really was. She ate Froot Loops every day . . . which is why I don't care for the cereal to this day. Each day I saw her, she greeted me with the broadest smile, and I just adored her even though I knew she was very ill. On the eve of her death, she wanted to give me a picture of both of her hands. In an attempt to draw both hands, she traced her left hand twice because she was right-handed. Therefore, I received a picture with two left hands! It was a special picture that I still have in my nursing archives and will always cherish. My patient passed away the day after I received the picture. Believe me, it was one of the most heart-breaking experiences, having to see the special joy of a child's spirit and to lose it so quickly. I knew, because of my frequent tears during this affiliation, that pediatric nursing would not be my choice of work.

After leaving Cincinnati, I experienced my first airplane flight home. Also, I received my very first job offer from Children's Hospital because of my meritorious nursing clinical work there! So, I left this rotation with great joy and sorrow . . . something we often experience during our tenure of nursing.

Mary Carmichael remembered:

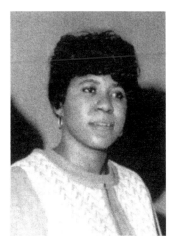

When we were at the Children's Hospital in Ohio, I fell in love with one of my patients named Jimmy. He was a cute, little, red curly-haired, two-year-old. He was in the hospital because of complications from gallbladder disease. He was a sick little boy with lots of tubes that had been inserted. I had always believed that gallbladder disease was an adult disease, but little Jimmy showed me otherwise.

Also, when we were in Ohio, the "Afro Wigs" were popular. I think all of us purchased one, and we all walked around looking like Angela Davis; we were cool.

Mary Carmichael. Courtesy of Carolyn Evangeline Henderson.

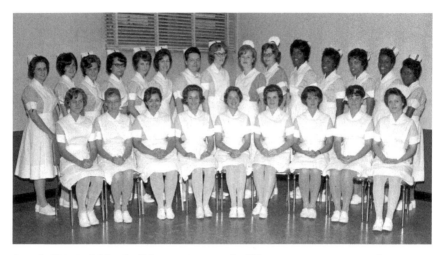

Lincoln Hospital School of Nursing integrated affiliation experience in psychiatry at Eastern State Hospital, Lexington, Kentucky, 1965. Back row right to left: Lincoln students Penny Davis, Jeronica Williams Hardison, Patricia Martin Blue, Jimmie Ruth Gore Persley, and Shirley Ann Oliver Scott. Courtesy of Carolyn Evangeline Henderson.

The students' affiliation experiences, in addition to providing them with excellent clinical learning experiences and prospective job opportunities, facilitated their professional, social, and emotional development. Students developed lifelong skills, for example, the art of playing cards! For many students, Durham had been their first time on their own and the farthest they had traveled from home. Additionally, the affiliation experience provided some students with the opportunity to take their first flight or bus ride. Students were introduced to various cultural activities, had opportunities for sight-seeing and participating in excursions to beaches and roller-skating rinks, and interacted with different ethnic and racial groups. Patricia M. Blue, who came from a small racially segregated town in Alabama, shared that her first exposure to integration was the dormitory she lived in during her affiliation in Lexington, Kentucky. She laughed at how both White and Black students were in awe of each other's culture. She has vivid images of Whites waving their hair with jello and Blacks "frying their hair" with straightening combs and curling irons. From my own psychiatric affiliation in Crownsville, Maryland, I have vivid memories of enjoying noted Blues singer Bobby Blue Bland while on the beach in Annapolis. My first roller-skating experience was in Washington, D.C. It looked as if it would be easy, but I never mastered the skill of staying upright; thus, I had many bruises on my return to the dormitory. Nursing students had opportunities to socialize with military personnel on the Ft. Meade Base. Students were bussed to the base. Many relationships were formed on these excursions. These trips to Army bases were similar to those that students in earlier years had taken to the USO on Fayetteville Street in Durham and to Camp Butner in Butner, North Carolina.

Through the 1970s students continued to have affiliation experiences in pediatrics and psychiatry. In 1970, the students additionally had their obstetrics and pediatrics experience at Watts Hospital in Durham. Lincoln Hospital transferred its obstetrics service to Duke Hospital in 1970.

NATIONAL LEAGUE OF NURSES ACCREDITATION

The Board of Nursing continuously focused on the professional standard and image of nursing. As a mechanism for raising the status of nursing schools and training, the Board of Nursing, in the mid-1950s, recommended that nursing schools seek National League of Nurses (NLN) accreditation. NLN accreditation would signify excellence and serve as a stamp of approval for the nursing program. Lincoln sought to comply but did not complete the application process for NLN accreditation. In an interview with Ms. Z she expressed that the expense was too great. The application fee was $250-plus, and the expenses of the labor and follow through for NLN visits were to be borne by the institution. On reviewing the application booklet dated 1957, I could see that the requirements were very specific and required detailed attention to all the standards for curriculum, admission, course plans and hours, and many other aspects of the school's operation. This, in my opinion, would have required hiring someone who could give their full attention to this process, and the resources were not available. The faculty was already responsible for instruction, the supervision of students, and patient care, which stretched them beyond their limits. It is noteworthy that Watts Hospital School of Nursing was the first three-year diploma program in North Carolina to be accredited by the NLN, in 1956. This school continues to operate as of the writing of this book.

STUDENT ACTIVITIES

Students admitted to Lincoln in the mid-1940s benefited tremendously from a new support system. New students were assigned "big sisters." This support network was especially important during those first six months. Thus, the bonding began. As informal mentors and mentees, big sisters were expected to share the expectations for behavior and support their "little sisters" in various ways. For example, there were many places that were off-limits: Club 55 on Highway 55, Mr. Pratts on Pine Street, the Goodwill Club, the College Inn and P&W Pub on Fayetteville Street (which was literally across the street), and students could not linger on Pettigrew Street. It was dangerous to be caught in these places; you could be sent home. Big sisters shared clothes, food, boyfriends (not intentionally), helped with assignments, and guided their little sisters in the "ways of Lincoln" to prevent them from getting into trouble. They offered study tips, as well as tips on how to get along with certain instructors. They also helped relieve their little sisters' anxiety about taking care of the patients. The intimacy of caring for patients, especially male patients, was an entirely new adventure for most of the students. Gwendolyn C. Jones Parham (RN '58) recalls the following of her experience as a little sister:

> As a preclinical nursing student I perceived my first encounters with the instructors and superiors to be harsh, unfriendly, and punitive. For the first time in my life I felt uncomfortable in a school setting. However, I did what was required of me and successfully completed the preclinical period.
>
> The upper-class students were very supportive and friendly, and I am very grateful to my big sister Cassie Nixon for her sensitive and caring personality. The second year at Lincoln took a new direction for me. I had overcome my fears and decided that I could and would continue on in my quest to become a nurse (I really didn't have any other choice). The instructors and hospital nurses expected us to perform nursing care without hesitation or errors.
>
> As I reflect on my professional career, I am grateful to Lincoln Hospital School of Nursing for laying the foundation upon which I have been able to grow professionally in so many ways. This foundation has led to my ability to persevere in difficult situations, to problem solve, and to function in a variety of professional settings with competence and confidence. What I think made Lincoln unique was the presence of strong role models who set high standards of excellence and who were good examples of professionalism. It is with pride that I say that I am a graduate of Lincoln Hospital School of Nursing.

The 1948 issue of *The Scalpel* relates an experience of another Lincoln student, Andre Doris Ruff. She apparently was a member of the Class of 1950, but we could not confirm a graduation date.

Upon my arrival at Lincoln School of Nursing, I found the atmosphere more hospitable, but still I felt very jittery. Fortunately for me the freshman dormitory was full; therefore, I was carried to the upperclassmen's dormitory. After meeting my roommates, I was greeted by Misses Muriel Harris, Lois Clements, and Zella Perry, who introduced themselves as seniors. The very word "senior" made my knees knock and my legs feel like jelly, but after meeting them this queer feeling disappeared into thin air. These girls were so amiable and congenial that I felt I hadn't made the wrong choice in choosing "nursing" as my career.

Later in the week at "Meeting the Gang," I met the whole class of seniors and as a whole they were the most entertaining group of girls I had ever met. As time passed our acquaintances grew profoundly, and I feel that they will be invaluable and everlasting.

PROFESSIONAL DEVELOPMENT ACTIVITIES

At all times, professional behavior was expected from the students. The rules regarding the behaviors of nurses and the courtesies to be accorded doctors and administrators also included upper-class students. Etiquette and decorum required that preclinicals and lower-class students open the door for upper-class students and let them enter first. These acts showed respect for rank and status.

The professional development of the students was enhanced by opportunities to participate in the various student organizations, which included class officers, Student Government (Student Council), the Big Sister pro-

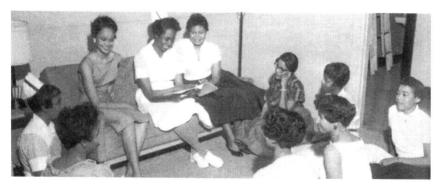

Student Government/Student Council. Reprinted from *The Nightingale*, 1958. Courtesy of Marion Glen Miles.

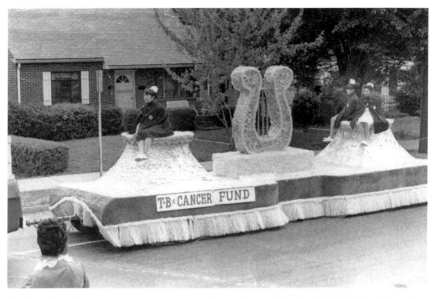

Student Float in community parade. Students pictured: *Lottie F. Hall, Alice Harrell Young Tharrington, and Myrna Watson Hughes, Miss Lincoln 1967.* Courtesy of Myrna Watson Hughes.

gram, yearbook production, and the North Carolina State Student Nurses Association, which was formalized in 1950. These organizations gave many students the opportunity to learn, practice, and expand their social and leadership skills. Lincoln students became very involved in the North Carolina State Student Nurses Association. In 1957 Gwendolyn Cooper Jones Parham (RN '58) and Celestine Patricia Rascoe Maness (RN '58) attended the National Student Convention in Chicago, Illinois, and Ruby Bell Jewel Borden (RN '59) attended the National Student Nurse Convention in Atlantic City, New Jersey. Miron Andrews Wilkerson (RN '63) was elected Vice President of the Student Nurses Association from Region V, which included Durham and Chapel Hill, North Carolina.

Lincoln graduates have continued to participate on the state and national levels in these professional organization as well as organizations representing specialty practice areas. Many of these affiliations are identified in the "Voices" of their stories that accompany each chapter.

Lincoln Hospital School of Nursing had a tradition of participating in professional activities. In fact in 1941 Ms. Beulah Jackson, one of Lincoln's nursing instructors and later the director of nursing, was treasurer of the Colored Nurses of North Carolina Organization.

(continues on page 140)

Saundra Obie B. Clemmons, RN '67, BSN, MSN, FNP

My name is Saundra Obie Clemmons. I entered Lincoln Hospital School of Nursing, in Durham, North Carolina, in the fall of 1964, straight out of high school, as Saundra Paulette Obie. I graduated in 1967 as Saundra Obie Best.

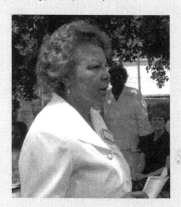

I was born about sixty-five feet from where I currently live, in Person County, North Carolina, to Bernard Chester and Chestina Tuck Obie, the oldest of seven children. I was delivered by a lay midwife, Miss Florence Wade. There was a sister born two years before me, however, she died at the age of three months, so by default I became the oldest child.

Courtesy of Saundra Obie B. Clemmons.

I grew up on a farm in Person County, where we raised tobacco, corn, wheat, and soybeans as major crops. My father tried other crops as well, such as cucumbers and peanuts. We also raised pigs, chickens, ducks, and dairy and beef cows for our own use. I grew up fulfilling the role of a son until my brothers came along and were big enough to help. I also assisted my mom with cooking, washing, canning, and caring for the younger children as well as working in the tobacco and corn fields.

I attended an all-Black elementary school (Bethel Hill, then North End), Person County High School, and Lincoln Hospital School of Nursing (LHSN). In high school, I was a member of the National Honor Society, the Future Nurses Club, and was the feature writer and photographer for my high-school newspaper (*The Panther*). I enjoyed reading, writing (including poetry), and participating in French and Home Economics classes. I graduated in 1964 as salutatorian of my class.

Although Dad only went to the eighth grade and Mom only to the tenth, education was important to my family; in fact, my mother got her GED and an associate's degree in criminal justice after I left home. All of the children completed college. There are doctorates (including MDs), three master's degrees, and numerous bachelor of science degrees within immediate and second-generation offspring.

Church was also a big influence during my years growing up. We attended Sunday School each Sunday, walking two to three miles, one way, to church. Church and God continued to be important during my years at Lincoln, from participating in weekly Vespers to attending local community churches such as St. Joseph African Methodist Episcopal and White Rock Baptist.

During the time that I was in high school (1960–1964) career choices were limited for women, especially in rural schools. One could be a teacher, a nurse, or a secretary. I believe I chose nursing because of the influences of my mom, my grandmother (Nannie Paylor Obie), two Black public-health nurses (Mrs. Kathryn Lawson and Mrs. Albright), and Mrs. Salome Jeffers Miles, my eleventh grade homeroom and English teacher and Future Nurses Club advisor.

I chose LHSN after being denied entrance into the Women's College of Greensboro, North Carolina, supposedly for not having taken geometry in high school. Because I wanted my siblings to go to college, I felt an obligation to get out of the way, so as not to be a burden on my parents. I applied to a two-year then three-year school. I don't regret attending and graduating from Lincoln because the school and classes were small and therefore we received more individualized attention. There was a sense of family among the graduates that continues today through our biannual reunions.

At Lincoln we were taught by Mrs. Lucille Zimmerman (LZ) Williams and our various instructors how to be professional in our dress and appearance and in our actions. They taught us to be the best nurses we could be and to be patient advocates. A sense of integrity was instilled in us. We were shown how to be well-mannered young women.

My career has been filled with various positions. I graduated from LHSN on September 13, 1967. I went to work one week later at Sibley Memorial Hospital, in Washington, D.C. For three months I worked on the GYN unit. Other positions include: staff nurse at the Veteran's Affairs Medical Center, Washington, D.C.; emergency, intensive care, and mobile intensive care nursing; supervision (head nurse and house supervisor), Quality Assurance/Improvement; JCAHO Coordinator; special projects and clinical nurse specialist at Person County Memorial Hospital, in Roxboro, North Carolina; and a joint clinical instructor appointment with Person County Memorial Hospital and Piedmont Community College, also in Roxboro.

While working full time at Person County Memorial Hospital, I attended Piedmont Community College, in Roxboro, North Carolina, and North Carolina Central University (NCCU), in Durham, where I earned the bachelor of science degree in nursing in 1983. I continued my studies at the

University of North Carolina at Chapel Hill and obtained the master of science degree in nursing in 1989 and entered a post-master's family nurse practitioner (FNP) grogram, graduating in 1995. From 1995 to March 2000 I worked part-time as an FNP, Board Certified with Person Family Medical Center and Beckford Medical Center, in Henderson, North Carolina. While at NCCU I received the Allegra Ward Award for perseverance, and I was a Robert Wood Johnson Scholar (with a full scholarship) at UNC-Chapel Hill.

On March 6, 2010, I began employment at the North Carolina Board of Nursing, in Raleigh, North Carolina, as an investigator. Since that time I have attended National Certified Investigator Training and have become certified. My position there involves investigating allegations of violations of the North Carolina Nursing Practice Act. This may involve site visits, chart reviews, medication records and systems audits, licensee and witness interviews, writing reports, and testifying at Administrative Hearings. Additionally, I conduct investigations with various other boards and agencies, such as the Medical Board, Pharmacy Board, local police, the military, and the State Bureau of Investigation.

It had been a desire of mine to be elected to the Board of Nursing, but I never imagined that I would be employed by the Nursing Board. This opportunity came about through networking and through the grace of God. Even though I am happy with this opportunity and my job, I still miss direct patient care and working in the clinical areas. I have worked at the board for a little over ten years and anticipate being there for several more years.

I am a member of various professional organizations, including the American Nurses Association, the North Carolina Nurses Association (NCNA), the Chi Eta Phi (XHO) Nursing Sorority, and the Sigma Theta Tau Honor Society. I have been very involved, holding various offices on a district level, in the NCNA. I have also held several offices at the chapter level in Chi Eta Phi, Rho Phi chapter.

I remain involved in church activities at Prospect Hill Baptist Church, in Roxboro, N.C., including the Usher Ministry and the Choir Ministry, and I am the assistant financial secretary. I am also the leader of the Health Ministry and over the years have coordinated health fairs for the church with the help of some of my Lincoln and Chi Eta Phi sisters.

I can, truthfully, say that I have had a blessed life and career. I owe it all to God and to my training at Lincoln Hospital School of Nursing in Durham, North Carolina.

In 1948 the North Carolina State Nurses Association (NCSNA) Board of Directors voted to recommend that the association admit Negro nurses to membership and issued an invitation to the members of the North Carolina Association of Negro Registered Nurses, Inc. In 1949 the Negro nurses voted unanimously to dissolve the North Carolina Association of Negro Registered Nurses, Inc. and became members of the NCSNA. Since that time Lincoln graduates have consistently participated in the NCSNA, holding local and state offices in the organization. Among the many who have served are: Joan Miller Martin Jones Mathews (RN '62), the first Black Treasurer and second Black President of District 11; Lydia Ruth Flintal Betts (RN '35), President of District 11; Evelyn Pearl Booker Wicker (RN '63), Board of Directors, District 11, State Home Health Committee, North Carolina Nursing Association; Mary Lee Richardson Baldwin (RN '66), Chair of Commission Services, NCNA (the first Black nurse to be on this board); Carolyn Evangeline Henderson (RN '71), Chair, NCNA Commission on Nursing Education; Saundra Obie B. Clemmons (RN '67), District II, Board of Directors, and NCNA delegate for a number of years; and Gloria Taylor Cheek King (RN '67),

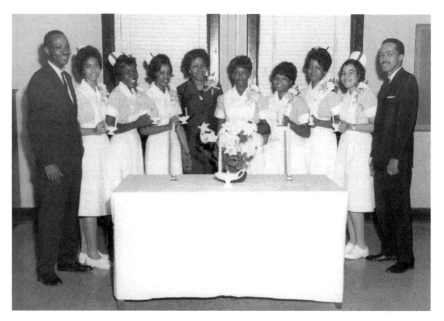

Santa Filomena Inductees, 1966–1967. Left to right: *Dr. Charles Johnson, Rebecca Mitchell Carter, Pauline Langston Edwards, Beverly Miller Harris, Mrs. L. Z. Williams (director of nursing), Alice McClain, Reatha Young Knighton, Lenora Graham Gerald, Loretta Gail Flateau Chestnut, Miles Mark Fisher III.* Courtesy of Carolyn Evangeline Henderson.

President, NCNA Delegate. Many alumni have been recognized for their outstanding contributions and service to the state organization.

The LHSN Alumni Association has encouraged its members to join the State Nurses Association and the American Nurses Association as the official organizations with which the alumni associate through membership. These organizations have established several recognition programs over the years; one of the more recent recognition programs is the Great 100 Nurses program. Several Lincoln graduates, including Mary Richardson Baldwin, have been recognized as one of the Great 100 Nurses, a recognition bestowed on a registered nurse for her or his leadership and involvement in the organization. Mary is also a Mary Lewis Wyche Fellow.

The Santa Filomena Student Nurse Honor Society was another source of highly regarded recognition. Leadership, scholarship, and service were the underpinnings of this organization; LHSN became involved in the 1960s. The students were selected by the faculty, and induction ceremonies were held yearly. Many of these nurses have gone on to outstanding professional careers.

YEARBOOK

The LHSN Yearbook is a prized possession of the Lincoln graduates. Much of the information captured in this book comes from the yearbooks produced between 1946 and 1963. Ms. Z introduced the first yearbook, which was to document the history of LHSN at that period in time. Participation in the design, organization, selection of activities, and fundraising was a challenging and rewarding experience for students and faculty. The yearbooks captured the highly valued social activities and organizations of the nursing program. They featured the current classes, instructors, social and religious activities, professional associations/organizations, and staff of Lincoln Hospital and the School of Nursing, as well as community supporters via their advertisements. Students were expected to solicit contributors and sponsors to help fund the yearbook's production. Classes shared responsibility with faculty advisers for the coordination and production of the yearbooks. The yearbook was titled *The Scalpel* through 1957, after which it was titled *The Nightingale* for two editions, 1958 and 1959. I was not able to discern why the name changed.

Lois Clements Brown Thorpe (RN '48), in a conversation before her death in 2011, described how she and her classmates raised money by selling hot dogs to help finance the first yearbook. Later, other classes used the same

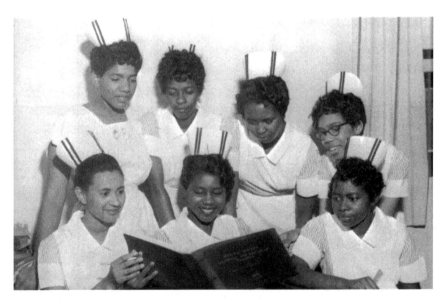

Yearbook editorial staff, 1959. Front row left to right: *Bobbie Jean Hightower Fair, Rose Lee Outerbridge Harrell, Maurice Otelia Blount Snead.* Back row left to right: *Cleo Marie Dunn Bell, Edwina Marie Sellers Colbert, Ruby Jewel Bell Borden, Margaret Louise Wilson Smith.* Reprinted from *The Nightingale*, 1959. Courtesy of Marion Glen Miles.

fundraising activity to help finance their yearbooks. The yearbook captured memorable events in the students' lives. A description of Lois's first day at Lincoln headlined the first yearbook in 1946.

My First Day at Lincoln
    On August twenty-fourth, nineteen hundred and forty-five about six o'clock p.m., I arrived on the campus of Lincoln Hospital bag and baggage. Upon my arrival, I was encountered by a smiling young lady whom I later came to know as Miss Cave. She showed me to my room and offered her assistance. When I thanked her and refused, she did a disappearing act. Alone and enclosed within the four walls of my little room, I began to make plans for this great adjustment that I knew must be made—that of living so close to so many different individuals, and I do mean different. Miss Perry, a young lady from Bluefield, West Virginia, who had moved across the hall just ahead of me, came over to say hello. These were just two of the twenty-five eager girls who were on the campus before the day was ended.

About thirty minutes after my arrival, I decided to introduce myself to my fellow classmates, and this I did. You can imagine the confusion of twenty-five "giggling getties," getting acquainted at once. Once again, Stokes Nurses Home was filled with the laughter of eager young women resolved to set foot on the ladder of ambition to seek the profession of their choice. The night of the twenty-fourth brought with it a birthday party given by Miss Othello Cave and Miss Alice Williams in honor of their roommate, Miss Rosebud Roderick [Beverly], that turned out to be a "know-me-better" informal. Here, we played cards, told jokes, and ate refreshments that had been so thoughtfully prepared.

At ten o'clock, completely exhausted from the experiences of the day, I crept down the stairs to join my roommates. We undressed, got into our own beds, and I was indeed thankful that mine was not the upper bunk. Thus, this is the story of our arrival on campus that we now call "Home."

TEA TIME

Could you picture a 2013 student nurse dressing up for tea time in the dormitory or student union? Sunday afternoons were reserved for tea in the parlor to provide Lincoln students an opportunity to engage in stimulating conversation, develop the art of listening, and practice modeling social graces. Some viewed this as an unnecessary chore, while others embraced the activity. Many students had deficiencies in social graces due to limited exposure in their backgrounds prior to Lincoln.

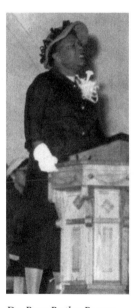

Ms. Z wanted to assure that all students had the proper etiquette for interacting on both the personal and professional levels. She often engaged people from the community to come into the school and address such topics as communication, proper attire for different occasions, dining etiquette, walking and sitting with good posture, and so on.

A person frequently called upon was Dr. Rose Butler Brown, who was a prominent figure in the city. She was the wife of the minister at Mount Vernon Baptist Church on Roxboro Street in Durham and a professor at North Carolina College. JoAnna Neal Dowling, (RN '62) remembers her experience:

Dr. Rose Butler Brown. Guest Speaker on professional etiquette. Courtesy of North Carolina Department of Cultural Resources.

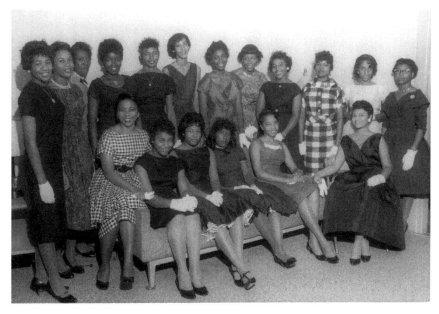

Tea in the parlor.

Upon entering Lincoln I experienced a culture shock. Lincoln served two
purposes: one being for my formal education in nursing and the other
being as a charm school. I remember having to dress up in a black dress
and white gloves for an afternoon tea to formally meet my classmates and
some of the faculty. We were taught proper etiquette, manners, and dress.

I didn't realize then how valuable the training would be to me later in
my career. Lincoln gave me the comprehensive education and experience
to successfully begin my nursing career, which I grew to appreciate more
and more as time passed.

CORONATIONS/PROMS/DANCES

What an honor to be crowned Miss Sweetheart or Miss Lincoln. These coronation ceremonies were grand occasions that began in the 1930s and continued for the life of the school. The queens were selected by individual classes.
Much time, energy, and excitement were spent in the preparation, decoration, and coordination of the actual ceremony. What dress to wear? To bor-
row? Who would be the escort? The actual crowning was usually done by
some dignitary from Lincoln or the community. The queens were striking.

(continues on page 146)

JoAnna Neal Dowling, RN '62, BSN

I was born in Charlotte, North Carolina, to Clarence and Azilee Neal, the second of three daughters. I attended West Charlotte Senior High School and graduated in May 1959. Following graduation, my parents realized I had not applied to any colleges. They sat me down one afternoon after work and asked about my intentions. Being the sensitive and thoughtful child that I was, I told them I planned to work for one year to save money for school. My reason was that my older sister, Marianna, had just completed her freshman year at Johnson C. Smith University and I didn't want to put a strain on them. My younger sister still had four years to go. They told me that was their concern, not mine. My mom said, "If

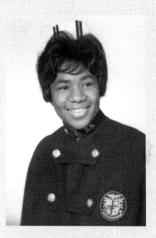

Courtesy of JoAnna Neal Dowling.

you don't continue your education, once you stop, it will be difficult to go back." I had taken core business and science courses in high school and I was torn between choosing a career in clerical work or nursing.

My mom was a beautician with her own business but had really wanted to be a nurse. However, circumstances prevented her from realizing that dream. She often spoke of Lincoln Hospital School of Nursing being one of the best nursing schools for Blacks at the time. She had even met Ms. L. Z. Williams, the director of nursing at Lincoln. Mom went into action and called Ms. Williams to ask about the requirements to enter the school. Ms. Williams gave her the date for the next pre-entrance exam. My parents took off work and drove me to Durham to take the exam. After a few anxious weeks, I got the results that I had passed, and I was soon on my way to my incredible journey to becoming a professional registered nurse.

Upon entering Lincoln I experienced a culture shock. Lincoln served two purposes: one being for my formal education in nursing and the other being as a charm school. I remember having to dress up in a black dress and wearing white gloves for an afternoon tea to formally meet my class-mates and some of the faculty. We were taught proper etiquette, manners, and dress. The classes and clinical schedule were intense. I remember my classmates and I walking down Fayetteville Street at 7:00 a.m. on cold mornings to North Carolina College (now North Carolina Central University) for our chemistry class with Professor McMillan.

I didn't realize then how valuable the training would be to me later in my career. Lincoln gave me the comprehensive education and experience to successfully begin my nursing career—a fact I grew to appreciate more and more as time passed. After successfully passing the North Carolina State Board Examination in the fall of 1962, I was off to Baltimore, Maryland, for my first job at Johns Hopkins Hospital in a General Medical/Surgical Unit. I then moved to New York to live with relatives. My first job there was at a long-term-care hospital and I was assigned the head nurse position. After a year, I went to work at Mount Sinai Medical Center, a very large teaching hospital. I knew I had found my niche. While working on a surgical floor I would do private duty nursing at other hospitals all over the city. I had always wanted to work in another country, so I went to Bermuda and worked at the hospital there for five years. After returning to New York, I went back to school and earned a bachelor's degree in health-care administration.

The last thirty-five years of my career were the most accomplished and rewarding. Following my return from Bermuda I went back to Mount Sinai and started to work on the Dialysis and Kidney Transplant Unit. It was small and new and as it grew, I grew. I participated in new trends and procedures. I earned my nephrology nurse certification and moved up to leadership positions ranging from supervising to teaching new RNs, technicians, and nursing students. I also trained patients to do their dialysis at home.

Renal nursing included newborns to geriatrics, critical care to ambulatory care. I learned every day and I was rewarded every day.

When I retired and while receiving all the recognition certificates and plaques, I stood surrounded by my nursing colleagues, the medical staff, and, yes, my beloved patients. It was then that I gave thanks to my parents for all of their sacrifices and to all the instructors and graduate nurses at Lincoln for the best education and training. This allowed me to have the most successful and rewarding nursing career ever. God bless the memories of Lincoln Hospital School of Nursing.

The proms were fun, too. Students, though dressed formally, could "let their hair down," albeit in a "ladylike" fashion. The senior reception and the prom were yearly events sponsored by the junior classes. The Big Nine, as the Class of 1959 was known, was suspended and sent home for going to the Goodwill Club for their pre-prom party, an off-limits establishment. This is the reason for the month's delay in graduation of the Class of 1959 after returning from their psychiatric affiliation in Tennessee. *Rules* were *expected* to be followed or there were consequences. To the students these were considered harsh consequences! Mary Pointer was a member of that class and shares this memory (see her story on the facing page).

(continues on page 150)

Mary Williams Pointer, RN '59

I was born in a rural town in eastern North Carolina. My parents were farmers, share croppers, to be exact, with twelve children—six boys and six girls. I was the fifth oldest child. My father was a Primitive Baptist minister, and both my parents instilled rules and values in all of us. These values have paid off, and I have carried them with me throughout my adult years. We were also taught to help one another; this led to my coming to Lincoln Hospital School of Nursing, my way out and my saving grace. It was either farming or getting an education.

Upon graduating from Frederick Douglass High School, my older sister, a teacher, volunteered to be responsible for my educational expense. Not wanting her to pay for four years of education, I opted for one year, becoming a licensed practical nurse. My sister suggested that if I added two more years to the one year, my career choices would be greater. She was correct.

Attending Lincoln Hospital School of Nursing helped me to develop confidence and great pride. The first day we put on our starched uniform and went to class at North Carolina College (now North Carolina Central University), all heads turned. Our shoes and shoe laces had to be clean and white, no run-over shoes or runs in stockings, minimum make-up, and no perfume or jewelry (except a watch with a second hand).

Administering nursing to the patients was very rewarding because they were so appreciative. Our instructors had our best interests at heart and motivated us to achieve high standards. Lincoln nurses were highly sought after and employees were not disappointed in our performance. A few memories include: being crowned Miss Lincoln in 1958; singing at Christmastime with the Duke and Watts School of Nursing students; and my whole class being sent home for one month, pushing our graduation back to October 1959. (We decided to attend a social club against the advice of our nursing director.)

Upon graduation, I embarked on a very successful career, with more than forty years of professional experience, in research (Duke University Medical Center); hospital rehabilitation (UNC-Chapel Hill); clinics (Lincoln Community Health Center and North Carolina Central University, Infirmary); and outreach (Community Health Coalition). Lincoln Hospital School of Nursing prepared me to become a head nurse at Durham Veteran Administration Medical Center after being employed there for only six months. My leadership and administrative roles allowed me to become a clinical consultant supervising LPNs and NAs, implementing new guidelines and procedures, setting up and managing a Cancer Detection Clinic (headed by Dr. Donald Moore), and collaborating with Operation Breakthrough. My expertise with community outreach involved writing grant proposals and securing funding from the American Cancer Society, Susan G. Komen Breast Health, the National Institute of Health (Diabetes Disparities), Cancer Support Groups (Duke Endowment), and others. Other professional experiences included my work at Holy Family Catholic Hospital in Atlanta, Georgia. During my busy career I managed to take courses at North Carolina Central University toward my bachelor of science degree in nursing.

After retiring, I experienced a yearning and a desire to reach out to still another phase of nursing. In 2001 I enrolled in the Parish Nursing Program offered at Duke Divinity School and successfully completed the program in one year. This led to a church ministry at CARR United Methodist Church, Cedar Grove, N.C. (sponsored by the Duke Endowment). The rewards were endless. Parish nursing promotes the whole person within the faith community, and it considers the spiritual aspect to be at the center of the practice. It also addresses the physical, emotional, and social aspects. Parish nursing taught me the importance of spirituality in healing and in patients' well-being.

THANK YOU, LINCOLN, for my foundation and for a wonderful career in nursing.

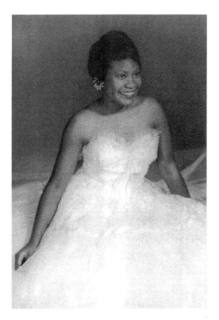

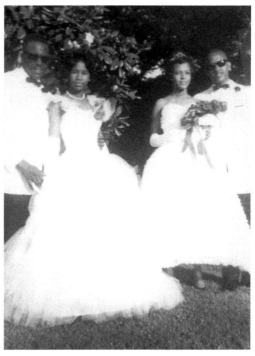

Mary Williams Pointer, Miss Lincoln 1958. Reprinted from *The Nightingale,* 1959. Courtesy of Marion Glen Miles.

Miss Lincoln 1965 coronation. Left to right: *Mary Richardson (Baldwin) and Charles Baldwin, Geneva Vann Dees (Miss Lincoln 1965) and guest.* Courtesy of Mary Richardson Baldwin.

148

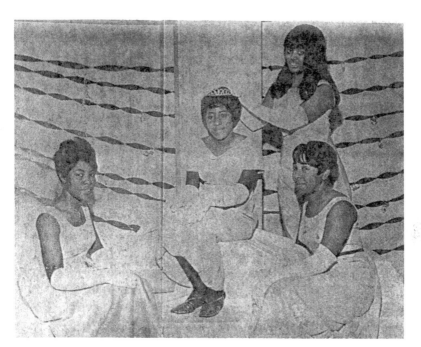

Myrna Watson Hughes, Miss
Lincoln 1967, crowning Shirley
Vereen, Miss Lincoln 1968.
Her court left to right: Vivian
Barnes, Ms. Vareen, Ms.
Watson, Lottie F. Bolding (Hall).
Reprinted from *The Carolina
Times*, June 1, 1968. Courtesy of
Myrna Watson Hughes.

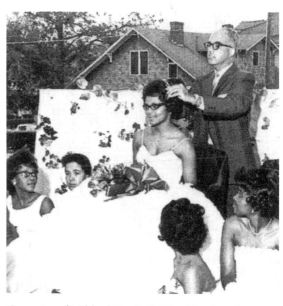

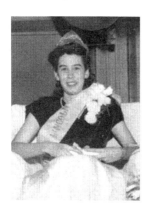

Crowning of Mildred Kindred, Miss Lincoln 1963,
surrounded by her court, crowned by Frank Scott,
hospital director.

Lois Smith Morris, Miss Lincoln
1946. Reprinted from *The Scalpel*,
1946. Courtesy of Lois Smith Morris.

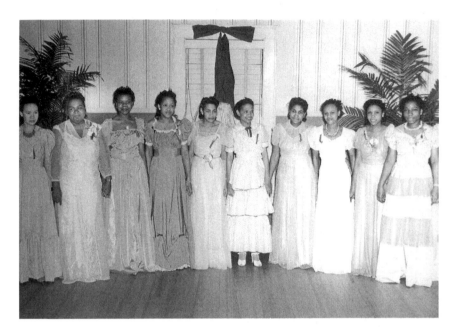

Dressed for prom, class of 1943. Left to right: *Vivian Rudd Parks, Marian Walden Smith, Lillian F. Cuffie, Gladys Williams Britt, Cornelia Jackson Hardie, Ms. L. H. Houston (class advisor), Janie Goodman Cooke, Susie Virginia Carrington Buie, ___ Holmes (left before graduation), Mildred Dert.* Courtesy of Janie Cooke.

ACTIVITIES

Playtime

The hospital lawn was a beautiful setting for numerous activities, both for Lincoln Hospital and the School of Nursing. How many can remember May Day and wrapping the Maypole on the beautiful hospital lawn? Young women in colorful, pastel dresses moving to the music with long streamers was a foreign exercise to some. For others, it had been an annual field-day event in elementary and high school signifying the beginning of spring. Other outdoor games included badminton and croquet on the front lawn of the nursing residence and the hospital lawn. How many played croquet on the front lawn? Esta Segars recounts many days competing with her classmates, and anyone else who came by. She loved it. She was good. Another favorite pastime was playing cards and board games, which included Pitty Pat, Scrabble, Monopoly, Chinese Checkers, Dirty Hearts, Go Fish, Checkers, Pi-

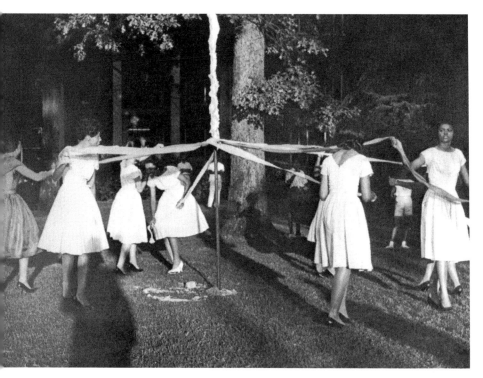

Wrapping the May Pole. Reprinted from *The Scalpel*, 1962. Courtesy of Patricia Martin Blue.

nochle, and Bid Wiz. If you didn't know how to play, someone was always willing to teach you. Mostly everyone enhanced their card playing skills on affiliation. Many Lincoln graduates are still expert at these games today and have formed card clubs and frequently host parties and tournaments. Mary Carmichael talked about dancing in her dorm room. Dancing was another favorite pastime.

> We often had dance contests in the dorm. We would form a circle and, boy, we would dance up a storm, and as your city was called (Kinston, Goldsboro, etc.) we would get in the center of the circle, and everyone would try to out dance each other.

> Common dances were the Jitterbug, Hully Gulley, the Charleston, the Shag, and "Walking the Dog."

Choir

Whether they had beautiful alto and soprano voices or couldn't carry a tune, students were required to sing in the student choir. This was considered another enrichment experience. However to some students it meant more structured time and less freedom. Regardless, students participated— some grudgingly, others willingly—because choir was a carryover from their home church experiences. There were many practices before events in which the choir performed. Many alumni have fond memories of the Christmastime Choral Communion between Lincoln, Watts, and the Duke School of Nursing, which was held at Duke. The choir was coordinated by personalities from the city. Some students participated in church choirs in the city as time permitted.

The Choral Communion program at Duke University, December 14, 1955. Courtesy of Patricia Rascoe Maness.

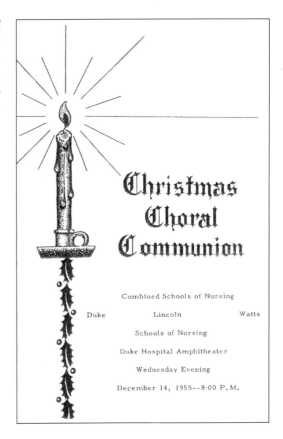

𝕮𝖍𝖗𝖎𝖘𝖙𝖒𝖆𝖘
𝕮𝖍𝖔𝖗𝖆𝖑
𝕮𝖔𝖒𝖒𝖚𝖓𝖎𝖔𝖓

Combined Schools of Nursing

Duke   Lincoln   Watts

Schools of Nursing

Duke Hospital Amphitheater

Wednesday Evening

December 14, 1955--8:00 P.M.

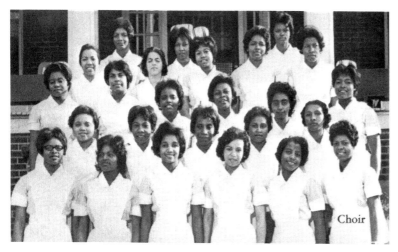

Lincoln Hospital School of Nursing choir. Reprinted from *The Scalpel*, 1962.
Courtesy of Patricia Martin Blue.

Ministry of Worship

Minister-Dr. James T. Cleland

coln-Cassie Nixon   Duke-Carol Brady
    Annie L. Thomas   Agnes Logan

        Watts-Judith Rumley
            Yvonne Yeargin

Ministry of Music

.e-   Lincoln-
ector-Dale Sprague   Director-William Reeves
ompanist-   Accompanist-
atricia Harlan   Patricia Rascoe

        Watts-
        Director-Mrs. Eugenia Umstead
        Accompanist-Joan McLeod

Ministry of Service

ts -   Lincoln-   Duke-
ty Egerton   Geneva Armstead   Frances Olsen
cy Gambill   Carolyn Jones   Gwynne Tuckwood
gy Tew   Sarah Saunders   Edna Quinn
    Williams   Mary Yancey   Judy Hudson

Order of Worship

Prelude
Call to Worship

Congregation: The First Noel
                                      Joy to the World

Duke Choir----------- --------------I Wonder As I Wander
                                     Infant Holy, Infant Lowly

Lincoln Choir------------------- --------Holy Art Thou
                                         Carol of the Bells

Congregation: O Come All Ye Faithful
                                      Away in a Manger

Watts Glee Club----- ----------- --- ------Bethlehem

            The Sacrament of Holy Communion

The Explanation
The Invitation
The Communion Hymn----- Break Thou The Bread of Life
The Words of the Institution
The Prayers
The Distribution of the Elements

Congregation: Silent Night
                                      Blest Be The Tie That Binds

Benediction

Guests and students are invited to a Social Hour immediately following this Service, in the Hanes House
Recreation Room

Games

Basketball Team

As if students did not get enough exercise on the long halls of the hospital or on their walks to classes at North Carolina College, there was the LHSN basketball team. Yes, Lincoln won at least one game. Gloria King, a 1967 graduate, stated that she attempted to play basketball on the school league but was too blind without her glasses to be effective! The *Dispatch*, a hospital newsletter that began in the 1960s, reported the scores for a game between Lincoln and DeShazor's Beauty College, located on Fayetteville Street. The Durham Business College, also located on Fayetteville Street, was another worthy opponent. Students also had the opportunity to attend sporting events at North Carolina College (NCCU) when their schedules permitted.

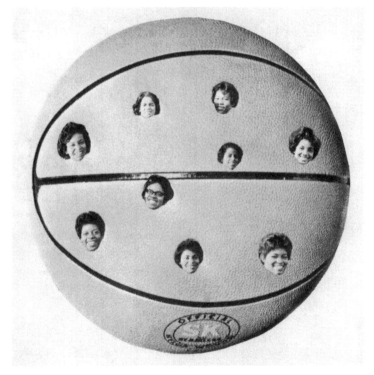

Basketball Team, Scalpel, *1962*
Top row left to right: *Carolyn Levister Harris, Norma Roberts Lipscomb, Ann Gooding Davis.* Middle row left to right: *Mary Lassiter Howell, Margaret Kindred Hunt Capehart, Gertrude Carson Meadows, Lila B. Millard.*
First row left to right: *Emily Jean Carrington, Geraldine Richardson*

Religious Influences

Most students came to Lincoln from deeply religious families. Students at Lincoln represented many faiths and denominations; however, the most common denomination was the Baptist faith. Church attendance provided spiritual guidance and a social outlet. The city of Durham was rich in religious culture and traditions. The early graduates of the 1930s spoke primarily about work, classes, church on Sundays, and Vespers at North Carolina College. Ophelia Dowdy Barnes (RN '48) shared her experience of going to Vespers at NCC on Sunday afternoons and having assigned seats. At Lincoln, Wednesday nights were reserved for Vespers in the nurses' home. Between 1947 and 1950, Reverend Cannon, a Presbyterian Minister, presided at Vespers. Unless you were on duty, you were expected to be there. According to Clara Miller Harris (RN '45), if you were not at Vespers on Sunday evening, then you had a meeting on Monday morning.

> Students worked half days on Sundays, either from 7:00 a.m. to 1:00 p.m. or 1:00 p.m. to 7:00 p.m. If you didn't go to work until 1:00 p.m., then you got dressed and went to church at White Rock, St. Joseph, or Saint Titus. These churches were located on Fayetteville Street and were within walking distance of Lincoln. The minister at St. Joseph would make sure that students were out by 12:00 noon or 12:15 p.m. so they could get back to the campus in time for lunch because on Sundays an evening meal was not served. At the midday meal, a little brown bag with a sandwich and an apple or some fruit was given to the students for their supper.

> Other churches students attended include Kyles Temple on Dunston Street under the leadership of Rev. George Tharrington, Covenant Presbyterian near Merrick Street, Oak Grove on Colfax Street, Russell Memorial on Alston Avenue, St. Joseph AME on Fayetteville Street, and Holy Cross Catholic Church on Alston Avenue. In fact several students were married in the Catholic Church. Some alumni have made these churches their homes. Gloria Taylor Cheek King (1967) commented,

> I attended White Rock Baptist Church during my training at Lincoln. White Rock was within walking distance of the school and it was also of my faith. I loved the Sanctuary Choir and they also had a wonderful male chorus. The infamous Rev. Dr. Miles Mark Fisher was the Pastor. His son, Rev. Miles M. Fisher III, was the Chaplain for the nursing school and the basketball coach.

She continues to worship at White Rock.

Through social, religious, and team-building experiences students developed a bond that supported them amid the challenges of the course work, the clinical work, the faculty, and their new home. Carrie Stone Reavis (1965) describes it this way:

> Life at Lincoln was not fancy but meaningful, and most students were purpose-driven and educationally inspired; supported and impressed by voices from the administrative faculty and hospital staff; energized and refreshed by participating in community events; spiritually strengthened by weekly reverent requirements; mentored and nurtured by inherited big sisters; restrained, approved, and questioned by a forceful but caring housemother; taught by others the art of frying and dying hair the Lincoln way; learned winner's luck at being a card playing ace. I embraced this sisterhood of education, friendship, networking, trust, and respect at Lincoln to become empowered to be the "Best of the Best" in professional nursing.

THE EXTENDED LINCOLN FAMILY

Students were supported in various ways by all the departments and employees in the hospital. They formed special relationships with members of the dietary, housekeeping, laundry, laboratory, and ancillary staff, as well as with licensed practical nurses, orderlies, aids, and certainly all of the staff nurses with whom they interacted on the floors. The students' new family extended to the community. The community in which Lincoln was located was called Hayti and was an area of bustling activity. The Hayti area was known for the houses of the well-to-do Blacks and Black-owned businesses that were located on Fayetteville and Pettigrew Streets. On Southside, there were churches (as previously mentioned), businesses such as doctors' offices on Fayetteville Street and surrounding streets (e.g., those of Dr. Leroy R. Swift, Dr. Charles Watts, Dr. Robert E. Dawson, Dr. James Cleland, Dr. Bowen, Dr. D. B. Cooke, Dr. Robert E. King), the Stanford L. Warren Library, and the Biltmore Hotel. On Pettigrew Street, there was the P&W Grill and Pratt's. On Pickett Street, you could find barber shops, beauty salons, the Regal Theater, the Donut Shop, Garrett's Pharmacy, John's Diner, Yarboro Dees Pool Hall, Birdland Social Club, W. D. Hill Recreation Center, and rooming houses—all within walking distance of the nurses dorm and school. Later, Pages Store, Weaver's Dry Cleaners, and The College Inn opened. The College Inn really was off-limits, but many students secretly

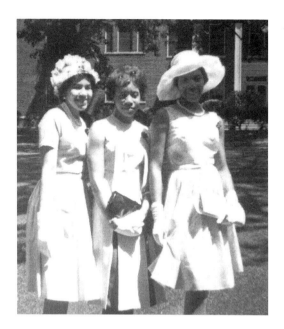

Dressed for church. Left to right: *Loretta Gail Flateau Chestnut, Dellamar Inez Davis Washington, Christine Stokes.* Courtesy of Mary Richardson Baldwin.

frequented it. This was a gathering place for some of the locals (single and married!) and for athletes from North Carolina College.

Community support through the churches, individuals, schools, and businesses was important to the well-being of the hospital and the School of Nursing. Other individuals in the community fed, nurtured, and mentored students, as well as paid them to babysit. Mr. Wingate maintained the grounds around the nurses' residence and the hospital, and they were immaculate. Imagine being exhausted and ready for sleep at 7:00 a.m. after completing an 11:00 p.m. to 7:00 a.m. shift in the hospital and having to try to block out the noise as Mr. Wingate mowed the lawn. He always had the friendliest and brightest smile as he went about his tasks. But on those particular days, so early in the morning, there was nothing friendly or bright about his smile to students trying to sleep. In fact, it was downright sickening to many of us! But, he redeemed himself. He lived across the street from A. B. Duke Nurses Home and he and his family were very supportive of the nursing students. Many meals were enjoyed at his table.

Mrs. Elizabeth W. Thorpe (RN '48) sang the praises of Mr. Hopper, the only orderly for a very long time. He ran the laundry (he was responsible for the nurses' starched, white uniforms), fired the boiler, drove the van, and maintained the morgue. Once the nurses had given their after-death care,

(continues on page 160)

Jocelyn Thompson Hodges, RN '58, BSN, BA
My Story
A LIFE OF BLESSINGS AND THANKFULNESS

I am Jocelyn Thompson Hodges, a member of
the graduating class of Lincoln Hospital School
of Nursing in 1958. There were five girls and four
boys in my family, and we lived and worked on a
farm in Bladen County, North Carolina. Education
was very important to my parents. All nine of us
graduated high school and eight of us completed
college. Religious education was also important
to my parents. Consequently, Sunday school and
church were a must every Sunday.

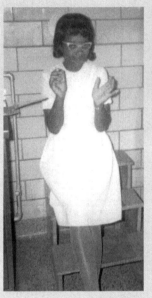

My first memories of my paternal grandmother
were that she was sickly and hospitalized frequently. I loved going to the hospital to see her and
helping her as much as I was allowed. I realized
early that my passion was to help sick people. My
love for nursing was developed at that time. My
father was also hospitalized during my high-school
years, and I was allowed to stay in the hospital
overnight with him. After staying in the hospital
with my dad I knew nursing was the career I
wanted.

Courtesy of Jocelyn Thompson
Hodges.

Following graduation from high school, I was
determined to go to nursing school. Lincoln Hospital School of Nursing was my
first choice for the following reasons: 1) Lincoln was the best three-year program,
based on its literature; 2) My sister lived in Durham and I would not have to be
away from all of my family; 3) My parents could not afford to pay tuition for a
four-year college education at that time; and 4) Durham was not that far from
home.

Nursing school was challenging to say the least, but I enjoyed the challenges,
classes, classmates, instructors, and the patients. I was not a particularly smart
student and I had to study, study, and study along with shedding some tears
and praying. The education I received at Lincoln was second to none. I had the
knowledge and skills to function as a prepared, proficient nurse.

I graduated from nursing school and passed the State Board Exam. This I call
blessing number one: my dream of becoming a registered nurse was realized.

I had always wanted to join the military and become an Army nurse. But
I felt that I needed to get work experience first. I was employed at Cape Fear
Valley Hospital in Fayetteville, N.C., in 1959. This was a small hospital with
segregated facilities. Having heard about Michael Reese Hospital, in Chicago,
Illinois, I applied and was accepted as a staff nurse. This hospital provided

avenues that I could pursue, and I could also enjoy big-city life. After working there for three years, I applied to the military and moved back to the east coast. I was denied acceptance into the military because it was determined that I had a heart condition; this was shocking to my ego. But, I refused to let a negative experience direct the course of my life. I applied for employment at the Veterans Administration Hospital System and was hired almost immediately. Employment at the VA hospital was paramount to me since I could not get into the military. I call this blessing number two: being able to take care of the men and women that had served in the military to protect our country during peace and war.

In 1965 I was married and in 1967 God blessed us with a beautiful daughter who is the apple of our eyes. This I call blessing number three: marriage and family.

In 1966 I started employment with the VA Hospital Systems in Baltimore, Maryland. Most of my work has been in medical, surgical, and neurology nursing as the charge nurse on the midnight tour. The need to continue my education was always apparent. I enrolled in night classes. Blessing number four: accomplishments. I obtained a diploma in nursing, became certified in medical nursing, received a bachelor's degree in sociology, received the Veterans Affairs award for Excellence in Nursing, and became a member of Chi Eta Phi Sorority. I received citations from President Clinton and Vice President Gore at my retirement.

My tenure at the VA lasted thirty years and six months. And, what a rewarding and fulfilling experience! The circle had now closed, in 1996. Blessing number five: God allowed me to finish my employment at the VA as a positive team player respected by my peers, co-workers, and patients.

I then started a new circle, which included part-time work with a research drug company at the University of Maryland and the gastrointestinal (GI) Lab at the VA Hospital, in Baltimore. Blessing number six: I still have marketable skills with which to find employment.

My travels have taken me to London, England; Paris, France; Cape Town and Johannesburg, South Africa; Mexico; Canada; and Hawaii, Alaska, and many eastern, midwestern, and western states. Blessing number seven: learning through travel, joy and relaxation.

Officially, I retired from public nursing in 2003 when my husband's health began failing and I needed to be available to assist him. This time also allowed me to develop other skills and growth in other areas: computer skills, arts and crafts, and involvement in church activities. Blessing number eight: still able to help him and learn new skills.

My daughter married in 2000. We gained a son and in 2003 we were blessed with a grandson, the apple of all our eyes. Blessing number nine: additions to our family.

I realize that I did not make this journey alone. Blessing number ten: the most important blessing—Giving God thanks. THANK YOU, GOD, THAT YOUR MIGHTY HANDS HAVE LED AND GUIDED ME EVERY STEP OF THE WAY. THANK YOU, GOD! THANK YOU, GOD!

he would open the morgue on the old side of the hospital. Many students remember taking bodies up an incline to the morgue on the roof by the labor room. Skill was required to push the stretcher up the incline without an accident.

A humorous memory of Mr. Hopper was shared by Patricia Martin Blue (RN '65). Mr. Hopper took her class to a Science Fair at Duke Hospital and forgot to return for them. One student had enough money to pay bus fare for all of them. The students were fully dressed in uniform on public transportation on their return to Lincoln. They were campused because being in uniform in public was against the rules. They resented this punishment because it was not their fault.

Many students came to know people in the community and established lasting friendships. Mary Carmichael (RN '71) shared the following story:

> During one of my clinical rotations at Lincoln I was assigned to a female patient. She was scheduled for surgery and was very emotional, crying and really afraid of the outcome. I gave her lots of tender loving care, and we bonded. She started calling me "Stokley," you know, after Stokley Carmichael. She had an uneventful recovery, and we became very good friends. She attended my graduation. She was a longtime resident on Otis Street off Fayetteville Street. After graduation, I would visit her for the weekend, and she would be excited to have me visit her and treated me as a daughter. We communicated often until her death. She was sweet, intelligent, humorous, and it was a joy to be in her company. I cannot recall her ever calling me Mary; it was always "Stokley."
>
> She loved Lincoln Hospital and the nursing students. If I recall correctly, she was a graduate of NCCU.

This chapter began with a class poem from 1948, which was a reflection on the students' three years at Lincoln. The following piece of writing by Mary Louise Williams Pointer (RN '59) recaps the events of a day in the life of the student nurses at LHSN in the 1950s. As you'll see, there were not too many changes from the 1940s.

A Day in the Life of the Student Nurses at Lincoln Hospital School of Nursing (1950s)

At 6:00 a.m., the bell would chime, rung by our house matron, Mrs. Mason. We would scurry to the bathroom to get dressed for class, held at North Carolina College (now North Carolina Central University).

By 7:00 a.m., the students would be in line at the hospital cafeteria for a hearty breakfast. By 7:30 a.m., the preclinicals (the first-year nursing students) would walk to North Carolina College (NCCU) for 8:00 a.m. classes. One of our professors was Dr. L. T. Walker, a coach at the time, who was instrumental in touching the life of Lee Calhoun. Lee was an Olympic winner in 1956–1957 who represented North Carolina College. At 12:00 noon all classes were completed and again we would walk back to Lincoln Hospital Nursing School, where lunch would be waiting.

Once lunch was over, students would return to the dormitory rooms and change into the nurses' uniforms. The uniforms were spotless and heavily starched (done by the hospital laundry), shoes had to be polished with white shoe laces and clean white stockings (free of runs). Nursing caps were placed atop the head (long hair tucked neatly in a bun, other lengths kept above the collar). A watch with a second hand was the only jewelry allowed (students were not allowed to marry at that time; therefore, no engagement or wedding rings were worn).

At 1:30 p.m. (sharp) the students would assemble in the classroom (downstairs in the dormitory) for clinical nursing courses. Twice a week the students were taken to the hospital (by the instructor) and assigned patient care. This included checking urine for glucose, taking blood pressures and temperatures, sterilizing thermometers, bedpans, and emesis basins, giving back rubs, filling water pitchers, and reading to patients. Nurses were taught to stand when physicians approached the desk at the nurses' station. All nurses and staff were addressed by their last names.

At 4:30 p.m. the nursing students were finished for the day and dinner was served. During the sunlight hours, students were allowed to walk up and down Fayetteville Street but were forbidden to walk on Pettigrew Street. We were also forbidden to ride in cars; so, our means of transportation were walking or riding the city bus (#5). Of course some of us defied that rule.

Vespers was every Wednesday night at the dormitory. All students were encouraged to participate in singing with the students at Duke and the Watts School of Nursing in the Duke Amphitheatre (at Christmastime), entertaining patients and staff. These were memorable occasions.

An award was started in the 1950s for the best all-around student (based on performance on the ward and in the classroom). Ruby Jewel Bell (Borden) (Class of 1959) was the first student to receive that honor, and her name was placed on a plaque. This plaque hung in the foyer of the nursing dorm.

Students participated in pageants. I held the crown for Miss Lincoln in 1958.

(continues on page 164)

Mary Lee Richardson Baldwin, RN '66, BSN, MPHA

I was born to a teenage mom and raised by a maternal aunt and an uncle who at eighty-eight years old still sneaks and chews (Levi Garrett) tobacco. From this beginning, raised on a dirt road joining farms, I grew up with four uncles, two aunts, my sister Rosetta, and a total of nineteen cousins, all of us participating in killing hogs, barning tobacco, picking cotton and cucumbers, pulling corn, and going to church.

My first official job was driving a school bus forty-five miles round trip because there was no Black school for us to attend. I ended up being the only bus driver that wrecked her bus when a wasp went up my dress and I jumped a ditch and ended up in a corn-field. Johnston County Memorial Hospital afforded me the opportunity to enter nursing school after winning a county writing essay on "Why I Wanted To Continue My Education." A three-year education scholarship was paid as long as my grades were above average.

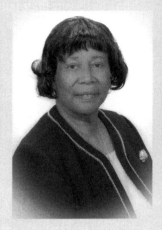

Courtesy of Mary Richardson Baldwin.

During my developmental years there was a sense of family, church, community, and a strong work ethic from strong personalities that were there to guide me and pay close attention to my life. From these fertilizing roots, I embarked on my lifelong journey of trying to determine who I would become. As the now ninety-year-old mother/aunt would say to me when she left me on the stoop at Lincoln Hospital School of Nursing, "Do your best because you don't know who is watching you and if you can't do what you are supposed to do YOU can come home and barn tobacco!" I prayed at that moment, "Please God, don't let me go back to that life."

We were poor in money but rich in love and tradition. This tradition kept me humble and true to being the best I could be. Lincoln provided me with friends for a lifetime. I entered with the Class of 1966. We started with twenty-two students but there were only eight by the end of the first semester: Dellamar Davis, Linda Loftin Woodson, Rebecca Mitchell Carter, Pauline Langston Edwards, Loretta Flateau Chestnut, Alice Jean McClain, and Sarah O'Lene Jinwright. A bond developed among us very early. We called ourselves the "Sensational Eight" and continue to meet every other year some place on the east coast.

Lincoln taught me that being a nurse required the skills of a follower, a leader, and a stickler for details as well as being able to recognize quality care and the importance of meeting patients where they were. We cared for poor patients that could not be cared for on the other side of the tracks. I saw doctors and nurses that looked like me. I also recognized the type of nurse I wanted to pattern myself after and certainly there were some nurses that had issues. As a student I worked from 11:00 p.m. to 6:30 a.m. then would go to Pharmacology class at 7:00 a.m., followed by medical/surgical class, then go to bed, get up and study for a few hours, then back to work at 10:45 p.m. (Barning tobacco didn't look so bad.) But through it all, perseverance, professionalism, crying, and prayer prepared me for the world outside of my Lincoln tradition.

After leaving Lincoln, I went to work in a tertiary hospital. It brought on a world I had almost forgotten, that is, being told I was not qualified because I didn't have a degree. This, when I saw White nurses that also did not have degrees being hired in leadership roles. So, with my husband's support, I obtained a BSN degree and was appointed to a head nurse position. I was ready. One morning, I was approached by the nursing supervisor and informed that a physician had written a letter stating that I needed to be taken off the floor and made a head nurse. I was not sure what he wanted in a head nurse. The supervisor then said, "Well, we can't keep a charge nurse so we thought we would try a Black nurse." My response was, "You just get out of my way and I will show you what a Lincoln Hospital nurse can do." About three years later the nursing director of the Hospital (a Lincoln nurse) hired me as the first Black supervisor of Ambulatory Care (all public clinics).

It was God's grace through prayer that allowed me to complete a BSN and a master's in public health. When I tried to enter the BSN program at North Carolina Central University in Durham, North Carolina, my SAT scores were not high enough, so I called the chairman, Helen Miller, and she said, "Girl come on down and sign up for class." I was determined not to disappoint her. I took the MSAT and again I did not meet requirements. This time I talked with Professor Moses Carey, and he had me sign up for nine hours, and I passed all the courses. Wow, what an accomplishment for someone from Middlesex, North Carolina.

My struggles at the tertiary medical center continued as other Black nurses realized that there was a pattern of Black nurses needing degrees to achieve leadership positions. We had city rallies, gained support from the Durham NAACP, and established the Concerned Black Nurses Committee. A national committee was appointed and it uncovered some problems, but the administration chose to diffuse our efforts by eliminating positions.

Through all of these struggles, this Lincoln Hospital School of Nursing graduate was hired to return to the grounds where she started—Lincoln Community Health Center (where Lincoln Hospital once stood). I returned to oversee the nursing care and monitor the quality of care provided. For twenty-one years I provided care to the uninsured and underserved. During those years, my husband and I had to raise two small grandchildren. From those fertilizing roots, I had to give back and help save the people that I love very much.

What a journey. I have networked with the state nurses associations, the community, the National Black Nurses Association, formed the prostate support group and breast health support group at Lincoln Community Health Center, mentored nurses, and encouraged those who were interested in the profession to follow their dreams. This profession has taught me to be qualified through formal knowledge but also to be truthful and straightforward in my dealings with others. Nurses want leaders to be open, fair, caring, and goal oriented.

Thanks for the opportunity to share my journey. I wish to thank all those persons that participated in my journey, and I hope that I have given back in some way. Thanks to the authors that had the vision to document these facts.

During our senior year, we were sent on affiliation (attending classes in specialty areas not available at Lincoln Hospital School of Nursing). Our assignment for psychiatric nursing was at Crownsville Mental Hospital, in Crownsville, Maryland, where in addition to studying and working with the mentally ill, you learned how to play pinochle and shoot pool. We lived on campus; therefore, there were no other activities in and around Crownsville. Sometimes relatives from Washington, D.C., and Baltimore, Md., would pick some of us up and take us to Washington for a tour of Howard University. Also, we were able to visit Johns Hopkins Hospital in Baltimore.

Our affiliation for pediatric nursing was in Nashville, Tennessee, at Hubbard Hospital. Classes were held at Meharry Medical College and Tennessee State University. Most afternoons we would watch Wilma Rudolph (a 1960 Black Olympic winner and the first American woman to win three gold medals) practice on the track at Tennessee State.

Our return to Durham, North Carolina, was the beginning of the end at Lincoln Hospital School of Nursing. It was getting ready for graduation (even though our class was delayed for one month), applying for employment, and preparing for the State Board Examination.

Our experiences at Lincoln Hospital School of Nursing were exciting, enjoyable, and memorable. It was an experience that will be treasured for a lifetime. It was the best thing that could have happened to most of us. It prepared us for employment and job opportunities in which we excelled in all phases of nursing and that spanned many nationalities throughout the United States and Abroad.

Our lives as Lincoln students were touched by all of these people. There is no one particular event that stands out, but all were important in our lives as students. They are included here to generate memories of our individual experiences with them.

THE CHANGING FACE OF HEALTHCARE AND NURSING

While the internal climate at Lincoln remained fairly stable, the external climate was changing rapidly. The challenges facing the hospital and the School of Nursing were interdependent and had mutual impacts. Since 1925 Lincoln Hospital had been operating within the same facilities, and they were in need of repair and remodeling. Several key events/movements occurring in health care and hospital management had indirect effects on the school. The sources for the following were extracted from various documents including *Highlights in Nursing in North Carolina, 1935–1976,* and Annual Reports of the Board of Trustees meeting minutes.

1) The passage of the Social Security Act in 1935 by the United States Congress had broad-reaching effects. It created provisions for the aged, blind, dependent and crippled children, maternal and child welfare, public health, and the administration of unemployment compensation laws. These programs were funded by the North Carolina General Assembly. Lincoln became active with the Crippled Children Program. Student nurses and staff nurses were trained to work with these special populations.

2) The North Carolina Medical Care Commission was established in 1945 to administer a program of state financial support for hospitalized indigent patients, survey the hospital needs, administer federal funds for hospital construction and/or expansion, administer a loan program for students in the health-care profession, and administer a hospital licensing program.

3) In 1947 Congress passed the Hill-Burton Act, and the North Carolina General Assembly appropriated $600,000 in matching funds for a program of hospital and health-care-facility construction in the state, which was to be administered by the North Carolina Medical Care Commission. Loans were also made available to students of dentistry, medicine, nursing, and pharmacy. An immediate impact was felt throughout the state, which saw an expansion of health facilities and an increased demand for nurses. A few Lincoln nursing students received loans from this program.

4) In 1949 hospital facilities at Lincoln and Watts were in need of repair and remodeling. Claude Munger, a consultant, recommended that Lincoln and Watts be remodeled, and based on his recommendations the hospitals' respective boards of trustees approved plans for construction and remodeling.

5) In 1950 Lincoln Hospital was donated to the County of Durham, and shortly thereafter the county returned Lincoln Hospital to the board of trustees through a lease for the sum of $1.

6) New construction began on both Lincoln and Watts Hospitals in 1951, and in 1953 Lincoln Hospital had an opening ceremony on the lawn. Dignitaries from across North Carolina, city and county government officials, members of the medical community, nursing students, and citizens participated in this momentous event.

7) In 1955 North Carolina had four schools that offered a bachelor's degree in nursing: UNC in Chapel Hill, Duke University in Durham, A&T College in Greensboro, and Winston-Salem State Teachers College in Winston-Salem.

8) The Board of Nursing and other professional nursing organizations recommended that all schools of nursing seek NLN accreditation.

9) UNC Chapel Hill was the first baccalaureate school to be accredited by the NLN.

10) In 1957 LHSN began the NLN accreditation process. It was never successful in completing the process probably due to finances, its patient census, and faculty recruitment issues.

11) In 1960 any hospital receiving Hill-Burton funds was required to open its staff and facilities to both Blacks and Whites.

12) In 1964 Guidelines for Nursing Education in North Carolina were formulated by an independent group of nurses. The guidelines called for two levels of basic nursing preparation within academic institutions and a time allowance of between three and five years for all nonaccredited schools to show movement toward NLN accreditation.

13) In 1965 the North Carolina Nursing Practice Act was rewritten, and legislation was passed by the General Assembly to include provisions for mandatory licensure, new definitions of nursing practice, and flexibility in programs for nursing education.

14) Watts suffered from overcrowding, whereas Lincoln suffered from poor occupancy. Integration meant that Black citizens, who once had only Black hospitals from which to receive care provided by Blacks with dignity and respect, now had choices. Duke and Watts Hospitals were now integrated institutions that had modern, state-of-the-art facilities, advanced technology, equipment, and care modalities along with adequate professional staff. Black patients could go to Duke and have private physicians, Black or White, as their primary care providers. Duke Hospital was established in 1930, twenty-nine years after Lincoln Hospital opened its doors, and became a thriving hospital in a short time, most probably due to the financial support of private philanthropists.

Collaborative ventures were set up between Lincoln and Duke Hospitals. Lincoln had a large charity load, which interns and resident staff from Duke and other Black institutions served. These interns and residents were supervised by attending staff on their respective specialty services. From its early days, Duke Hospital admitted Negro patients but housed them on segregated units.

Students at Lincoln lived through World War I, the Great Depression, World War II, the Cuban Missile Crisis, the Civil Rights Movement, and the Vietnam War. Lincoln nursing students were not permitted to become involved in civil rights activities for several reasons. Sylvia Overton Richardson, director of nursing education and assistant director of nursing services, explains it this way: "This was not a written decision on the part of Mrs. Williams but a practical one: Students needed to be in class and they needed to be on duty to receive people if there were traumatic or critical situations. This had both a financial and educational impact."

THE CLOSING CURTAIN

All of the above developments in some way influenced the changing tide at Lincoln. In addition to the civil rights unrest, LHSN began to face serious challenges with the Board of Nursing. Student first-time passing rates on the board exam between 1963 and 1967 were low. The NLN tests were also used as a tool for measuring student achievement. Student performance on these tests was also low. In those areas of the hospital where the census was inadequate, in terms of number and patient diversity, the students seemed to be challenged. Conversely, in areas where students had received supplemental experiences on affiliations, their performances on tests were better. Visitors from the Board of Nursing in 1967 identified several areas wherein Lincoln Hospital and School of Nursing were not meeting Board standards. Discrepancies existed between the written curriculum plan and how it was being executed. The hospital census and patient mix were inadequate to provide sufficient learning experiences. Faculty and students were interviewed, and students expressed concern about the ability of the school to provide the experiences they needed to be successful on the board exam. The administration was given one year to improve and comply with the standards. The hospital and School of Nursing administrators developed a response plan for overcoming the deficiencies. A year later, in 1968, at the Board's visit Lincoln had corrected two of the deficiencies but had been unsuccessful in attaining

(continues on page 170)

北 Carolina Board of Nursing

P. O. BOX 2129

RALEIGH, NORTH CAROLINA

June 23, 1969

Mrs. Lucille Z. Williams, R.N.
Director of Nursing
Lincoln Hospital
School of Nursing
Durham, North Carolina

Dear Mrs. Williams:

At its meeting on June 12, 1969, the Board of Nursing reviewed the March 12, 1969 survey report of Lincoln Hospital School of Nursing. Data in this report were reviewed in the light of: stated stipulations under which Lincoln Hospital was returned to the List of Accredited Schools of Nursing on August 31, 1967; the Nursing Practice Act; and the Standards for Educational Units in Nursing.

Information in the survey report indicated that Lincoln Hospital has complied with two of six stipulations stated by the Board as necessary for the program to meet minimum Standards for Accreditation.

A further study of this report revealed specific areas of non-compliance with the Nursing Practice Act, Section 90-171.7, Requirements 3 and 4 and Standards for Educational Units in Nursing as follows:

I. Students, page 6, Standards for Educational Units in Nursing

Special attention is called to item 1:(b) and 2:

"1:b - admission--there must be evidence of admission policies in keeping with the purposes of the educational unit in nursing and achievement expected of students. Screening must include an evaluation of emotional and physical health status as well as scholastic attainment and personal characteristics.

"2 - There must be evidence that the established criteria are implemented."

Information in the survey report indicates that admission policies are not implemented.

Letter from State Board of Nursing about noncompliance with standards, June 23, 1969. Courtesy of Duke University Archives, Rare Book Room.

II. **Curriculum**, page 7, Standards for Educational Units in Nursing

   a. Paragraph 2

"Instruction is a planned process through which teacher and student interact with selected environment and content so that the response of the student gives evidence that expected learning has taken place. Wherever and whenever students are scheduled for learning opportunities, faculty must control the teaching, directing, and supervision of all learning experiences."

The type and amount of instruction provided for the obstetric course is not in keeping with this requirement.

   b. Paragraph 3 and Items 1-4

"The faculty must present a design of instruction in keeping with the stated purposes of the program. Inherent in the stated purposes of all basic programs in nursing must be the goal of preparing students to become licensed practitioners of nursing. Any proposed major change of the curriculum must be submitted to the Board for approval prior to implementation.

"1. Learning opportunities must be planned in logical sequence so that prerequisite knowledge is provided prior to the experience to which it is basic.

"2. Course descriptions must show:

(a) objectives indicating types of skills and understandings expected of students, and

(b) descriptions of content, learning environment activities, placement, allocation to time and methods of evaluation.

"3. Schedules for students must provide for optimal educational achievement.

"4. Faculty shall present evidence of an ongoing plan for evaluating the curriculum as it relates to the total program and projecting needs for revision."

A design of instruction with minimum printed materials was available for review during the survey. However, non-compliance with curriculum standards is evident in that the plan of instruction is not implemented as designed.

The failure of the program to meet, at a satisfactory level, the "goal of preparing students to become licensed practitioners of nursing" is documented.

the affiliation agreements that would provide students with better learning experiences. At this time the school was directed to reduce the number of students admitted such that the total school enrollment did not exceed forty. The LHSN attrition rate, hospital patient-care needs, and increased financial burden created an insurmountable obstacle given the timetable for change. The last class entered Lincoln in the fall of 1968 with twenty-one students, of which fourteen graduated in 1971. In 1969 all admissions to the school were suspended. Ms. Z and Mr. Suitt presented a strong case for continuing the school, and requested more time to make the necessary changes, but to no avail.

Parallel to this activity in the School of Nursing were challenges facing the hospital. The building was in need of repair, the census was low, and Durham was debating the value of renovating Lincoln and Watts Hospitals: Could there be one hospital for all the citizens of Durham? Could Lincoln Hospital sustain the medical programs with its dwindling census? The Civil Rights Act of 1965 had made it clear that Medicare and Medicaid funds awarded to hospitals could not be used in a discriminatory manner. Consequently, as stated earlier, patients could go wherever they wanted for their care.

Two Bond elections had been held regarding the continued operation of the two hospitals. In 1960 Durham voters rejected the first $15 million Bond referendum. However, in 1968 the citizens approved the $20 million Bond referendum for construction of an entirely new hospital to serve all citizens of the community—Black and White. So what about the nursing schools? Watts Hospital School of Nursing had served young, White women; Lincoln had served young, Negro women.

Several questions can be posed about the closing of LHSN. First, was Lincoln unfairly judged by the board with regard to passing rates? In many instances there were a number of first-time failures on the Board, but there were also successes on first-time writings of the Board exam. However, graduates passed on subsequent attempts. Second, should LHSN have had more time to remedy its deficiencies? Perhaps the reality that Lincoln was not operating on the same playing field as Watts Hospital School of Nursing and some of the other White nursing schools is part of the equation. At this time Lincoln was the only Negro Diploma Program in North Carolina. St. Agnes had closed in 1961, Good Samaritan had closed, and Kate Biting in Winston-Salem had transitioned its last two classes to Forsyth Hospital School of Nursing. Jubilee in Henderson had lasted only a short while, and

North Carolina Board of Nursing

P. O. BOX 2129

RALEIGH, NORTH CAROLINA

July 2, 1969

Mrs. Lucille Z. Williams, R.N.
Director of Nursing
Lincoln Hospital
Durham, North Carolina

Dear Mrs. Williams:

Our records indicate that on June 24, 1969, you received the letter notifying you of the recent action taken by the Board relevant to the accreditation status of the Lincoln Hospital School of Nursing.

In addition to the action taken, the Board recommended that future plans for the enrollment of students into this program be suspended indefinitely.

This recommendation is made because of the current situation at Lincoln Hospital School of Nursing, including:

      a.   failure to comply with minimum requirements and standards for educational units;

      b.   the failure of students from this program to perform satisfactorily on the licensing examination;

      c.   the apparent inability of the faculty to implement a sound program within the existing framework of the institution.

Please contact us if you have questions relevant to the action and/or this recommendation.

Sincerely,

(Miss) Mary McRee, R.N.
Executive Director

MMcR;pj
cc: Miss Lelia Crockett
     Mr. Larry Suitt
     Mr. W. C. Harris, Jr.
     Dr. Eloise R. Lewis

Letter from State Board of Nursing, suspending admissions indefinitely. Courtesy of Duke University Archives, Rare Book Room.

Julia Simpson Armstrong, RN '38

Julia Simpson Armstrong was born on January 23, 1913, in Bennettsville, South Carolina. Her father was a mechanic and her mother was a cook. She had four siblings, attended high school in Asheboro, North Carolina, and currently resides in Durham. Her church affiliation is Baptist.

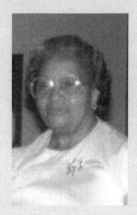

Courtesy of Evelyn Booker Wicker.

Mrs. Armstrong shared that she conceived of her desire to become a nurse due to the influence of her grandmother, who was a midwife and delivered babies in the home. She further related that her mother placed value on getting a college education, as this was an avenue by which one could secure a better job and income. Knowing that money was scarce, she set out to plan her entry into nursing. Through her grandmother's midwifery duties, she was able to observe medical care in the home, and she secured jobs as a baby sitter and cashier, which allowed her to earn money to pay her tuition.

While there were other schools of nursing to choose from—for example, Saint Agnes in Raleigh, North Carolina—she chose Lincoln Hospital School of Nursing in Durham because of its close proximity to Asheboro, where her family lived.

As a student at Lincoln, Mrs. Armstrong experienced a bit of college life. She took courses at North Carolina College (now North Carolina Central University). Professors from North Carolina College would also come to Lincoln to teach courses.

L. Richardson Hospital School of Nursing in Greensboro had closed. Third, the Board of Nursing espoused the idea that nursing education should be placed in a collegiate setting. The Board of Nursing was segregated until the appointment in 1968 of Mrs. Helen S. Miller, who was then chair of the Public Health Nursing Program at North Carolina College. The point is that the Black diploma schools of nursing did not have a voice, even though the professional organization was integrated during this time.

During her training, Mrs. Armstrong got practical experience by working in the office of a gynecologist. This was her first paid nursing job, for which she was paid $25 a week.

As her career expanded, she worked with the government's Rapid Treatment Center (Syphilis treatment). Later she returned to Lincoln Hospital and experienced a work environment led by then director of nursing Pattie Carter.

After getting married and working at Lincoln Hospital for about four years, she became pregnant. Following the delivery of her child she became a stay-at-home mom. After eight years or so, Ms. Armstrong returned to Lincoln Hospital as a night supervisor. She found the job satisfying and gratifying as the administration and staff were supportive of her. The patient populations, as well as the staff, were predominately African-American. At Lincoln, she felt that she was able to work with many distinguished physicians in an environment of collegiality and mutual respect.

With the consolidation of Lincoln and Watts Hospitals in 1973–1974 into Durham County General Hospital, a change in professional relationships occurred. Mrs. Armstrong was placed in an environment where she was required to deal with a different set of values. The environment became one in which White and Black nurses provided service to all people. As she was still a supervisor, the challenge to promote fairness was always present. She remained at Durham Regional Hospital until 1983, when she retired.

Mrs. Julia Simpson Armstrong's story was adapted from an "Informant's Profile" and an interview with Evelyn Wicker, RN, MPH for her doctoral dissertation titled "Factors That Have Influenced the Career Development and Career Achievement of Graduates From Lincoln Hospital School of Nursing." Dr. Wicker did a follow-up interview in 2010. At that time, Mrs. Armstrong was ninety-seven years old.

Could the fate of LHSN have been different? In hindsight, the answer appears to be yes, but we will never know. Watts Hospital School of Nursing survived. Could Watts and Lincoln Hospital School of Nursing have merged just as Lincoln Hospital and Watts Hospital merged? Could LHSN have merged with NCCU and its undergraduate nursing program? A final question that begs attention is whether Lincoln students and the school had equal opportunity for success? In retrospect, one could speculate that adequate economic and political resources could have stemmed the tide. But ultimately, as professional nursing programs became increasingly college- and university-based, the closing of the school may have been inevitable. The closing of LHSN signaled the end of Negro diploma schools of nursing in North Carolina. The challenge to secure sufficient qualified faculty coupled with the financial constraints, increasingly strict regulations, a lack of professional nursing advocacy and support, and a lack of political support led to the demise of these schools. The challenges became insurmountable. Following the closure of the school, Lincoln Hospital continued to maintain inpatient and outpatient clinical services. In 1971 Lincoln Community Health Center, a federally funded neighborhood health center, officially opened, occupying the basement and lower level of the hospital. The mission of the health center was to serve the underserved population in Durham and the surrounding county. The newly created Durham County Hospital Corporation, whose responsibility was to plan and orchestrate the one hospital initiative, had a ground-breaking ceremony in 1972. On October 3, 1976, Durham County General Hospital opened. On October 10, the first patients were transferred to its beds. This merger had a profound effect on the Durham community. It represented a tremendous loss to the Black community; gone was a long-standing health-care institution, an educational and training institution, and a source of pride and role modeling for future Black leaders. A few Lincoln Hospital nurses transitioned to leadership roles in the new hospital. Lincoln nurses have expressed the bittersweet emotions they experienced around this time of transition. And yet the merging of these two hospitals occurred because both were facing insurmountable challenges. To continue on the path they were taking would have meant their sure demise. The citizens of Durham and community and medical leaders had spoken: one hospital was the best way to address the future health-care needs of the city's citizens.

Both hospitals, Watts Hospital and its School of Nursing and Lincoln Hospital and its School of Nursing, had flourished because of the collaboration and cooperation between the White and Negro communities. The arrangement had been mutually beneficial to both communities. Communicable diseases were rampant in both communities, and the diseases knew no boundaries. The earlier spirit of collaboration and respect between the medical and community leaders served as a model for addressing the challenges of the merger and transition. The positive leadership of both entities helped ease the transition of two culturally diverse groups and enabled them to

Lucille Lawrence, RN '58

I was born in Morganton, North Carolina, in 1935, one of four children. My father worked in a furniture store and my mother was a domestic worker. I had always wanted to be a nurse. I went to Lincoln because I had a cousin who attended Lincoln and was employed there as supervisor of the operating room, Mildred Crisp, a 1940 graduate. After I graduated from Lincoln in 1958, I worked there my entire career (including the merger with Durham Regional Hospital): first as staff nurse, then as a head nurse at night, and then as assistant night supervisor with Ms. Armstrong. Upon the move to Durham Regional Hospital in 1976, I was appointed the 11:00 p.m.–7:00 a.m. night administrator for the hospital. I maintained that position for sixteen years from 1976 until my retirement in 1994. I will always praise and respect my school. Lincoln Hospital School of Nursing prepared me well for my life journey.

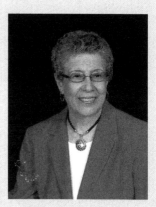

Courtesy of Lucille Thomas Lawrence.

meet the challenges and embrace the changes. Clearly this could have been an explosive situation.

Mrs. Julia Simpson Armstrong was one of the Lincoln nurses who made the transition. During one of my interviews with her, she shared that with the consolidation of Lincoln and Watts Hospitals, in 1976, there came a change in professional relationships. She was placed in an environment that required her to deal with a different set of values. The environment became one in which White and Black nurses served patients of all races. The challenge to promote fairness was always present. She remained at Durham Regional Hospital until 1983, when she retired.

Another firsthand account of this merger comes from Ms. Lucille Lawrence, a 1958 graduate:

When we moved to Durham Regional Hospital (DRH) the atmosphere was very different from Lincoln: there were more people, more diversity, and the climate was somewhat racially charged. Several of Lincoln staff moved

176 Voices: Lincoln Hospital School of Nursing, 1903 . . .

to DRH in leadership positions and the questions were being mumbled, why did Lincoln nurses get those positions? The response to those questions from some of the physicians was "Not to worry, they will come with the positions but they will not keep them." Lincoln nurses maintained those positions, performed admirably, and survived. Over time the atmosphere/climate improved, however it felt like someone was always trying to find fault with the Lincoln nurses. As a result of the merger, the benefits for the staff improved. The salaries were adjusted upward to be more comparable with the Watts employees, but one questioned whether they were really equivalent. Mr. [Larry T.] Suitt, the last administrator at Lincoln, moved to DRH as a senior administrator. Dr. Thelma Brown, RN, the last director of nursing at Lincoln Hospital, moved to DRH as a senior nursing administrator. Ms. Lawrence believed that Mr. Suitt and Dr. Brown strongly advocated for the equal treatment (positions, salaries, and benefits) of the former Lincoln staff as they were integrated into Durham Regional Hospital. Mr. [Larry T.] Suitt held the title of senior vice president when he retired in 1999.

Carolyn Evangeline Henderson transferred to Durham Regional Hospital in a staff educational development position. She was responsible for helping to prepare the staff for the move and transition.

While some Lincoln nurses and staff transitioned to Durham County General Hospital, the story does not end there. In fact, Gwendolyn Cooper Jones Parham recalls that when the Lincoln Community Health Center first opened in 1971, she was one of the first clinical nurses employed there. She reminisced about her first day, greeting the first patient enrolled in the center. She was the supervisor for the Home Health Care section and was involved in training nursing assistants. She recounted the intensive efforts of Dr. Charles Watts in securing funding for the Center and in hiring Dr. Evelyn Schmidt. Since then, other Lincoln nurses have directed nursing at the Lincoln Community Health Center. Lincoln nurses Patricia Martin Blue and Mary Richardson Baldwin functioned in the roles of director of nursing and quality assurance coordinator, respectively, for almost forty years. Lincoln nurses have also served in key leadership roles at Duke Hospital and Durham County Hospital Corporation (previously Durham Regional Hospital), many being the first African American nurses to do so. We take the time to recognize these nurses because these institutions take us back to the roots of our entry into professional nursing. Other Lincoln nurses have served equally important roles in other institutions, as the "voices" provided throughout this book reflect. The Lincoln legacy continues as it began.

Patricia Martin Blue, RN '65, BSN, MPH

I am a sixty-nine-year-old graduate of Lincoln Hospital School of Nursing (LHSN), Class of 1965. I was born in Childersburg, Alabama, where I lived "in poverty" with my mother, stepfather, and half-brother. My childhood was filled with personal pain related to rejection by my biological father and the hard discipline of my mother. I learned at an early age to deny self and gain approval through hard work, sacrifice, and a positive spirit.

The core principles and values that stemmed from my childhood were reinforced at Lincoln, continued throughout my personal and career development, and are with me today. These principles and values are: always remain humble, be committed, work hard, be honest, persevere, maintain a loving spirit, and always help others whenever you can.

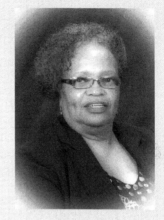

Courtesy of Patricia Martin Blue.

Nursing was not a chosen career for me. My high-school teachers encouraged me to consider a health-care career because of my academic abilities in math and science.

My first career choices were a pediatric physician and an interior designer. Neither of these choices was affordable for my parents. Nursing was an affordable possibility but would require my family to endure even greater financial hardships. I was not convinced that nursing was a career choice at all until a partial summer of domestic work *really* let me know that I didn't want the earning level or the work! I hurriedly completed the admissions requirements for Lincoln and came to North Carolina with much fear and trepidation; I had never spent a night away from home prior to this experience.

The three years I spent in training at Lincoln were filled with joy, pain, excitement, new experiences, hard work, and love. As student nurses, we worked eight-hour shifts on all three shifts. I worked on days off and earned $8 per shift. We would get off duty at 6:00 a.m. for breakfast and go to Pharmacology class at 7:00 a.m. These and other hardships and challenges caused us to form a bond of family/sisterhood that has endured throughout our lives. The Lincoln graduates reunite every two years to celebrate our family, thanks to the hard work of the LHSN Alumni Association. Kudos to members of the Executive Committee for taking the lead in keeping this family/sisterhood together, informed, and involved.

At Lincoln social life and recreation was very limited and controlled. We had one late leave each week, until 11:00 p.m. on Friday night. Guests could visit on the weekend, until 9:00 p.m., but had to remain in the common sitting areas. The dress code was monitored, both professionally and socially. Uniforms and skirt lengths were measured in inches from the floor. One of my classmates was actually released from the nursing program because she refused to lower her hemline.

Church and religious participation were integral parts of my home and school life. At home I was required to walk five miles to attend church every Sunday. At school we were required to participate in Vespers every Wednesday evening and to sing in the choir whether we could sing or not. The choir leader said to me, "Just work your lips, don't sing!"

Strict adherence to moral, ethical, academic, and professional standards was expected at Lincoln. Noncompliance with these rules, regulations, and codes of conduct was not tolerated. For example, twenty-three students entered the nursing program with me but only ten graduated. In another instance, some of my classmates and I attended a Science Fair at Duke University and the school transporter failed to pick us up. The school dress code did not allow us to ride public transportation in our uniforms. We were in uniform, but since we had no way to get back to school, we rode public transportation back to campus. The director learned of our actions and grounded us for a month! I felt this was very unfair, so I called my mother to inform her that I was leaving the program. My mother made it clear that I would accept the punishment and continue the program— which, of course, I did.

My need to escape the rigorous code of conduct at home and the nursing program is reflected in my job and career choices after school. My graduate education and many of my jobs have been in public health, which is a broad field and supports a high-level of autonomy. Many of my leadership roles have been in newly formed jobs that required creativity and development. In other words, I looked for opportunities that supported my need to be autonomous and creative and that had minimal rules and regulations.

Upon completion of the nursing program in 1965, I got married. My husband and I had two children, a son and a daughter, three grandchildren, and one great granddaughter. My husband and one grandson are deceased. After my husband's death, I found that remaining socially active was a must for me. In 2008, I formed a seniors' single group known as the "Sensational Platinum Singles." Not only does the group keep me socially active, its members have also made life fun again.

My church affiliation is Baptist. I am a member of Greater St. Paul Missionary Baptist Church. I work with the AIDS/HIV, Parish Nurse, and Seniors ministries of the church.

Since leaving Lincoln in 1965, I have earned a bachelor of science degree in Nursing from North Carolina Central University, in Durham, North Carolina; a master's degree in public health from the University of North Carolina School Of Public Health, in Chapel Hill, North Carolina; and become licensed as a nursing home administrator by the State of North Carolina. My nursing career includes experiences as a staff nurse for eight years in maternity care, labor and delivery, full-term and premature nurseries, and postpartum care at Lincoln and Duke University Hospitals, Durham, North Carolina; community health director of nursing for ten years, Lincoln Community Health Center, Durham, North Carolina; long-term care associate director of Carol Woods Retirement Center for ten years, Chapel Hill, North Carolina; community health director of operations for two years, Wake Health Services, Raleigh, North Carolina; and clinical operations director at Duke Outpatient Clinic and Duke Family Medicine Clinic for twelve years, Duke University Hospital, Durham, North Carolina.

I was a delegate to the House of Representatives for the American Association of Homes for the Aging for two years, a member of several boards that included the Durham County Board of Health, Adult Day Care, and the Home Health Advisory Board, and past president of the Nursing chapter of the North Carolina Central University Alumni Association. I have also received a number of other recognitions for my professional work as well as for my work in the community and the church.

At sixty-nine years of age, I am still looking for unique experiences and ways to enjoy each day and make useful contributions to my brothers and sisters with minimal rules and regulations.

REFERENCES

Board of Nursing Communication to Lincoln Hospital, L. Z. Williams, RN. June 23, 1969. p. 10. Duke University Archives, Durham, N.C.

Bulletin. 1931. Lincoln Hospital of the School of Nursing. University of North Carolina at Chapel Hill Library, Chapel Hill, N.C. Cp610.73 L73b 1931.

Clemons, Della Marie Harris. Interview with the author. October 21, 2010.

Gordon, Elizabeth. Interview with the author. June 2011.

Harris, Clara J. M. Interview with the author. 1998.

Highlights in Nursing in North Carolina, 1935–1976. 1977. A 75th Anniversary Project. North Carolina Nurses Association, Raleigh, N.C.

Johnson, G. "Nursing as a Profession." *Davis Nursing Survey* 17, no. 4 (April 1953): 101.

Lawrence, Lucille. Interview with the author. September 29, 2012.

Letter to all Departments from Lincoln Hospital Directors. April 10, 1970. Duke University Archives, Durham, N.C.

Lincoln Hospital School of Nursing Application for National League of Nursing Accreditation. 1957. Lincoln Hospital School of Nursing Archives, Durham, N.C.

Lincoln Hospital Trustees Hold Annual Meeting. 1948. Administrative office files publicity periodicals, 1948–1956. Duke University Archives, Durham, N.C.

McCullum, Ethel B. Interview with Dorothy Esta Dennis Segars and the author. March 13, 2011.

Minutes of Meeting of North Carolina Association of Colored Graduate Nurses. 1941. North Carolina State Archives, Raleigh, N.C.

Morris, Lois S. Interview with the author. August 2011.

Notes on North Carolina Board of Nursing Consultant Visit to Lincoln Hospital Between 1967 and 1968. p. 9. Duke University Archives, Durham, N.C.

Oliver, Julia. Interview with the author. March 2011.

"Philosophy of Lincoln Hospital School of Nursing." *Bulletin.* 1959. Lincoln Hospital School of Nursing. Lincoln Hospital School of Nursing Archives, Durham, N.C.

Regulations for Schools of Nursing in North Carolina. 1948. Joint Committee on Standardization. North Carolina State Archives, Raleigh, N.C.

Report of Attrition. 1960. Excerpts from the Board of Nursing to Lincoln Hospital School of Nursing. Duke University Archives, Durham, N.C.

Rhynie, Sarah M. Interview with Dorothy Esta Dennis Segars and the author. March 2, 2011.

Richardson, Sylvia O. Interview with the author. September 2011.

Sullins, Della Mae Davison. Interview with Dorothy Esta Dennis Segars. October 2011.

The Dispatch 2, no. 2 (1960). Lincoln Hospital School of Nursing Archives, Durham, N.C.

The Scalpel. 1946. Lincoln Hospital School of Nursing yearbook. Lois Smith Morris, Durham, N.C.

The Scalpel. 1948. Lincoln Hospital School of Nursing yearbook. Lincoln Hospital School of Nursing Archives, Durham, N.C.

Thorpe, Elizabeth W. Interview with the author. March 1971.

Wilson, E. H., and S. Mullally. *Hope and Dignity: Older Black Women of the South.* 1933. Reprint, Philadelphia, Penn.: Temple University Press, 1983.

Chapter Four

Continuing the Legacy

AT THE TIME OF THIS WRITING, it has been four decades since Lincoln Hospital School of Nursing (LHSN) closed its doors. The youngest graduates of the school, the Class of 1971, are now sixty-five; the oldest known living graduate is one hundred and four. Although all the Lincoln graduates have reached their retirement years, many have not retired. Some are employed in part-time roles as educators, consultants, administrators, and entrepreneurs; others are volunteering their time for church and community activities and in other venues. The tradition of familial sisterhood and community service lives on in the hearts and deeds of the Lincoln graduates who continue to serve their communities.

Can you imagine being one hundred and one years old and still providing community service in the church, interacting with young children in school, or participating in a firing range with police recruits? No? Then meet Mrs. Josephine Demmons McBride, a 1936 graduate of LHSN. The June 18, 2010, headline of the *Virginia Pilot* in Norfolk, Virginia, reads, "At 101 Years Old She's A Real Pistol"; another headline read "Norfolk's Newest Deputy." Mrs. McBride, in 2010, completed the competitive firing range course at the police academy in Norfolk, Virginia, and as a result was appointed honorary sheriff. In the spring of 2011 several Lincoln alumni visited her and were treated to a scrumptious homemade meal including dessert prepared and served by Mrs. McBride. On August 25, 2012, several Lincoln alumni traveled to Virginia Beach, Virginia, to share in her birthday celebrations; she was a proud one hundred and four years old. At 3:45 p.m. she sauntered into the home of her daughter, Josephine McBride Nobles, stopped in the dining room to look at her birthday cakes, and did a Chubby Checker Twist into the kitchen to greet her family. She was stunningly attired in a smart green suit with a hint of yellow, the colors of Chi Eta Phi, one of the many professional organizations with which she is associated. Anxiously awaiting her arrival

Josephine Demmons Mcbride, RN '36

My birth parents, John and Eliza Chambers, lived in Belton, South Carolina, where I was born on August 27, 1908. There were four children before me, two boys and a set of twins (a boy and a girl). The girl died at birth. I was told that my mother passed away when I was two years old; therefore, I don't know much about her. My father remarried soon after my mother died. With his new wife and four children, he moved from city-to-city or town-to-town, and then to a farm in Belton County, where they farmed for several years. They were blessed with a girl, Elizabeth Chambers.

Our education was limited due to the distance we had to travel. When the older boys grew up they left the farm, leaving no one to help my father; consequently he moved to Anderson, South Carolina, and then to Winston-Salem, North Carolina.

For some reason, my sister, Elizabeth, and I were left in Winston-Salem with my stepmother. She soon returned to Belton, South Carolina, and sent me to my oldest brother in the town of Lowndesville, South Carolina. By this time my education was lagging behind, and my desire to go to school was becoming only a dream. However, I knew that an angel guided me day-by-day and would make a way for me. Today I give thanks to God for Ms. Ross, a classmate's mother, who introduced me to my adoptive parents, W. C. and Ethel Demmons, of Greenville, South Carolina. They cared for me, sent me through high school, and then on to Lincoln Hospital School of Nursing (LHSN) where my dream to become a nurse would be fulfilled. Lincoln Hospital School of Nursing was chosen because my parents had a friend there, Ms. Kennedy.

It was a hot day on July 1, 1933, that I began my journey along with others who joined me at LHSN. Miss Pattie H. Carter, who was our beloved superintendent, was awaiting us. She was very kind, loving, and motherly, and she inspired us to continue our three-year journey.

On September 20, 1933, thirteen of us entered a little room where we were to begin our class-work. The first week was spent getting acquainted with our new subjects and hoping that we would pass the preliminary period.

The class was organized with Miss Gertrude Bullock as president, Miss Elizabeth Ethengane as secretary, and Miss Pearl Winbush as treasurer. Finally, the big day arrived when we were given our uniforms and caps. This meant

were her children, nieces and nephews, grand, great grand, and great-great grandchildren, friends, a special adopted daughter, and Lincoln alumni, including Janie Cooke (RN '43), Eleanor Matthewson Ruffin (RN '49), Shirley Bryant Southerland (RN '60), Dorothy Esta Dennis Segars (RN '68), Gloria Taylor Cheek King (RN '67) Lottie Fleming Bolding Hall (RN '69) and yours truly, Evelyn B. Wicker (RN '63). Two other special guests were Fostine Riddick, a supreme basileus in Chi Eta Phi Sorority, Inc., and Sydney Lorraine

that we had passed the preliminary period. We crashed out on the neighboring community of Lincoln Hospital as "The Nurses of 1936."

In March 1934, Miss Bullock, a contestant from our class, was selected and crowned as "Miss Lincoln." She held that honor for three years.

The months continued to go by, and again we found ourselves facing the second semester's exams. The report from the examination brought us joy because we had passed without difficulty with creditable grades. The months passed swiftly and at last we were ready to take our final exams.

Again we conquered what we thought could not be done. Over the course of the three-year journey, several interesting persons entered our travels with the aim of making us better suited to tackling the many obstacles in nursing. Miss Henerietta Forrest became our new superintendent of nurses. She greatly inspired us and made our dark days seem brighter.

When I graduated in 1936, I was employed by Lincoln Hospital after passing the State Board Nursing Exam. I was given a position as a head nurse and then as a night supervisor. I worked at Lincoln Hospital for one year, and then I wanted to move. I accepted a position at Norfolk Community Hospital in Norfolk, Virginia, under Ms. Thelma Gibson, the director of nurses, and Mr. W. C. Mason, the administrator. I was hired as a head nurse in a 25-bed hospital. The hospital grew and in a few years it became a 198-bed building where I became one of the day supervisors. At that time the State Board did not require nurses to have a bachelor of science or advanced degrees; therefore, many times I would assist as director of nursing, and eventually I was promoted to that position.

I think going to Norfolk Community Hospital was not by my direction but was God's will. In Norfolk, I found Bute Street First Baptist Church as well as many friends. Soon after, I married Elbert McBride and gave birth to twins, Joseph and Josephine. I have received awards for counseling high school students, nursing students, and mentoring students at my church. Other honors that I have received came from my sorority (Chi Eta Phi) and the Civic League and include the ICON Award (the Hattie McDaniel Award). I completed the Citizen's Police Academy Program in 2010 in my leisure time. I also completed a Police training course and was named Honorary Deputy Sheriff for the city of Norfolk.

To God be the glory for all that He has done for me!

McCree, my eight-year-old granddaughter. Both Mrs. Janie Cooke and Mrs. Eleanor Matthewson Ruffin (a school nurse for thirty-five years) recognized Mrs. McBride as being very influential in their nursing careers. She was their supervisor when they started their careers at Norfolk General Hospital in Norfolk, Virginia. With tears in her eyes and surrounded by an overwhelming spirit of love, devotion, and thanksgiving, Mrs. McBride was awarded a resolution from the LHSN Alumni Association presented by Lottie F. B. Hall,

At Josephine Demmons McBride's 104th birthday celebration. Lottie Hall (left), Josephine Demmons McBride with Sydney L. McCree, eight-year-old granddaughter of Evelyn Booker Wicker. Courtesy of Floyd Wicker Sr.

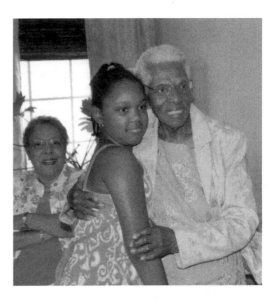

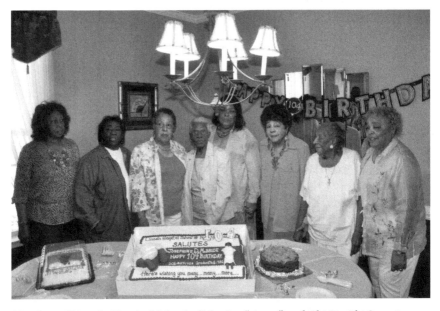

Members of Lincoln Hospital School of Nursing "sisters" and Chi Eta Phi Sorority honoring the life and achievements of Josephine Demmons McBride on her 104th birthday, August 20, 2012. Left to right: Evelyn Booker Wicker, Dorothy Esta Dennis Segars, Lottie Fleming Hall (president LHSNAA, Inc.), Ms. McBride, Gloria Taylor Cheek King (presented special cake), Eleanor Matthewson Ruffin, Janie Cooke, Shirley Southerland. Courtesy of Floyd Wicker Sr.

association president. This resolution was a demonstration of the respect and the sisterhood bond shared by Lincoln nurses. What a legacy. Highlights of the extraordinary life of this Lincoln nurse are depicted in her story (see pages 184–185). But Mrs. Josephine Demmons Mcbride is just one of many Lincoln nurses to be the first to achieve extraordinary accomplishments.

Just as Lincoln nursing students came from places up and down the eastern corridor, many have returned to those areas. Until the mid-1960s graduate nurses could practice without being licensed as a registered nurse (RN);

Yetta Hardy Clark, RN '68, CRNA

Lincoln Hospital School of Nursing (LHSN) prepared its graduates to serve in all facets of nursing. The relationship between LHSN and North Carolina Central University (NCCU) exposed its students to liberal studies as well as to the sciences. This exposure insured that Lincoln students were competitive with students from other programs and prepared to adequately serve the public. The director of the nursing program, Mrs. L. Z. Williams, worked tirelessly to develop a program second to none in its time. Lincoln students did internships in pediatric nursing at Saint Christopher's Children's Hospital in Philadelphia, Pennsylvania, and did psychiatric internships at Kentucky State Psychiatric Hospital in Lexington, Kentucky.

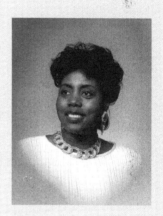

Courtesy of Yetta Hardy Clark.

The instructors on the campus of LHSN were academically prepared and cared about the students. The clinical program was rigorous and as any LHSN graduate could verify, it was not for the faint of heart. Upon graduating from LHSN, I discovered I was prepared to work in any professional nursing environment.

The instructors at LHSN had a profound influence on my life. Their professionalism and dedication to education will always be with me. I chose the field of anesthesia as my lifelong profession because of the influence of "Pinkie." She was the certified registered nurse anesthetist (CRNA) at LHSN who performed her job with such extreme precision and confidence that I knew this special area of practice was for me.

Finally, the educational experience I acquired at LHSN allowed me to compete for admission to the Nurse Anesthesia Program at Wake Forest University North Carolina Baptist Hospital. I was blessed to be the first African American graduate and the second non-White graduate.

I am still practicing nurse anesthesia and applying the knowledge I gained while a student at LHSN. Thank God for Lincoln Hospital School of Nursing!

Thereasea D. Clark Elder, RN '48, MPH

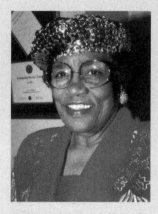

I, Thereasea Clark Elder, am a retired nurse who helped integrate Mecklenburg County's Public Health Nursing Department. I am a graduate of historic West Charlotte High School in Charlotte, North Carolina, and I continued my education by studying to fulfill my childhood dream of becoming a nurse. I studied nursing at Lincoln Hospital School of Nursing, in Durham, North Carolina, and graduated in 1948. I received additional education at Howard University in Washington, D.C.; Freedom Hospital School of Nursing, in Washington, D.C.; University of North Carolina at Chapel Hill, N.C.; Livingstone College in Salisbury, N.C.; and Johnson C. Smith University in Charlotte, N.C.

Courtesy of Thereasea Clark Elder.

    I began my career at L. Richardson Hospital in Greensboro, N.C., and later went to work at Good Samaritan Hospital in Charlotte, N.C., where I enjoyed a rewarding nursing career for more than fourteen years. I then went to work for the Mecklenburg County Health Department, where I integrated the Public Health Nursing Department. After serving for thirty years as a public health nurse, I retired in 1989. However, I continued to serve my city, state, and nation by remaining active in many causes, with a special emphasis on health care. I spearheaded the revitalization of the Rockwell neighborhood located in North Mecklenburg County, and the neighborhood park has been named the Thereasea Clark Elder Park to honor me. I founded the Charlotte-Mecklenburg Black Heritage Committee and the Greenville Community Historical Society, and I am responsible for the placement of several historical markers commemorating the achievements of Black citizens in Mecklenburg County. Two special markers commemorate Good Samaritan Hospital, which was the first privately funded, independent hospital in

many stayed at Lincoln as graduate staff nurses while studying for the board exam and honing their nursing skills. Once they had successfully completed the board, many moved on. Some moved back to their hometowns, while others moved to big cities to work in more modern institutions where they were to enhance their technical skills. As Lincoln nurses moved into their career paths, many became the first to break through the barriers to what was once impossible for Negro/Black nurses. Many became the first head nurse, administrator, nurse educator, or advanced clinical practice nurses

North Carolina built exclusively for the treatment of Blacks. The hospital once stood on ground now covered by the Bank of America Stadium in uptown Charlotte, North Carolina. The other is a monument at the Pearl Street Park that bears a marker identifying it as "the first Negro playground and first African-American park in Mecklenburg County."

I serve on several local, regional, national, and international boards and commissions that include, but are not limited to, the Mecklenburg County Human Relations Commission; the National Council of Negro Women; the National Association of Negro Business and Professional Women's Clubs; the League of Women Voters; the Mecklenburg County Cancer Prevention Coalition; and the Charlotte Housing Strategy Stakeholders Committee.

I was married to the late Willie Elder for over thirty-nine years and am extremely proud of my two sons, Ronald Carl Elder and Cedric Clark Elder, who are both prominent engineers. I have three grandchildren and three great grandchildren. I have been a lifelong member of Second Calvary Missionary Baptist Church where I have served faithfully as president of the Missionary Society, chairperson of the Ministry of Health, and chairperson of the Building Fund Committee.

The love of education was instilled in me at an early age by my parents, the late Booker T. and Odessa Clyburn Clark. Though lacking formal education themselves, my parents were able to send six children to college. Their sacrifice and God's grace have been the inspiration behind my efforts to create numerous scholarships to help young people further their education.

Among my many awards is the Order of the Longleaf Pine, North Carolina's highest civilian honor. My life history is archived in the Smithsonian National Museum of African American History as part of the StoryCorps' Oral History Project. In June 2009, I accepted the Maya Angelou/Elizabeth Ross Dargan Lifetime Achievement Award at the Maya Angelou Women Who Lead luncheon.

Nurse ◇ Trailblazer ◇ Humanitarian ◇ Extraordinaire ◇

in areas where their employment was once prohibited. Many of us experienced blatant racism in our nursing careers as we branched into hospitals and practice arenas that had not been friendly or embracing of Negro/Black nurses. As a new Black nursing supervisor in Ambulatory Care at a notable tertiary medical facility, I was frequently mistaken for a LPN mainly because of my color. It was a shock to the educational coordinator conducting orientation when I was introduced as the supervisor of the outpatient department. It was interesting to observe her body language. It was 1973 and I was

(continues on page 191)

Carlita LaVerne Hall Merritt, RN '64

I, Carlita H. Merritt, was born on February 5, 1938, in McLean, Virginia, and am a graduate of the Class of 1964 from Lincoln Hospital School of Nursing (LHSN), in Durham, North Carolina. I retired from the federal government in 2004 after thirty-five years of service.

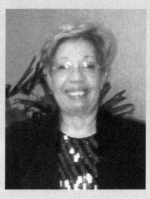

From the age of nine my passion was to become a professional nurse. My request for Christmas every year was a nurse's kit. All of my sisters, brothers, and playmates had to be my patients.

Upon graduating from LHSN in 1964, I sought employment at Arlington Hospital in Virginia. Much to my surprise and

Courtesy of Carlita Laverne Hall Merritt.

enjoyment, I was employed as the first African American nurse on an all-White med-surgical unit (North 2). When I went to seek employment at Arlington I was asked if I had any experience as a nursing aide; I promptly replied to the secretary, "No, I just graduated from an accredited professional school of nursing." My interview was with the director of nursing, who hired me and promptly gave me specific instructions; I was to be addressed as Miss Hall and I would be eating my meals in the professional section of the cafeteria. I ate all of my meals alone in the professional section of the cafeteria.

After passing the State Board of Nursing Examination, I was employed at the Mt. Alto Veterans Hospital, in Washington, D.C. During my tenure there I assisted in the move to the newly built Veterans Hospital on Irving Street. My departure from the Veterans Hospital was not due to discrimination but to privilege. The Veterans nurses were rewarded with the best assignments. I noted that I received the same treatment in assignments as the White nurses did. I resigned from the VA Hospital and was employed at Freedman's Hospital, in Washington, D.C., and was promoted to head nurse.

In 1968 I married Lavell Merritt, Major (U.S. Army Retired) and we had two children: Lavell Merritt Jr., who now has a PhD in Philosophy, Parks, Recreation, and Tourism Science and LaVerne Merritt Vowling, a doctoral candidate in psychology.

In 1976 I was employed as an occupational health nurse in Washington, D.C. During my career as an occupational health nurse, I worked for nearly every government agency in the federal system. I was the first African American nurse promoted to nurse manager at the Park-lawn Building with a population of 11,000 employees. The staff accomplished some very exciting first health-care initiatives in the system. The following are examples of some of these accomplishments: first to organize a comprehensive lactation program; first to set up an AIDS screening program in partnership with the Public Health Service of Montgomery County, Maryland; first to implement a pilot program for practical nurses in occupational health in which standards of work for that position were developed.

My last assignment was at the U.S. Attorney's Office in Washington, D.C., which also was a very exciting and rewarding position.

Lincoln Hospital School of Nursing trained all of its nurses well, especially me. The director of nursing and the teaching staff were exemplary. To quote my daughter, LaVerne, "WHEN THAT SCHOOL CLOSED, THE MOLD WAS BROKEN."

GRATEFULLY SUBMITTED,

Carlita LaVerne Hall Merritt

the first Black nurse employed as an administrative supervisor of a department. While working as a staff nurse at the same institution years before, physicians on the unit would approach any White person before recognizing me. It became a game for me because as the only RN on the floor I knew that sooner or later the physician, out of necessity, would have to approach me for nursing orders or whatever the case may be that required the skills and knowledge of the professional nurse. In the 1960s, after integration, many Black nurses were recruited to work in hospitals once forbidden to them. These hospitals soon realized that to employ a Lincoln nurse was to employ an RN with special skills. This includes employment and service in the military, health-care institutions, and nursing organizations as well as other specialty areas of practice. Today the Lincoln tradition lives on through alumni who continue to esteem themselves in practice as well as in community service and our alumni organization.

DEVELOPMENT OF THE ALUMNI ASSOCIATION

The Alumni Association was established in 1938 and has remained active since the school's closure. The "voices" of a few living graduates from the 1930s and correspondence between the alumni groups and the administration of the School of Nursing and Lincoln Hospital attest to the dedication, loyalty, and support of the organization, which has been translated into visible community projects celebrating the students and the school. Two sources of information have verified how the Alumni Association originated. First, Ms. Della Mae Davison Sullins (RN '37) shared in a conversation with Dorothy Esta Dennis Segars that the Alumni Association was in the process of being organized in 1937 and had been completely established by 1938. According to Ms. Sullins, the first president of the Alumni Association in Durham was Ms. Caroline Allen Dunn (RN '29). Within the past four years the street on which Ms. Sullins lives has been designated the Della Sullins Street. Ms. Sullins did not disclose this information herself; Dorothy Esta Dennis Segars, Recording Secretary of the Alumni Association at that time, noticed her address change and later confirmed that the street was indeed named after her.

Second, an article in the *Carolina Times* affirmed that the Alumni Association was in operation in 1938. The article highlighted a dance for the Class of 1938 graduates following the graduation ceremony, which was sponsored by the Alumni Association. The article identifies three graduates: Ms. Julia Marie Simpson Armstrong, from Asheboro, N.C.; Ms. Catherine B. Dixon, from Roanoke, Va.; and Ms. Carrie M. Henderson, from Greenville, S.C.

The constitution and bylaws of the Alumni Association were developed early on, however, the earliest documentation of these laws appears as the revised edition of 1963. The objectives of the association were as follows: 1) to "promote improvement in professional work and increase fellowship among the graduates of Lincoln," 2) to "create an interest for the advancement of the training school program," and 3) to "cooperate with the North Carolina State Nurses Association and the National Nurses Association in promoting professional educational advancement of Nursing."

The next revision of the constitution and bylaws occurred in 1975, and this change focused on maintaining the bond and sisterhood and thereby keeping the legacy of Lincoln alive. The objectives of the association became twofold: 1) "to promote ongoing education among its members in order to improve the standards and quality of services rendered," and 2) "to

Della Mae Davison Sullins, RN '37, BSN, MSN

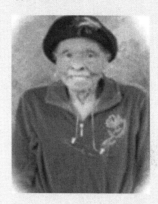

I was born October 13, 1917, in Charlotte, North Carolina. My father was a cab driver and my mother was a housewife. I attended Lincoln around the age of nineteen, still a teenager, and graduated in 1937. I have many fond memories of Lincoln. We were expected to respect the upperclassmen. As part of our initiation, we had to iron their uniforms and always open the door for them, a design of their own. Student life included going to St. Joseph Church down the street and creating our own leisure activities. In the dorm we played records on the old record player, had sing alongs until it was quiet time, and played cards. We

Courtesy of Della Mae Davison Sullins.

did each other's hair in our rooms even though there was a place on the first floor for doing hair. My most difficult challenge while in school was getting up early; we had to be on duty by 7:00 a.m. and had to go back to the hospital to cover staff shortages.

Excerpts of my nursing career include the following:

I was the first nurse in the state of Alabama to receive the bachelor of science degree in nursing from Tuskegee Institute; this also means that I was the first Black nurse to receive that institution's bachelor of science degree. Later I attended Indiana University in Indiana and obtained my master's degree. The major part of my practice centered around Tuskegee Institute. I began my career as a staff nurse at the Veterans Administration Hospital in Tuskegee and progressed up the ladder to assistant chief nurse. I also taught nursing at Tuskegee Institute and assisted in setting up the nurse aide program at the Veterans Administration Hospital. I have been involved in numerous activities in the community and have received many honors and recognitions.

create, promote, and maintain interest and fellowship among the graduates." The constitution and bylaws were revised to redefine the objectives of the alumni, to establish a central registration of alumni members, and to establish periodic meetings of the chapter's executive officers. The Lincoln Hospital Alumni Association was incorporated in 1976.

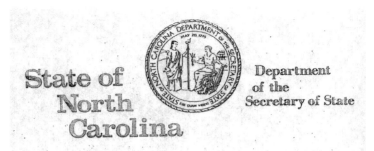

To all to whom these presents shall come, Greeting

I, Thad Eure, Secretary of State of the State of
North Carolina, do hereby certify the following and
hereto attached (3   sheets) to be a true copy of
ARTICLES OF INCORPORATION

OF

LINCOLN HOSPITAL SCHOOL OF NURSING ALUMNI ASSOCIATION

and the probates thereon, the original of which was
filed in this office on the · 29th   day of   october.   19 76 ,
after having been found to conform to law.

In Witness Whereof, I have hereunto set my hand
and affixed my official seal.

Articles of Incorporation of LHSNAA, Inc., October 29, 1976. Courtesy of
Carolyn Evangeline Henderson.

In 1993 there was a proposal to revise the constitution and bylaws to include licensed practical nurses and registered nurse graduates of other
schools. The idea behind the proposal was to assure the perpetuity of the
Alumni Association and the Lincoln legacy. This discussion was tabled for
a later date. Between 2003 and 2005 the issue was revisited; LPNs were not
granted membership, however, RNs who were distantly located from their
alma mater could become associate members. As the constitution and bylaws had provided for honorary members in 2005, the alumni honored Mrs.
Margaret Kennedy Goodwin, a longtime Lincoln Hospital radiology technician, as an honorary member in 2005. Mrs. Goodwin was a staunch advo-

Margaret Kennedy Goodwin

Mrs. Margaret Kennedy Goodwin was born in 1912, the daughter of Margaret Lillian Spaulding, sister of C. C. Spaulding. The Spaulding and Kennedy families were always involved with Lincoln Hospital as true advocates as well as a serving Board of Trustee members. In discussing Lincoln Hospital and how it got its name Mrs. Goodwin replied, "Lincoln was named for Abraham Lincoln because he signed the Emancipation Proclamation to free the slaves." For now this explanation is accepted as plausible.

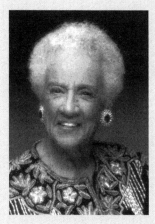

Courtesy of Alice Harrell Young Tharrington.

Mrs. Goodwin began her career at Lincoln in 1938. When she was twenty-six years old, her husband died and she needed to work to support her two-year-old daughter (Marsha Goodwin Kee). The female employee who was running the Radiology Department (name unknown) left, creating the need for a replacement. Mrs. Goodwin said, "I was that somebody and I went to stay until they found someone to run it and I stayed forty-five years!"

Mrs. Goodwin was a chemistry major in college. Having grown up around Lincoln and Dr. Aaron Moore, who was her uncle, this seemed a natural fit for her. She went to school with the interns at Duke and Watts and did a residency there and then went to Pennsylvania and became certified in radiology. She then returned to Lincoln and began teaching radiology interns and lab technicians, accepting students in residency training, and preparing them for state and national registry boards. She remained there until her retirement.

Mrs. Goodwin was always supportive of the nursing students, teaching them about radiology as they moved patients in and out of radiology. She has attended the graduation and reunions of Lincoln alumni consistently throughout the years. She was inducted as an honorary LHSN alumni at the 2005 Reunion.

cate of the hospital, and she loved the School of Nursing. She was always in attendance at the alumni affairs, supporting their efforts. She died on January 27, 2010.

At one time the Alumni Association had three chapters, located in Washington, D.C., New York City, and Durham, North Carolina. These chapters were formed because they had the largest concentrations of Lincoln nurses. Every two years the reunion was rotated and hosted by one of the chapters. Each chapter operated independently in terms of its programs and fund-raising events, however, each chapter was expected to provide a detailed accounting of its activities during the reunion. Specific details of each chapter are forthcoming.

A decrease in membership owing to the death or advanced age of many members led the New York and Washington chapters in 2005 to merge with the Durham chapter. After the chapters merged the constitution and bylaws were changed to reflect this merger. Since the merger, there has been an expansion of the executive committee to include at-large members from the former chapters as well as members outside of the local chapter. This expansion has made quarterly meetings essential, in order to facilitate members' participation in decision making.

The latest revision of the constitution and bylaws occurred in November 2011. This revision made provisions for the merger of various committees and some positions to reflect the changing dynamic of the organization and the aging of the alumni as a whole. Alice Harrell Young Tharrington (RN '68) chaired the constitution and bylaws committee.

Membership Composition and Dues

The alumni organization is supported through annual dues of $35; initially, for many years dues were $5. The fiscal year runs from January 1 through December 31 and the election of officers occurs biannually. The number of active members has ranged from thirty-four to seventy-five members. Currently the active membership numbers forty-one.

The Durham Chapter

The Durham Chapter has been the mainstay of the Alumni Association since being organized in 1938. The support of the alumni while the school was operational took many forms. Some of the ways the Alumni Association has demonstrated its commitment are in the form of fund-raising projects which supported the purchase of furnishings, equipment, books and other materials for the school. The alumni also helped to defray expenses for graduation ceremonies, provided luncheons for students and participated in graduation ceremonies.

The Alumni Association has initiated and awarded two special recognition awards at some of the reunions; the Alumni of the Year award and the

(continues on page 198)

Alice Harrell Young Tharrington, RN '68, BS

I graduated from Central High School in Gatesville, North Carolina, in May 1965. Gatesville is a rural town near Ahoskie and Elizabeth City in the northeastern part of the state. I attended Lincoln immediately following graduation from high school, and I graduated from Lincoln in 1968.

My immediate family consisted of my mother and father, four brothers, and one sister, who was the oldest and four years older than me. We were very poor but we were very close and knew we could not live without each other even though we had the normal sibling rivalry.

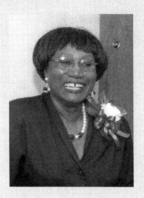

Courtesy of Alice Harrell Young Tharrington.

I picked cotton, chopped in the field, worked in my teacher's home cleaning up, and did any other jobs I could do. From about the age of eleven or twelve I stopped going to school every day because those old enough to work had to stay home to pick cotton. I never got behind, though, because one of my girlfriends who didn't have to work would send me my assignments to keep me informed. She would send it by my brothers who were too young to work. For two summers before graduating from high school I worked in Wildwood, New Jersey, as a chambermaid at a very nice motel.

I decided I did not want that life forever, so in my mind I made plans to get an education and leave home as soon as possible. When I found out that Lincoln was less expensive than college and that it only required three years of study, I began to pursue that school and nursing. That's why I went to Lincoln.

After graduating from Lincoln, I decided to get my bachelor of science degree in nursing (BSN). I attended North Carolina Central University to accomplish that goal. I became very frustrated with the nursing program and decided to get my BS in health education, graduating in 1977.

In 1971 I married Billy Young of Durham, North Carolina. My roommate from Lincoln, Carolyn Martin, introduced us. We were married for eighteen years before he passed away. From that union we have one son, Tyrone Young. Tyrone has a wife, Lisa, and one son, Winston. In 1999, ten years after Billy died, I married Lynwood Tharrington (who has three married sons and six grandchildren).

I worked for eight years in the hospital setting and twenty-five years at the American Red Cross, where for twenty-two years I supervised the aperesis lab. I also volunteered to teach health classes in the evenings. Following my retirement I started a business teaching CPR and first aid. I am currently still running this business, which is very fulfilling and making a difference in the lives of those who achieve certification.

Marion G. Miles, RN '54

I grew up in Northern Durham County, North Carolina, in an area named Rougemont, which was predominately Black. During my teenage years, it was suggested that I continue my education after high school. My mom suggested nursing school. She stated, and I quote, "Study to become a nurse, because people are always sick." After sending out general applications to nursing schools and visiting the School of Nursing at Lincoln Hospital and meeting with the director of nursing, Mrs. L. Z. Williams, I decided to attend Lincoln Hospital School of Nursing.

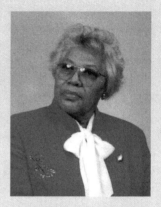

Courtesy of Marion Glen Miles.

I arrived at Stokes Nurses Home at Lincoln Hospital School of Nursing in September 1951 and was assigned to a room with three other roommates. We slept on bunk beds and I was fortunate to get a bottom bunk. We had to share the desks and dressers, but all of us were compatible and adjusted very well. Our classes were taught on the campuses of Lincoln Hospital and North Carolina College (now North Carolina Central University). Courses such as nutrition, chemistry, microbiology, and biology were taught at North Carolina College. Nursing educators and doctors taught the other classes at Lincoln Hospital. In the second semester of our first year, we began to get hands-on experience with patient care, such as giving baths, cleaning rooms, making neat beds, and communicating with the patients and staff. Over the three-year period, we received special training in all the departments of the hospital,

Nurse of the Century award. These two awards are based on overall service to the organization that contributes to achievement of the alumni objectives. Alumni of the Year recipients have included Carolyn Henderson (RN '71), Ruby Jewel Bell Borden (RN '59), Marion Glen Miles (RN '54), Pauline Langston Edwards (RN '66). The Nurse of the Century award, perhaps the most prestigious of the two, has been awarded only once, to Mrs. Clara Josephine Miller Harris (RN '45) in 2003. Mrs. Harris served as treasurer of the Alumni Association over forty years.

The members of the Durham Chapter have continuously participated in

including the operating room, obstetrics, medical surgery, and the emergency room. During my senior year at the school, I spent three months at Crownsville, Maryland Psychiatric Hospital for psychiatric nursing and Meharry School of Nursing for pediatric nursing.

During my study of nursing, I was taught the importance of understanding the patient's mental, physical, spiritual, and social needs. While in school, I was exposed to other activities to help me to become a well-rounded person. It was mandatory that we attend Vespers on each Wednesday night, which was held on campus. We were also encouraged to sing in the school choir, which was directed by Mrs. Virginia Alston. On occasion, at Christmas, we sang at other churches as well as at Duke Hospital. Students were also encouraged to attend a church of their choice. In my senior year, I was selected to be the speaker for the preclinical class and I capped the students during this service. I graduated in 1954. Nursing has been a very good career for me. My family consisted of my husband, three children, and me. Nursing allowed me to work the shift that suited my family. After graduating from nursing school, I continued to take courses that would enhance my career.

My work experience has been as a staff nurse, a head nurse, a nurse supervisor in a hospital setting, and a managing nurse in an industrial setting. I worked for forty years in the nursing profession and continue to volunteer in a hospital setting and in the community.

My accomplishments during my career include the following: Nurse of the Year, Lincoln Hospital School of Nursing Alumni, 1983; Leadership Recognition, National Council of Negro Women, Inc., 1986; Durham Academy Auxiliary, Durham Academy of Doctors, Dentists, and Pharmacists, 2007; Honoree for the Committee on the Affairs of Black People, 2008; The Order of the Long Leaf Pine, 2009.

social, professional, educational and community-service projects. Some examples include health screenings for prostate and breast cancers, diabetes, hypertension, and for the Healthy Carolinas initiative; annual breakfast fund-raisers, a benevolent offering for our sister alumni in the local community; community support projects in alliance with Lincoln Community Health Center, the Durham County Public Health Department, and the North Carolina Black Nurses Council, Inc.; establishing the endowed scholarship; obtaining the 501(c)(3) status and the historical preservation initiatives.

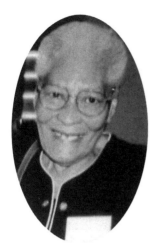 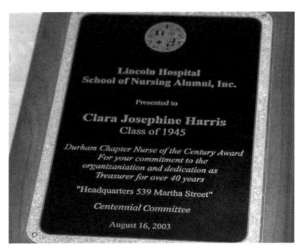

Clara Josephine Miller Harris, recipient of the Lincoln Hospital School of Nursing Alumni Nurse of the Century Award, August 2003. Photograph of Ms. Harris courtesy of Alice Harrell Young Tharrington. Plaque photograph courtesy of Beverly Harris.

In 2007 the Alumni Association re-established the "Miss Lincoln" award as a fund-raiser for scholarships. Miss Lincoln in 2007 was Ethelrine "Ethel" Pettiford Hennessee (RN '60). The Miss Vintage Lincoln of 2009 was Mrs. Carol Ann Russell Johnson (RN '71).

Alumni of the Durham chapter who have served as president include Caroline Allen Dunn (RN '29), Lydia Ruth Flintal Betts (RN '35), Julia Simpson Armstrong (RN '38), Ruth E. Parlor Amey (RN '45), Ruby Jewel Bell Borden (RN '59), Valeretta Roberts Bell (RN '59), Mary Richardson Baldwin (RN '66), Saundra Obie Best Clemmons (RN '67), Lottie Fleming Bolding Hall (RN '69), Gloria Taylor Cheek King (RN '67), and Carolyn Evangeline Henderson (RN '71). All of these alumni provided leadership for the Durham chapter from the 1950s and today. As of this writing, Lottie Fleming Bolding Hall (RN '69) is the president.

The New York Chapter

The New York alumni chapter was established in 1950. This chapter was probably the most active of the chapters during the early years in terms of leadership and financial contributions to the school. The New York chapter carried out numerous fund-raising drives and community-service activities. Annie Lee Phillips described elaborate dinner dances, theatre parties,

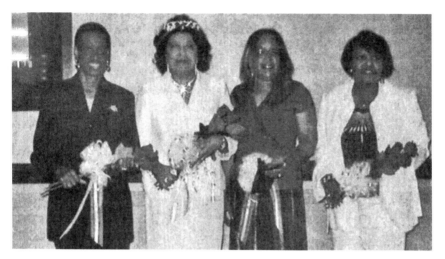

Ms. Vintage Lincoln 2007, Ethelrine "Ethel" Pettiford Hennessee. Left to right: *Linda Lofton Woodson, Ethelrine "Ethel" Pettiford Hennessee, Carolyn Martin, and Carrie Stone Reavis.* Reprinted from *The Herald-Sun, August 18, 2007.* Photo courtesy of Angela Ray. Clipping courtesy of Carolyn Evangeline Henderson.

planned engagements with personalities like Sammy Davis Jr., European and Caribbean cruises, and tours throughout the states. The New York chapter provided scholarships for Lincoln nursing students as well as numerous supplies and equipment for the School of Nursing library. It also contributed 50 percent of the cost of the NLN application fee for NLN accreditation. This fact is shared in a letter sent to the administrator of the hospital. The chapter became associated with the Hale House in New York, which began in 1969 as a home for unwanted children and children born addicted to drugs. As a result of some reported financial mismanagement of the home, the chapter severed this relationship. This was reported by the New York chapter at the eighteenth biannual reunion celebration in 2005. The house is now a center for educational enrichment and development for young children. The chapter also supported the "Nurses House" in New York, a home for nurses in transition. This chapter, like the Washington, D.C., chapter, dissolved in 2005 and its members became eligible for membership in the Durham chapter. The presidents of the New York chapter were Vivian Savage Nealy (RN '42), Nellie F. Collins (RN '52), Lucretia T. Thomas (RN '40), and Ruth Wade (RN '50). Annie Lee Phillips (RN '52), though not a president, was the business manager of the chapter and has vigorously promoted the association and its activities.

October 26, 1964

Mrs. Vivian S. Nealy, Secretary
New York Chapter
Lincoln Nurses Alumnae of Durham, North Carolina
31-40 105th Street
East Elmhurst, New York 11369

Dear Mrs. Nealy:

Mrs. L. Z. Williams has just shown me the very fine letter with the
enclosed check of $250 made payable to the National League for Nursing,
representing one half of the fee for accreditation for the Lincoln
Hospital School of Nursing.

We appreciate Mrs. Nellie Collins informing the New York Chapter of our
needs and we are most grateful to you for this very splendid contribution. The New York Chapter of the Lincoln Nurses Alumnae is certainly
one of our most loyal contributors. We cannot thank you enough for
this wonderful gift.

I think that the time has come or is certainly approaching where every
school of nursing will have to be accredited by the National League in
order to stay in business. This is going to be a hard struggle but I
certainly think that it is worth it. Although there is an acute short-
age of nurses, we owe it to the profession to graduate competent nurses
in order that they may successfully compete wherever they they are employed.

Please give my personal thanks to the entire New York Chapter and again we
wish to extend you a cordial invitation to visit us whenever you see fit.

Sincerely yours,

F. W. Scott
Director

FWS/aj

Acknowledgement letter from Frank Scott, director of Lincoln Hospital, to the New York alumni chapter of the LHSNAA, Inc. for their financial contribution toward the NLN accreditation application for the Lincoln Hospital School of Nursing. Courtesy of Duke University Archives, Rare Book Room.

February 21, 1957

Mrs. Lucretia T. Thomas, Secretary
New York Chapter
Lincoln Hospital Alumni Association
113-15 34th Avenue
Corona 68, New York

Dear Mrs. Thomas:

I have signed the Federal Tax Exemption form which you sent me
on February 11, 1957, and I am enclosing it herewith. I trust you
will find it in proper form.

We are very happy to know that the New York Chapter of the Lincoln Hospital Alumni Association is planning to raise funds for Lincoln Hospital School of Nursing.

We have recently fixed up both nurses' homes, and they are beautiful. In fact, the school was inspected about two or three weeks
ago by the Nurse Examiners' Board of Raleigh, North Carolina, and the
lady stated that she had not seen any nurses' homes in North Carolina
more beautiful than Lincoln's. We took out all of the old furniture
and disposed of it as junk, and purchased new modern furniture for
all the bedrooms. Last year, Dr. Donnell gave $2,000 for furniture
for the students' living room, and we have recently furnished a room
that the seniors used for a dating room. The old Stokes house was
furnished the same as the Angier B. Duke Nurses' Home for the graduate nurses. The room formerly used for a classroom has been changed
to an assembly room with new furniture. We have changed the old room
in the basement of the nurses' home that used to be used for a laundry
to a classroom for the student nurses. We have also taken out some of
the tubs on the second floor and installed tile showers. Asphalt tile
floors have been put down in both nurses' homes. As I say, they are
very beautiful.

We are still in need of funds to purchase some additional equipment and books for the nurses' library, and whatever amount you may
raise in New York will be used for this purpose.

Please remember me to all of our graduates in New York.

Wishing you all the success with the proposed dance, I am

Sincerely yours,

WMR/jlt   W. M. RICH, Director
Encl.

William H. Rich, director of Lincoln Hospital, to the New York alumni chapter of the
LHSNAA, Inc. describing updates in the nurses' home. Courtesy of Duke University
Archives, Rare Book Room.

Nellie (Ellis) Clemons-Green, RN '64, BS, MS

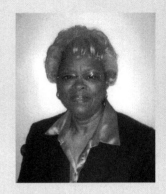

I, Nellie Olivia Ellis, the first of seven children born to Clyde and Olivia Ellis, was raised in Weldon, North Carolina. I attended public school, graduating as salutatorian from Ralph J. Bunche High School. At the early age of five, I had aspirations to become a nurse, and from then on math and science courses were at the top of my list as I prepared for a nursing career.

The family did not have a lot of money, so my parents suggested that I wait a year, get a job, and afterward enroll in a four-year nursing program. Having worked summers at Johns Hopkins Hospital and earning a fair salary, I felt this experience would lead to continued work without my having to enter school. My parents then decided they could afford entry into a three-year nursing program. We obtained from the state of North Carolina a list of all the nursing schools in the state. Lincoln Hospital School of Nursing (LHSN) was a viable choice in terms of location and cost. The application was sent, with no reply. My mom spoke to our local pharmacist, Dr. David Cooke, and he made a call to his son, Dr. David Cooke Jr., who just happened to be a practicing physician at Lincoln Hospital. On the Friday before the entrance exam was to be administered, word came that I was to report for the exam. I passed it and was off to Lincoln.

The time I spent at Lincoln was full of interesting experiences. My class of 1964 was offered the opportunity to do an affiliation at the Duke University Hospital pediatric department, and later we traveled to Lexington, Kentucky, for our psychiatric affiliation at Lexington State Hospital. While there, I received a communication from the Student Nurses Association inviting me to visit the Charlotte Memorial Hospital.

Courtesy of Nellie Ellis Clemons-Green.

The Washington, D.C., Chapter

The Washington, D.C., chapter was organized in 1971 with Geneva Smith Wade (RN '53) as president. Although documentation was not available, it is believed that the Washington chapter awarded the first Lincoln alumni scholarship to a nursing student at North Carolina Central University (name of awardee unavailable). The chapter hosted several biannual reunions. It is impressive that over the course of thirty years, the organization was guided by only three presidents, the other two being Evangeline Boone Harrell Rickman (RN '61) and Nellie Ellis Clemons Greene (RN '64). This chapter merged with the Durham chapter in 2005.

This turned out to be a blessing as I was offered my first job. Following graduation I traveled to Charlotte, North Carolina, to assume the position of staff nurse in their newly built intensive care unit.

After working for two years and getting married, my next stop was Cocoa, Florida, where I worked for the Brevard County Blood Bank in Rockledge. I was sent to their headquarters in Orlando for training. This was easy as the graduate nurses at Lincoln had already taught me the techniques of phlebotomy. My job was to obtain blood from the many donors. In the lab I processed the blood and supplied it to the local hospitals, as well as to the Kennedy Space Center. Three years later my husband and I traveled up the coast to Washington, D.C. A brief stint in private duty nursing as a contract nurse led to my entry into the field of occupational health nursing. This experience led to an offer for full-time employment with the federal government at the U.S. Department of State. This position provided me with many experiences, from extensive overseas travel with the Secretary of State to accompanying patients to their home countries such as Jordan and Sudan. I met many important people and dignitaries, including the Egyptian President Anwar Sadat, Israel's Prime Minister Golda Meir, and Joint Chief of Staff and later Secretary of State Colin Powell, as well as the legendary Pearl Bailey and Liza Minnelli and the basketball great Kareem Abdul Jabbar. This position provided me with the opportunity to obtain a bachelor of science degree in psychology from St. Joseph's College in North Windham, Maine, and a master of science degree in health sciences administration from Central Michigan University.

It was an honor to have been selected to work at the U.S. Department of State and to have been the first African American civil service nurse in the Medical Bureau. I retired from the position of health-care services nursing administrator after thirty-six years of government service. I spend my retirement singing in the choir at the Walker Memorial Baptist Church and serving on the boards for the Foreign Affairs Recreation Association at the State Department Federal Credit Union.

REUNION ACTIVITIES

Prior to the school's closing the Alumni Association conducted its annual meetings in conjunction with the graduation exercises. Since the school closed, biannual reunions have been held up and down the eastern coast and have included cruises and other excursions.

The first reunion was held in 1973 in Washington, D.C., and was sponsored by the Washington-Baltimore chapter.

The second reunion was held in 1975 in New York and was sponsored by the New York chapter. The highlight of that reunion was a tour of Manhattan and the initiation of the Miss Lincoln/Alumna award. Carol Ann Russell Johnson (RN '71) was presented with the award.

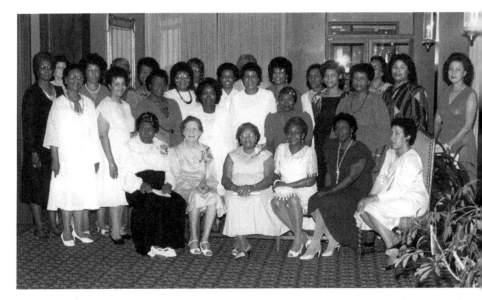

The seventh biannual reunion, 1985, Washington, D.C. Left first row seated: Beatrice Freeman Moss, a 1925 graduate, was honored as the oldest member in attendance. Courtesy of Mary Richardson Baldwin.

The third reunion returned home to Durham, N.C., in 1977.

The fourth reunion was held in 1979 and was sponsored by the Washington, D.C., chapter.

The fifth reunion was held in 1981 and was sponsored by the New York chapter.

The sixth reunion was held in 1983 and was sponsored by the Durham chapter. The old Lincoln Hospital building and A. B. Duke Nurses' residence had been demolished in 1981 and replaced with the new Lincoln Community Health Center. Dr. Evelyn Schmidt, the administrator of the health center, conducted a tour of the Lincoln Community Health Center for the alumni.

The seventh reunion was held in 1985 in Washington, D.C. Beatrice Freeman Moss (RN '25) was honored. She was the oldest graduate in attendance.

The eighth reunion was held in 1987 in New York.

The ninth reunion was held in 1989 and was hosted by the Durham chapter.

From 1991 through 2009, the biannual reunions have been held in Durham, North Carolina. The 1997 reunion was followed by a trip to West Africa.

Reunion memories—happy groups.
Courtesy of Mary Richardson Baldwin.

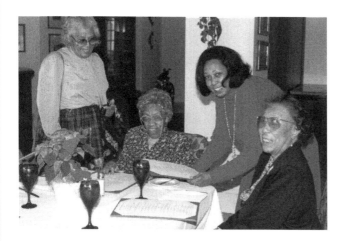

Left to right:
Marion Glen Miles,
Lucille Zimmerman
Williams, Evelyn
Booker Wicker,
Helen Neal Webb
Jones.

Left to right:
Margaret Louise
Wilson Smith,
Mary Williams
Pointer, Ruby Jewel
Bell Borden, Cleo
Marie Dunn Bell.

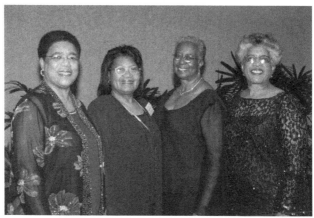

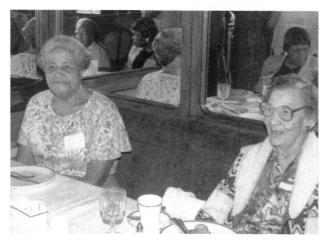

Left to right:
Mamie Maddox,
unidentified.

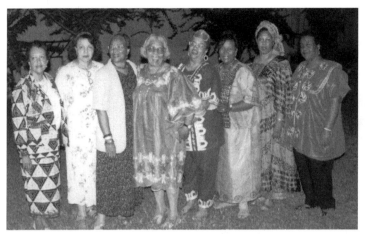

1997 Lincoln alumni trip to Africa. Left to right: Elsie Boyd Tyson, Sandra Obie B. Clemmons, Joan Miller Martin Jones Mathews, Marion Glen Miles, Patricia Martin Blue, Mary Richardson Baldwin, Evelyn Booker Wicker, and Jeronica Williams Hardison. Courtesy of Floyd Wicker Sr.

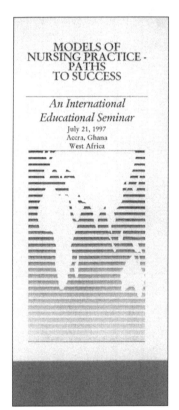

MODELS OF
NURSING PRACTICE -
PATHS
TO SUCCESS

*An International
Educational Seminar*
July 21, 1997
Accra, Ghana
West Africa

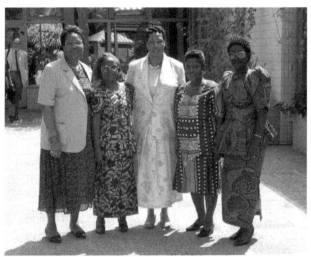

Brochure for "Models of Nursing Practice: Paths to Success" education seminar July 21, 1997, Accra, Ghana, West Africa.

Participants, left to right: Joan Miller Martin Jones Mathews; Joan Laryea, head of Department of Nursing, University of Ghana at Legon; Evelyn Booker Wicker; and Department of Nursing faculty. Missing from the photo are Patricia Martin Blue, Saundra Obie. B. Clemmons, and Mary Richardson Baldwin. Both courtesy of Floyd Wicker Sr.

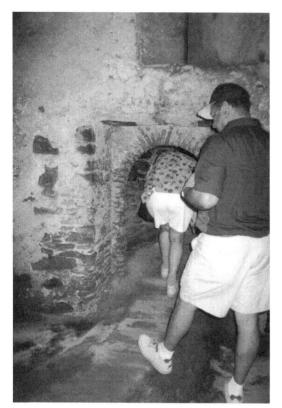

Elmino Castle, slave dungeon, passageway to the waiting ships. Courtesy of Delores Taylor.

The latest reunion at the time of this writing was held in 2011 and took place on a cruise to the Caribbean Islands. Themes for the reunions have varied over the years, but two predominate: "Love Has Kept Us Together" and "Capturing the Legacy, Retaining the Spirit."

Two monumental events have occurred in the last two decades: a trip to West Africa and the 100-year anniversary celebration of the School of Nursing. Following the Alumni Association meeting in 1997, the alumni went on a trip to West Africa. While in Africa, the alumni took excursions to Cote d'Ivoire, Benin, and Accra where we experienced historical enlightenment and spiritual kinship with our ancestral heritage. On tours to villages, we were exposed to the living conditions of the villagers, the spiritual worship of various idols and gods, the social strata, and libation ceremonies. Can you imagine walking through the slave castles and feeling the spirit of our forefathers, some of whom were held in captivity by ball and chain before being forcibly marched through the narrow opening in the wall to the gang plank where they boarded the ship for the middle passage to America and other countries? To actually stand in the dungeon of the castle, see the narrow passage, the beautiful white sand on the beach, and the bright blue ocean and appreciate such natural beauty and the ugliness associated with human degradation: for us, it was a life-changing event.

The more urban areas consisted of densely populated markets where we engaged in bartering, a common way of life. It seemed that everyone had a business venture at the market as well as on the street. These ventures, carried out by the extremely young to the aged, represented the entrepreneurial spirit of the African people. A lightbulb flashed! As descendants, we recognized some of the origins of our inborn traits, such as storytelling, shared caretaking, bartering, perseverance, creativity, responsibility, and attention to time. There seems to be a shared phenomena with regard to the relevance of time; the people appeared to be "in rhythm" with time as opposed to ascribing to the Western idea of "adherence to the set time."

The highlight of the trip was the collaborative nursing conference held in Accra, Ghana, with the University of Ghana at Legon. I helped coordinate this conference along with Ms. Joan Laryea, dean of the School of Nursing at the University of Ghana, while employed as director of career development in the human resources department at Duke University Medical Center. The conference was titled "Pathways to Leadership." The focus of the conference was on sharing leadership strategies for career development in nursing. Several members of the alumni participated in the conference: Patricia Martin Blue (RN '65), a licensed nursing home administrator representing health-care trends in long-term care; Mary Richardson Baldwin (RN '66), representing ambulatory nursing; Saundra Obie Clemmons (RN '67), representing legal issues in nursing; Joan Miller Martin Jones Mathews (RN '62), representing mentoring; and myself, Evelyn Pearl Booker Wicker (RN '63), conference leader and organizer. I shared excerpts from my dissertation titled "Factors Influencing the Career Development and Achievement of Graduates of Lincoln Hospital School of Nursing." While in Ghana we discussed the idea of establishing an exchange partnership with the University of Ghana at Legon. This idea was not realized, but two Lincoln scholars, Lavette Steele McGill and Dalisha Wade, have traveled to Dodoway in Ghana to work in a health clinic for a summer internship. These young ladies presented their experience through several poster presentations including one at a Lincoln Alumni Association meeting.

(continues on page 214)

Joan Miller Martin Jones Mathews, RN '62, BSN, MSN, EdD

1998 Distinguished Nursing Alumnus of North Carolina Central University In Recognition for Excellence In Nursing Practice, Education, And Research

I, Joan Delores Miller, was born on April 24, 1937, in Traphill, North Carolina, in Wilkes County, the third child and second daughter of Pearl Campbell and Thomas Calvin Miller. I lived with my maternal grandparents and extended family on a sixty-acre farm. My mother worked for a family in Elkin and my father was a hotel cook. They came home on Wednesday and Sunday afternoons, respectively, and went back to work early Monday morning. I would be excited on Saturdays when we would go to Elkin to shop, visit our parents, and go to the movies. Sundays were spent at church and visiting relatives and friends. Social activities included games, dancing, debates, picnics, and holiday parties.

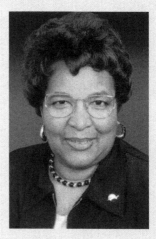

Courtesy of Joan Miller Martin Jones Mathews.

Education was emphasized in my family, as several family members were teachers and ministers. I began my education in a one-room school in Traphill. Because eight grades were taught in this room, I listened to the lessons for all the students and was able to pass two grades in one year. This school closed, and from fifth grade until my graduation in 1954, I attended Lincoln Heights High School in Wilkesboro. As class valedictorian, I gave my first major public speech from memory; no notes could be used.

During my freshman year at North Carolina College at Durham (now North Carolina Central University), I became interested in nursing and decided to transfer to Lincoln Hospital School of Nursing. My goal was to work as a federal government (AID) nurse in underdeveloped countries. In my junior year at Lincoln I withdrew because married students were not permitted to attend. In 1958, I received a diploma from the Durham School of Practical Nursing and ranked first in academic achievement in my class. I was employed on the Obstetric Unit at Lincoln Hospital. Lincoln Hospital School of Nursing began admitting married students and I re-enrolled and graduated in 1962. During the graduation ceremonies, I received two awards: the Excellence in Leadership Award and the Most Technically Competent Award. I received a commendation from the North Carolina State Board of Nursing for being one of two applicants to have the highest score (714 of 800) in obstetrics on the RN licensure examination in 1962. I was working on the Medicine and Surgery Unit at Lincoln

212 Voices: Lincoln Hospital School of Nursing, 1903 . . .

Hospital when Mrs. L. Z. Williams, Director of the School of Nursing, smiled and said, "Good Morning, Mrs. Martin, RN," and I realized that I had passed the State Board of Nursing Examination (the school received the scores before the graduates did). I was elated; I was a registered nurse! Thus, my career as a nurse truly began.

As the requirements for various career paths in professional nursing changed, I made changes as well. I continued my education as I changed positions in nursing. I obtained a bachelor of science degree in nursing in 1965 from North Carolina Central University; a master of science degree in nursing in 1971 from the University of North Carolina at Chapel Hill; and a doctorate of education in curriculum and teaching in 1997 from the University of North Carolina at Greensboro. I retired in 1999 from the University of North Carolina at Greensboro as a Clinical Associate Professor in Nursing, returned in 2000 as Adjunct Assistant Professor in Nursing, and was reappointed to serve in this capacity until 2011.

My experiences in nursing include visiting assistant professor in nursing, University of North Carolina at Greensboro, 1984–1997; assistant professor in nursing, North Carolina Central University, Durham, N.C., 1970–1984; instructor of medical-surgical nursing, Lincoln Hospital School of Nursing, Durham, N.C., 1966–1968; public health nurse I, Durham County Health Department, Durham, N.C., 1965–1966 and the summers of 1969, 1971, 1972, 1974, 1975, 1979; staff nurse, medical-surgical and gynecological nursing at Duke Hospital, Durham, N.C., part-time, 1980–1983, and Watts Hospital, Durham, N.C., May 1973–August 1973; staff nurse, medical-surgical, gynecological, and emergency nursing at Lincoln Hospital, Durham, N.C., 1960–1965, 1968–1970; and private duty nurse, part-time, Duke Hospital, Durham, N.C., 1976–1977.

During my career I have enjoyed working with students in classes and in various organizations, especially the nursing sorority. I am one of the beta sponsors for the Sigma Chi Alpha Beta chapter of the Chi Eta Phi Sorority at the University of North Carolina at Greensboro and have held this position since its chartering on February 27, 1999. I was also beta sponsor when Pi Beta chapter was chartered in 1971 at North Carolina Central University and served in that position until I moved to Greensboro in 1984. I have maintained mentoring relationships with many of my current and former students. Many send me announcements of their promotions, educational pursuits and successes, and personal and family achievements.

Lincoln Hospital School of Nursing emphasized participation in civic, professional, and community organizations. Lincoln Hospital was closely associated with and received support from the community. I embraced this behavior as demonstrated by my role in professional and community-service organizations. Among these organizations are the following: NCA&T State University School of Nursing Advisory Committee, North Carolina Association of County Boards of Social Services (vice president, 2010–2012); Guilford County Board of Social Services (vice chair, 2006–2007) by Guilford County Commissioners for two terms (1/4/01–6/30/07); American Nurses Association; Gamma Zeta chapter, Sigma Theta Tau National Nursing Honor Society; Lincoln Hospital School of Nursing Alumni Association (president, 1964, Ms. Lincoln Alumni 1976); Chi Eta Phi Nursing Sorority; and life member of the NAACP. I have held a variety of leadership positions in these organizations, such as president and committee chairperson. I have published articles in several journals and have completed a master's thesis and a doctoral dissertation. My public speaking has occurred in settings such as graduation ceremonies, civic and religious programs, and workshops.

Other awards and recognitions include educational scholarships, academic achievement awards, leadership awards, induction into the Golden Chain and Santa Filomena honor societies, citizenship awards, a Nurse of the Year for District 11 award from the North Carolina Nurses Association, and being nominated in 1991 for the M. L. King Service Award and Excellence as an organization advisor at The University of North Carolina at Greensboro. In 2009, I received Soror of the Year award from the South East Region, Chi Eta Phi Sorority for my contributions and leadership in nursing and the community. Since 1994 I have sponsored the Woodrow Jones Nursing Scholarship at North Carolina Central University.

I am describing the makeup of my family because I taught nursing using these different names. Students I taught at Lincoln knew me as Mrs. Martin, at North Carolina Central University as Mrs. Martin and later as Mrs. Jones, and at The University of North Carolina at Greensboro as Mrs. Jones, Dr. Jones, and Dr. Mathews. In 1956, I married Joseph H. Martin and had a Lincoln baby, Joseph H. Martin Jr. My son followed me into the health profession and is currently a physician in Atlanta, Georgia. Joseph graduated with honors from Howard University (Phi Beta Kappa) and received his medical degree from Duke University. Following my divorce from his father in 1980, I married Rev. Woodrow Jones Sr. in 1983 and moved to Greensboro, N.C. Reverend Jones died in 1994 following a two-year battle with cancer of the brain. In 1999, I married Louis H. Mathews, who is a retiree from the U.S. Air Force and U.S. Post Office. One of my nursing mentees, Lt. Colonel Elmontenal C. Allens, MS, RN, has adopted Louis and me as his parents.

As I stated at the beginning of my description of my nursing career, it really and truly began at Lincoln Hospital School of Nursing. Lincoln Hospital School of Nursing made it possible for me to have an interesting profession in nursing. I was able to be a leader in nursing and other organizations because of my excellent mentors and the support from colleagues and family to fulfill the predictions of the awards and recognitions received.

The centennial celebration of LHSN in 2003 was a historical milestone, marking 100 years of the legacy of the School of Nursing and its mission to train Colored, Negro, Black, African American Nurses. This celebration was a joyous occasion. It was held at the Sheraton Imperial Hotel and Convention Center, Research Triangle Park, in Durham, N.C., August 15–16. A combined greeting from presidents of the three chapters—Gloria T. King of the Durham chapter, Ruth Harrell Wade of the New York chapter, and Nellie Clemons-Green of the Washington, D.C., chapter—follows:

> To our Alumni Sisters, oh how time flies. One hundred years ago, LHSN was founded to train a core of nurses to care for the African American population in Durham and surrounding counties. Over 600 of us entered its doors and emerged as professional nurses. As professional nurses, many helped shape the existing health-care system locally, nationally as well as internationally. We emerged as leaders, teachers, trailblazers and mentors.
>
> This weekend, we gather for reflections, honor and celebration of the memories and legacy of our school. Many have come to share experiences, see old friends and reminisce about school days. Some are here to just give thanks that they are still here to see this day.
>
> Whatever the reason, we warmly greet you, share your joy and honor our successes.

The celebration was attended by the public, friends and family of Lincoln nurses, elected personalities, and city, county, and state officials. Excerpts from some of the congratulatory letters follow:

Mike F. Easley, governor of North Carolina: "Mrs. Easley joins me in extending congratulations on this auspicious occasion as you embrace your Centennial theme, 'Celebrating the Legacy . . . Retaining the Spirit.' We further send our best wishes for continued success."

Martha Barham, president, North Carolina Nurses Association, and Sindy Barker, executive director, North Carolina Nurses Association: "The North Carolina Nurses Association extends our warmest congratulations to the Lincoln Hospital School of Nursing in celebration of its

Facing page: *Celebrating the Legacy, Retaining the Spirit.*
LHSN centennial celebration, August 16, 2003, Durham, N.C.
Courtesy of Ruby Jewel Bell Borden and Jerry Head, photographer.

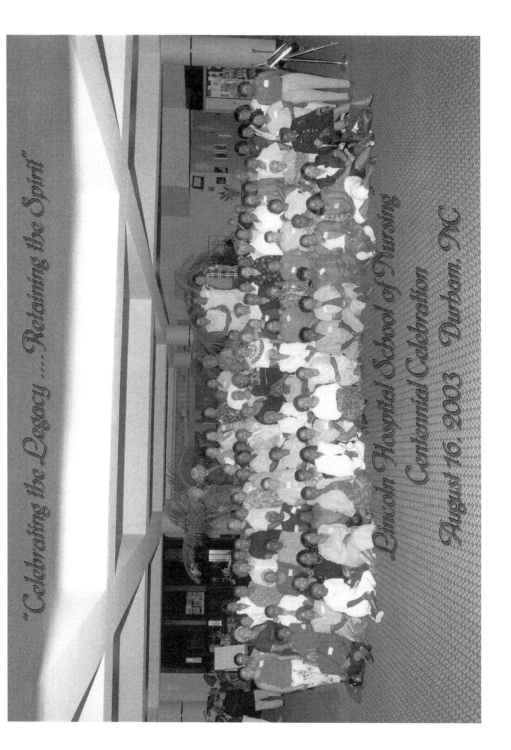

"Celebrating the Legacy .... Retaining the Spirit"

Lincoln Hospital School of Nursing
Centennial Celebration
August 16, 2003   Durham, NC

100th anniversary. Lincoln Hospital School of Nursing played such a prominent role in the early education of African-American nurses in the state. As you know, your history was closely interwoven in the historical documentary 'North Carolina Nurses: A Century of Caring.'

Lincoln Hospital School of Nursing benefited from a succession of competent and capable directors over the years. In looking back at the history, it is remarkable that the school only had six directors during its 68 years of operation. It is a testament to strong, committed leadership to see that Mrs. Pattie Carter and Mrs. Lucille Zimmerman Williams each served over 25 years in that role."

Peggy C. Baker, EdD, RN, Watts School of Nursing: "On behalf of the administration, students and faculty of the Watts School of Nursing, I would like to congratulate the Lincoln School of Nursing on your centennial celebration. The outstanding graduates of your program have long served Durham and many other areas in the delivery of nursing care; all are to be commended.

The legacy of the Lincoln School of Nursing lives today in the work of your graduates. The school was an important part of health care in Durham, graduating 614 nurses. May your celebration of this milestone be filled with wonderful memories, enduring friendships and dreams for tomorrow."

Betty P. Dennis, PhD, RN, associate professor, North Carolina Central University, Department of Nursing: "This year, Lincoln Hospital School of Nursing is marking an important accomplishment in nursing education and nursing practice. One hundred years have passed since its doors first opened to make a career in nursing possible for African Americans. Although the last class graduated in 1971, the return on investment has never ceased. The Lincoln Hospital graduates continue to distinguish themselves in many arenas. Strengthened by their early experiences in a nursing program that cared, was committed, and produced competent graduates, Lincoln nurses have excelled locally, nationally, and internationally. Their influence on health care is both direct and collateral. The more than 600 nurses who graduated have served to the benefit of many in innumerable ways. Over the years and today they remain engaged and continue to contribute to the health and well-being of clients, family, friends, and communities.

The impetus to create Lincoln Hospital School of Nursing has not been absolved. Inequities in health care services and the burden of poor health among African Americans persist. This celebration recognizes past accomplishments and importantly, it serves as an inspiration to today's nurses and nursing students to address continued healthcare needs.

Over the years, North Carolina Central University, Department of Nursing has had a special relationship with Lincoln Hospital School of Nursing. We treasure that connection. Therefore, it is with great pleasure that our students, faculty and staff offer our sincere congratulations on reaching this outstanding historical milestone."

Mary P. "Polly" Johnson, MSN, RN, executive director, North Carolina Board of Nursing: "Throughout its history, the Lincoln Hospital School of Nursing contributed greatly to the health care of the citizens of Durham and surrounding areas. Equally important, your school opened the doors of opportunity for Black women to develop nursing careers of excellence in numerous specialty areas, many of whom have received state, national and international acclaim for their leadership in the nursing profession. The Board of Nursing is pleased to have an alumnus of the Lincoln Hospital School of Nursing on our staff—Ms. Saundra Best. Also, we owe many thanks to Mary Baldwin, another Lincoln graduate, who served on the statewide Centennial Planning Committee for the wonderful 2002–03 celebration of nursing history in North Carolina."

Mary T. Champagne, FAAN, PhD, RN, dean, Duke University School of Nursing: "Congratulations to all 614 graduates of the Lincoln School of Nursing, to those here tonight, and to those who are no longer with us. Established in 1903 as one of the earliest schools of nursing in the country and in North Carolina, Lincoln nurses indeed have a proud heritage. You share with us at the Duke School of Nursing a common bond with the Duke family. What foresight Drs. Moore and Warren and Mr. Merrick had in convincing Mr. Washington Duke that a hospital to meet the needs of Black citizens was far more important than a monument. What intelligence educators Shepard and Latta had in establishing the Lincoln School of Nursing—as no hospital can provide care without nurses! And what wonderful courage was exhibited in naming the School the Lincoln School of Nursing—in North Carolina—in 1903!

The days of segregation are thankfully gone and the struggle now is social justice for all people. It is a goal that we all share and it clearly includes the right to health care for all people. Yet one can be sure, this was not the case for the greater part of the twentieth century. We all give thanks for the Lincoln nurses who were there, and with caring,

compassion, and expertise provided care for Black citizens. We give
thanks for those graduates who continue as members of our profession in
our current 'Jim-Crow-less society.'"

Evelyn D. Schmidt, MD, Lincoln Community Health Center: "The
Lincoln Hospital School of Nursing closed in 1971, but the graduates
continue to serve the Durham community. Many have served on the staff
of Lincoln Community Health Center. The present Director of Nursing,
Mary Baldwin, is a graduate of the Lincoln Hospital School of Nursing. It
is obvious that the mission of service was an integral part of the curriculum of the Lincoln Hospital School of Nursing.

Congratulations to all Lincoln Hospital School of Nursing graduates
during this 100th year celebration."

Capitol citations were received from Jeanne H. Lucas and H. M. Michaux
with the seal affixed and signed by Elaine F. Marshall, Secretary of State.

Jeanne H. Lucas, senator, 20th District N.C. Senate: "Whereas, the
school's legacy of service lives on in the contributions and accomplishments of its graduates, who have helped build Durham's reputation as the
'City of Medicine.'"

H. M. Michaux Jr., representative, 31st District N.C. House: "Whereas,
Lincoln Hospital School of Nursing has produced an Alumni Association
that has yielded an uncompromising love and devotion to it, making them
spiritually worthy of being anointed 'She's a Lincoln nurse.'"

Proclamations were received from:

**Ellen W. Reckhow, chairman, Durham County Board of County
Commissioners:** " . . . proclaiming August 16 as the 100th Anniversary of
Lincoln Hospital School of Nursing Day."

William V. "Bill" Bell, mayor, City of Durham: "NOW, THEREFORE,
I, William V. 'Bill' Bell, Mayor of the City of Durham, North Carolina, do
hereby proclaim August 16, 2003, as 'LINCOLN HOSPITAL SCHOOL
OF NURSING DAY' in Durham, and hereby urge all citizens to take
special note of this observance and further acknowledging the Lincoln
Hospital Nursing School Centennial Celebration as an official part of the
City of Durham 150th Anniversary Celebration."

This was the largest gathering of alumni to date. The evening celebration
began with a procession called the "Parade of Stars." Alumni were individu-

ally announced upon entry into the ballroom. The evening highlight was a video presentation titled "Parade of Stars: Capturing the Legacy," which I and other alumni produced. It was narrated by William "Bill" Hennessee, the husband of alumna Ethelrine P. Hennessee.

THE NORTH CAROLINA CENTRAL UNIVERSITY NURSING CONNECTION

The Lincoln Hospital School of Nursing alumni are interested in and dedicated to the entry of young African American women and men into professional nursing. They have focused concentrated efforts toward nursing at NCCU because of LHSN's long-standing relationship with the university. In 1930, Lincoln nursing students began taking courses on the campus, then known as North Carolina College (NCC). They have continued to seek advanced education there, first through the public health program leading to a certificate in public health, and then through the bachelor of science degree in nursing in the early 1960s under the leadership of Helen S. Miller. Mary Mills (RN '33) in 1946 spearheaded the development of the public health certificate program, the first nurse training program at NCC.

Lincoln nurses, many of whom are members of the NCCU nursing alumni chapter, have been long-standing active supporters of the Department of Nursing. Several of their more significant contributions include: 1) engaging in an alliance with the North Carolina Alumni and Friends Coalition, which was a collection of alumni of Historically Black Colleges and Universities (HBCU) in North Carolina, 2) certification of the nursing chapter of the NCCU alumni association as an official constituent chapter, and 3) the Helen S. Miller lectureship.

The NCCU Alumni and Friends Coalition, in the late 1980s, was instrumental in supporting the survival of the three HBCU nursing programs in North Carolina (Winston-Salem, A&T, and NCCU). The survival of these three programs was being severely scrutinized by the University of North Carolina system—primarily due to poor passing rates on the North Carolina nursing board exam. The efforts to support the schools were quite intensive and broad reaching. They entailed lobbying state legislators, making presentations to the Board of Governors of the University of North Carolina system, organizing marches, soliciting community support, and offering public testimony before the federal court in Washington, D.C. I remember riding to Washington, D.C., with two NCCU nursing alums (Mary R. Baldwin and Rosa S. Steele), reviewing the deposition I had made earlier in

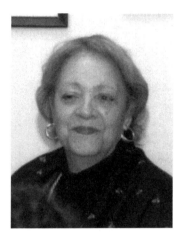

Carol Russell Johnson, first president of NCCU Department of Nursing alumni association and Ms. Vintage Lincoln 2009.

preparation for the U.S. court appearance. Speeches and presentations to the Board of Governors about the plight, inequities, and needs of these schools are documented in the Board of Governors Meetings records at the University of North Carolina system. As a result of multiple efforts on the part of numerous people, including the schools, these three schools survived and continued to thrive. Fast forward to 2013. These HBCUS continue to face similar challenges. Lincoln and NCCU alumni continue to support the struggle.

Alumni of the Department of Nursing organized an NCCU nursing alumni chapter. The first president of the NCCU alumni nursing association was Carol A. Russell Johnson, RN. She worked tirelessly to promote a sense of school spirit and to develop support for the nursing students. Another president was Patricia Martin Blue. Under her leadership, the Alumni Association was recognized as the first official constituent chapter of the NCCU alumni association in 1997. Charter members of this chapter are Patricia Martin Blue, Evelyn Pearl Booker Wicker, Carol Russell Johnson, Mary Richardson Baldwin, and Gloria King.

In 1998, with the cooperation and collaboration of Lincoln alumni, NCCU alumni, the Chi Eta Phi, Pi Chapter, Inc. and the Central Carolina Black Nurses Council, Inc., I was able to garner support to establish a lectureship honoring Helen S. Miller, the chair of the Department of Nursing at NCCU for many years. This lectureship was modeled after the Harriet Cooke Carter Lectureship at the Duke University School of Nursing. In the spring of that year the first Helen S. Miller Lectureship was held at NCCU. Helen S. Miller was a state and national nursing leader and was appointed to the Board of the North Carolina State Nursing Association in 1968, the first African American to hold this appointment. The mission of the lectureship is twofold: 1) to educate students and graduates in the latest trends, and 2) to raise funds to support the NCCU Department of Nursing. The lectureship invites outstanding nurse leaders to present topics related to current and future challenges in society and their impact on nursing education and practice. One of the first outstanding nursing leaders invited to participate was Brigadier General Clara Adams Ender (Retired). There are two awards associated with the lectureship, the Distinguished NCCU Alumnus of the Year award and the Helen S. Miller Scholarship award; both are awarded annually. The Distinguished Alumni Award recognizes outstanding community service, significant contributions to the field of nursing, and membership and financial support of the Alumni Association. Several Lincoln Hospital School of Nursing alumni have received the Dis-

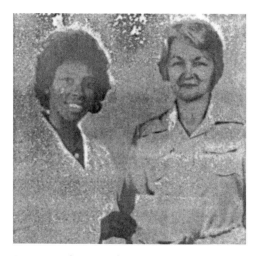

Laura Smith (right), first recipient of Lincoln Hospital School of Nursing need-based scholarship in 1976, presented by Dorothy Esta Dennis Segars (left). Courtesy of Dorothy Esta Dennis Segars.

tinguished NCCU Alumnus of the Year award: Mary Richardson Baldwin in 2000, Dr. Joan Miller Martin Jones Mathews in 1998, Dr. Evelyn Pearl Booker Wicker in 2002, and Gloria Taylor Cheek King in 2003. The scholarship is awarded to a current NCCU nursing student based on merit.

Since 1971 the Lincoln Alumni Association has directed its financial support to NCCU's Department of Nursing. Two mechanisms for providing financial support to nursing students were established: an emergency need-based scholarship and an endowed scholarship. The first recipient of the emergency need-based scholarship was Laura Smith in 1976. Laura was a diploma graduate returning to earn her bachelor of science degree.

In 2001 the Lincoln Hospital centennial was celebrated by the placement of a historic marker on the former Lincoln Hospital grounds. This marker, donated by the Durham Historical Preservation Society, assured the perpetuity of Lincoln Hospital's name. During the centennial celebration for Lincoln Hospital and the nursing alumni reunion the scholarship was transferred from the local level to North Carolina Central University. Recognizing the significant role that Dr. James E. Shepard, president of then North Carolina College, had played in establishing the School of Nursing, it seemed appropriate that our scholarship be established there. The alumni's goal was to endow this scholarship to support student nurse education.

To embark on such an ambitious undertaking, the organization needed to be classified as a non-profit. The organization was guided through this process and received its 501(c)(3) status on December 31, 2003. With this in place the organization could begin to solicit funds from businesses and corporations.

The first major task was assuring the perpetual legacy of the School of Nursing by placing a historic monument on the old Lincoln grounds, which are now occupied by the Lincoln Community Health Center. An initial meeting with Durham Mayor William Bell was held to discuss the vision of the organization and to garner support. Mayor Bell referred us to the Durham City manager, Miss Marsha Connors, whose guidance in helping us to obtain matching funds for the monument from the City and County was immeasurable.

With the funds in hand, the organization commissioned Durham Marble Works to secure the monument base. Liberty Arts, Inc. was commissioned to forge and sculpt the Nightingale Lamp, which was mounted on the top of the granite base.

The second phase of the organizations' mission was to endow the scholarship to be established at North Carolina Central University. An ad hoc committee spearheaded by the president of the Alumni Association included Ruby J. B. Borden (RN '59), Patricia M. Blue (RN '65), Pauline Langston Edwards (RN '66), Gloria J. Fulton (RN '56), Lottie F. Hall (RN '69) Carolyn E. Henderson (RN '71), and Dorothy Esta D. Segars (RN '68). The goal of this committee was to raise funds by offering for sale bricks that would be placed around the base of the monument. The bricks would offer a pictorial history of Lincoln and could include the names of all the graduate nurses, employees, friends, and supporters. Also included were arrays of Lincoln Hospital in its original and final form, the Stokes Nurses Home, and the A. B. Duke Nurses Home. The proceeds from this project would go toward endowing the scholarship.

Additionally, we approached two corporations, GlaxoSmithKline and Blue Cross and Blue Shield of North Carolina, for major funding. Gloria Taylor King (RN '67) wrote a grant proposal that was approved by the alumni organization and presented to GlaxoSmithKline for funding—our first attempt at utilizing our 501(c)(3) status. According to Mary Linda Andrews of GlaxoSmithKline, the decision was based largely on the development of the mentoring program that was part of the grant proposal. As chair-

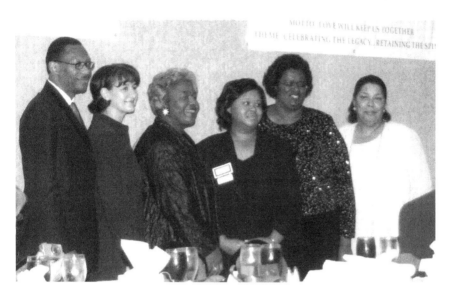

Angela Williams, the first Lincoln Scholar, at the 2005 biannual reunion celebration. Left to right: Dr. James H. Ammons, former chancellor of NCCU; Mary Linda Andrews, director of community partnership, GlaxoSmithKline; Carolyn Evangeline Henderson; Angela Williams, Lincoln Scholar; Lorna Harris, chair of NCCU Department of Nursing; and Gloria Taylor Cheek King. Courtesy of Gloria Taylor Cheek King.

person of the organization's Scholarship Committee, Carolyn E. Henderson, in consult with the other committee members, was responsible for the development of the criteria for the scholarship and the mentoring program. The committee consisted of Joan Miller Martin Jones Mathews, Evelyn B. Wicker, Sandra O. B. Clemmons, Annie L. Phillips, Ruby J. B. Borden, and Gloria T. King. As part of these criteria, which the organization approved, recipients of the scholarship are known as Lincoln Scholars. Thus the endowed scholarship, in partnership with GlaxoSmithKline, was funded in the amount of $100,000. Blue Cross and Blue Shield contributed $12,000. Other contributors were the City and County of Durham, Duke Health System, Duke University, and friends of Lincoln. The scholarship was officially endowed at North Carolina Central University on September 10, 2004.

At present, ten Lincoln Scholars have received scholarships totaling $1,500 per semester. Students become eligible in their junior year of nursing at NCCU. The first Lincoln Scholar was Angela Williams (2005 and 2007). Angela has since graduated and is a practicing nurse in Roxboro, North

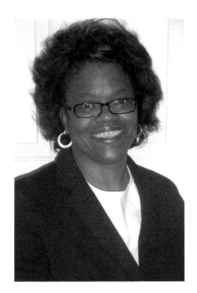

Carolina. The other Lincoln Scholars are Sonia White (2006), Darlisha Wade (2008), Lavette Steele McGill (2008), Michael Bannister (2009), Lidya Admassu (2009), Murtaza Haidermoto (2010), Allyson Kayescott (2010), Amber M. Waddell (2011), and Raya S. Wilson (2011). Previous to this initiative, Lincoln alumni served as mentors for NCCU nursing students following the establishment of the NCCU Nursing Alumni Association. Sonia White, a 2006 graduate, expresses her appreciation for the Lincoln Scholar program as follows:

Sonia White, NCCU Department of Nursing student, second Lincoln Scholar, 2006. Courtesy of Sonia White.

I was an over-the-traditional-age, commuting student, the mother of two active children, a wife, and a school volunteer. The Lincoln Alumni Scholarship helped me have time to focus more on my studies with less concern about how my bills would be paid! My mentor helped me through my senior year and kept me encouraged throughout a very challenging time as I began my nursing career. She gave me sound advice while not coddling me. Even though a number of years have passed, she remains, in my mind, a mentor and definitely a friend. Having Dr. Evelyn Wicker as a mentor has been priceless!

Lincoln alumni have been involved with NCCU in three capacities: as students taking courses while enrolled at Lincoln Hospital School of Nursing; as undergraduate students attaining the bachelor's degree; and as graduate students earning advanced degrees and certifications. Additionally several alumni have taught in the Nursing Department and been employed in the Student Health Service. Mrs. Helen Neal Webb Jones, RN, was the director of nursing for the Student Health Service until she retired. Several other Lincoln nurses have provided many years of service to the institution. Among these are Carol Russell Johnson, RN, BSN, Student Health Service; Emily Price, RN, assistant director of the Student Health Service; Joan Miller Martin Jones Mathews, RN, BSN, MSN, EdD, educator; Gwendolyn Cooper Jones Parham, RN, BSN, MSN, educator; Yvonne Goolsby Spencer, RN, BSN, MSN, EdD, educator and counselor, Department of Nursing; Evelyn Pearl Booker

---

Norma R. Roberts Lipscomb, RN '63

Norma R. Roberts Lipscomb was born on January 23, 1943, to Mr. Johnnie T. Roberts Sr. of Rougemont, North Carolina, and Mrs. Ollie Mack Roberts of Durham's Lebanon Township Community. She was the fourth of five children.

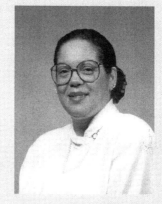

Courtesy of Carolyn Gill.

She received very humble beginnings in Durham, having attended the Durham City School System (now Durham Public School System). She was a graduate of the Hillside High School Class of 1960.

Her love and care for people led her to pursue a career in nursing. She attended and received her nursing degree from the former Lincoln Hospital School of Nursing and later received the bachelor's degree in nursing education from North Carolina College (now North Carolina Central University).

She began a rewarding and extensive career in nursing, having served the Durham health community as a registered nurse for many years. Later, she returned to school and received the master's degree in educational counseling from NCCU.

Because of her commitment to the nursing arena, which was her greatest joy, she returned to the profession to teach the freshman nursing classes at the former Watts Hospital School of Nursing for many years. She was the first African American on the faculty at that institution.

In her later years, she served in nursing administration at what is now Durham Regional Hospital. Upon retiring from the Durham community, Mrs. Lipscomb moved to Hackensack, New Jersey, where she headed a neurosurgical unit in a hospital there.

Later in 1995, having fought a courageous battle with colon-rectal cancer, Mrs. Lipscomb finished the race. She had kept the faith. She was awarded her sunset.

Wicker, RN, BSN, MPH, EdD, educator; Dorothy Esta Dennis Segars, RN, BSN, Student Health Service, Department of Nursing as a tutor/counselor; Doris Day Smith, RN, Student Health Service; Patricia M. Blue, RN, BSN, MPH, educator; Mary R. Baldwin, RN, BSN, MPH, educator; Carolyn E. Henderson, RN, BS, MSN, educator; and Gloria T. C. King, RN, BSN, MSN, student advisor and psychiatric mental health educator.

(continues on page 229)

Gwendolyn Cooper Jones Parham, RN '58, BSN, MSN

I was born Gwendolyn Melba Cooper to Terry and
Elizabeth Cooper on September 27, 1937, in Smithfield,
North Carolina. My father was a Black Seminole Indian,
which means that his father was a Seminole Indian and
his mother was an African American. He was born in
Marianna, Florida, and lived there on an Indian reser-
vation until he was fourteen years old. He and his father
migrated to North Carolina where he met my mother,
who was born in Raleigh. They were married in 1929
and eleven children were born to this union. My father
worked for the railroad in various capacities and my
mother was a housewife. They both completed the eighth
grade.

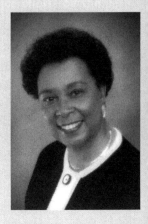

Courtesy of Gwendolyn Cooper
Jones Parham.

When I was a preschooler my mother and father moved
from Smithfield to Wilson. My mother was ill at the time
and had two other smaller children and four older ones.
I did not make the move, as I was left with close family friends who were also my god-
parents. They reared me as their only child until I graduated from Johnston County
Training School in 1955. I was a very active student, maintaining a high scholastic
average throughout my elementary, junior high, and senior school years.

My many extracurricular activities included the following: Singing in the school
chorus, participating in the 4-H Club, Girl Scouts of America, Dance Group, Honor
Society, Journalism Club, Student Council, School Band, Junior Varsity Basketball
Team, Spanish Club, and the Yearbook Committee. I was also Senior Class President
and the salutatorian. As you can see, my secondary school years were carefree, happy,
and gratifying. Little did I know that was soon to change.

I entered Lincoln Hospital School of Nursing in September 1955. I soon had many
rude awakenings. There were many first experiences for me. For example, I was in a
city where I learned about the existence of such things as illicit drug use, homosex-
uality, and civil rights unrest. I had been protected from most negative societal ills. I
was not exposed to sickness except for when I had strep throat and a kidney infection,
which sent me to Duke Hospital for treatment.

My strongest attraction to nursing was the recruitment advertisements about the
Army Nurse Corps that I had seen at school. I liked the uniforms and I was fascinated
by the possibility of being a flight nurse. Consequently, nursing became my choice as I
viewed this profession as a route to realizing my dream of becoming a flight attendant.

As a pre-clinical nursing student I perceived my first encounters with the instructors and superiors to be harsh, unfriendly, and punitive. For the first time in my life
I felt uncomfortable in a school setting. However, I did what was required of me and
successfully completed the pre-clinical period.

The upper-class students were very supportive and friendly, and I am very grateful
to my big sister Cassie Nixon for her sensitive and caring personality. The second year
at Lincoln took a new direction for me. I had overcome my fears and decided that I

could and would continue on my quest to become a nurse (I really didn't have any other choice). The instructors and hospital nurses expected us to perform nursing care without hesitation or errors. Thus, it was imperative that I pay careful attention to my classroom theory and the clinical laboratory procedures so that I could competently apply the information in the clinical practice setting. We were held accountable for being prepared, on time, and taking responsibility for our actions. These requirements prepared me for entry into the world of professional nursing as I embarked on my first job assignment. Following my graduation in 1958 I went to work at Duke Hospital. I was placed on a previously segregated ward housing all-White thoracic and general surgery patients. There, my rude awakenings continued, as I was the only "Colored" graduate nurse assigned to that unit. It was clearly communicated to me by the head nurse that I was not wanted and if I did not pass the state board exams I would not be allowed to stay. There were two other new graduates (Caucasians) who came at the same time but were treated with more dignity than I was. One failed the exam; the other one and I passed. My career at Duke was short-lived as I got married in 1959 and in 1960 gave birth to my first child, Jennifer. I then became a stay-at-home mom. By the time I was ready to return to work, I realized that I was pregnant with my second daughter, Lori, who was born in 1962. With two small children I decided that a school schedule was better for me than juggling a work schedule. I entered North Carolina College (now NCCU) in 1964 to matriculate in the bachelor of science in nursing (BSN) program for registered nurses. While there I was able to recapture the joy of going to school. Upon completion of the requirements for the BSN in 1968, I was hired by Durham Technical Institute as a nursing instructor, which launched my career as a nurse educator.

Following is a chronology of my places of employment as well as my responsibilities for each position held:

1958–1960: Duke Hospital, staff nurse and evening charge nurse on Thoracic and General Surgery ward. There I was responsible for providing pre- and post-operative care to surgical patients encountering the preoperative experience. I was also responsible for directing the care given by my team.

1968–1970: Durham Technical Institute (now Durham Technical Community College), instructor. I implemented a Nursing Assistant Program, which I developed and taught, providing many young men and women with the opportunity to acquire marketable skills to become self-sufficient. I also coordinated their job placement with Duke and Watts Hospitals, the Public Health Department, and other community health agencies.

1970–1972: Lincoln Community Health Center, family care nurse. My responsibilities included assisting the chief medical administrator, clinical administrator, and nursing administrator with the organization and implementation of health-care delivery to the first clients that were registered in the center. I also conducted classes that trained the first family care health aids for the center and supervised their work in the community.

1972–1998: North Carolina Central University. I advanced from the rank of instructor to that of a tenured assistant professor and assistant chairperson of the Department of Nursing. My responsibilities included curriculum development, research, and teaching many of the courses in the nursing major. My specialty was medical and surgical nursing, but I also enjoyed teaching the basic courses as well as courses in gerontology, research, leadership, and cultural diversity in nursing. Additionally, I functioned in many roles of leadership in the Department of Nursing as well as the greater university. For example, I have represented the department on several occasions at the National League for Nursing, the North Carolina Board of Nursing, and the Board of Governors of the University of North Carolina system by collaborating on the nursing curriculum and the status of the Department of Nursing regarding program performance and accreditation issues.

Professional affiliations of which I am proud include the American Nurses Association, National League for Nursing, National Black Nurses Association, North Carolina Nurses Association, Sigma Theta Tau Sorority (Duke University chapter), and Delta Sigma Theta Sorority (Durham Alumnae chapter).

My educational background is as follows:

Basic nursing diploma: Lincoln Hospital School of Nursing, 1958

Baccalaureate degree, BSN: North Carolina College (now North Carolina Central University or NCCU), 1968

Master's degree, MSN: University of North Carolina at Chapel Hill, North Carolina, 1977

Pre-doctoral studies: North Carolina State University at Raleigh, North Carolina, 1978–1979

Numerous Continuing Education Certificates at the local, state, and national levels.

I have been recognized by NCCU for my teaching excellence as well as for my contributions to the university, such as serving as a university marshal for many years and functioning in roles of leadership in the Faculty Senate.

As I reflect on my professional career, I am grateful to Lincoln Hospital School of Nursing for laying the foundation upon which I was able to grow professionally in so many ways. This foundation has led to my ability to persevere in difficult situations, to problem solve, and to function in a variety of professional settings with competence and confidence. What I think made Lincoln unique was the presence of strong role models who set high standards of excellence and who were good examples of professionalism. It is with pride that I say I am a graduate of Lincoln Hospital School of Nursing.

My greatest honors have been the meritorious evaluations given to me by my students and the university, as well as the verbal expressions of respect and thanks from my former students.

Currently I reside in Richmond, Virginia. Since my retirement in 1998 I have enjoyed singing in my church choir (Ebenezer Baptist Church), traveling throughout the United States, Europe, Africa, China, Asia, Turkey, and many of the Caribbean Islands, playing golf, and spending time with my family.

The history books will record Lincoln nurses as great improvisers and leaders who prioritize and problem solve with creative energy to get the job done. Limited supplies, equipment, and physical and personal acceptance and recognition did not deter a Lincoln nurse from her goal. Lincoln Hospital was always under financed and often short on staff, supplies, and equipment, but Lincoln nurses learned, despite these limitations, how to use what they had to give good care. In fact, these limitations served to make them more innovative and creative. They could work miracles; they used their creativity, problem-solving skills, and communication skills very well. Today, Lincoln nurses continue to have high standards, to work fearlessly, and to be self-directed with a strong sense of compassion and dedication. They exemplify loyalty, integrity, pride, humility, team spirit, commitment, and perseverance. They are disciplined, frugal, and friendly. As students they learned to be the patient's advocate, to listen with concern, to keep up with current events, to be optimistic, and to cultivate a love for all people. Lincoln nurses have contributed much and have had an impact on the local, state, national, and international health-care scenes, improving the lives of many people.

Alumni participation in professional development and continuing education activities reflects the value of and commitment to self-education instilled in us in school. The North Carolina State Nurses Association was organized into district associations in 1919 and these associations have continued. When the North Carolina Colored Nurses Organization dissolved and joined the NCNA, many Lincoln graduates became active in the association, and they continue to hold leadership positions at the local and state levels, representing nursing in many arenas. Alumni have also participated very actively in nursing sororities, including Chi Eta Phi Sorority, Inc., and Sigma Theta Tau, as well as in Black Nurses Associations, and in professional nursing organizations at the state, national, and international levels. These organizations exist to further the profession of nursing and nurses. The stories shared through the "voices" chronicle some of these accomplishments in leadership and professional extracurricular activities.

In 1983 Helen S. Miller and Ernest D. Mason, in their book *Contemporary Minority Leaders in Nursing: Afro-American, Hispanic, Native American Perspectives*, highlighted the careers of two Lincoln graduates, Della Raney Jackson, RN, and Capt. Mary L. Mills, RN, MA, CM, who have earned national and international recognition for their contributions to the profession of nursing and to health care in general. Since that time other graduates have achieved similar recognition. Some graduates have been published in

(continues on page 232)

Clara Mae Cobb-Fraling, RN '53, BSN, MSN, PhD

I, Clara Mae Cobb, was born in 1931 to Frank and Dora Cobb in Tarboro, North Carolina. The Cobb family included my sister, Mildred, my brother, Willie, paternal and maternal grandparents, aunts, uncles, and cousins. My father worked for the 7-Up Bottling Company. My mother was a seasonal peanut factory worker, a mail clerk, and a cake baker for local county residents. My mother was raised by her mother and Quakers in Lancaster, Pennsylvania. After the death of her father, my mother and grandmother moved to North Carolina to be near my grandmother's family.

I attended Eastern Star Baptist Church with my family. At age three my mother read to me from the Bible, showed me colorful pictures of flowers, animals, well-kept houses, and other interesting

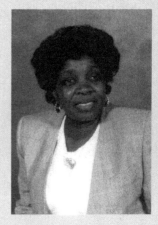

Courtesy of Clara Mae Cobb-Fraling.

subjects. At age four Mrs. Henrietta Foster Mebane, a Lincoln Hospital School of Nursing (LHSN) alumnus and my Sunday School teacher, discovered that I could read some basic words—for example, is, the, he, she, was, them—so she let me help other four-and five-year-olds read the weekly Sunday School card. Upon Mrs. Mebane's recommendation my mother took me to the first grade class. Mother was given a reading list (the Dolch) to teach me for one month and by September, I was in school!

Mrs. Mebane was the county's only Black registered nurse who visited the schools for Black students. In eighth grade I talked with her about Lincoln Hospital School of Nursing. She was always positive in discussions of what is expected of any nurse. I became interested in nursing and made the honor's list throughout my education at W. A. Pattillo Elementary and High Schools, graduating in 1950.

In 1947, my mother began taking me to visit the sick and shut-ins in our community. I started asking more questions about caring for the sick. I asked if we could visit some nursing schools close to home. She said, "You do not have to pick a school that is near home; you should select the one that teaches you what will take you through life." We visited four schools, but I was not satisfied with any of them. My mother and I then visited Lincoln in Durham, North Carolina. I found Lincoln different from the moment that we met the director, Mrs. Lucille Z. Williams, for a conference and a tour. Lincoln's smiling staff was introduced as we met them in the hallway. The facility looked clean and had no negative odors. Students, staff, and patients were groomed and professional. The hospital facility and the nurses' dormitories were clean and well kept. The director's communication skills during the tour and her honest interaction with my parents was impressive. I received materials, including information on what was expected, the facilities, and a summary of the curriculum (which would prepare me for the State Board Examination for licensure). I was impressed with the list of local religious facilities and with the opportunity to attend North Carolina College (now North Carolina Central University) for various classes. That comprehensive university offered academic programs that led to the certificate in public health. Attending LHSN would give me an opportunity to attend a nursing school that was affiliated with a college bearing a rich background in education taught by world scholars. That experience was so positive that my parents and I talked about Lincoln all the way home (three-and-one-half hours).

My decision to attend Lincoln Hospital School of Nursing was the greatest that I made and, as of this minute, I would not change Lincoln as my educational preparation for nursing. During my freshman year at Lincoln I was appointed by Mrs. Lucille Z. Williams to plan the weekly Wednesday evening Vespers for the group. Those plans were submitted to her every Monday. Those one-hour services were mandatory, consisting of guest speakers, drama groups, concerts, and individual topics selected by the student body. On graduation day I was awarded Dr. Robert P. Randolph's certificate for most dedicated student nurse at Lincoln Hospital from 1950–1953.

While at Lincoln I was able to help Catholic students at North Carolina College and I assisted Father Risacher in building the statue of the "Blessed Mary," which is still standing. That site was a part of my wedding in 1955. Holy Cross Catholic Church was important to me. I attended services daily for three years. I was married there and Lula Cowan McNair, my roommate, stood with us when we took our vows. Lincoln Hospital School of Nursing united me with a roommate that I highly respected as a dedicated nurse.

Since becoming a registered nurse through Lincoln, I have been involved in several assignments and received outstanding evaluations. I have been able to use the many skills received at Lincoln and have been invited to return to any position that I left. I have had a productive career in nursing. Following is a listing of some of my career experiences in psychiatric and general hospital settings: staff nurse, administration and education. Among my most notable positions are acting director of Crownsville State Hospital; numerous positions as supervisor; school teacher, elementary, secondary, and college (1965–2000), certification as elementary, middle, and high school principal; certification as science, math, and reading teacher; earning my bachelor of science degree in nursing, my master's degree, and a PhD. My dissertation is housed in the Library of Congress in Washington, D.C.

I am a member of the following sororities: Chi Eta Phi, Phi Delta Gamma, and the Top Ladies of Distinction, Inc., Baltimore chapter. I was inducted into W.A. Pattillo High School Hall of Fame and received the M. L. King's Citation from Pleasant Plains Elementary School.

The people skills I was taught at LHSN are still apparent to others. I believe that Lincoln has guided my daily life and growth. During the graduation ceremony I felt that I was being dedicated to nursing. I was willing to work hard for the career that I had selected. Lincoln prepared me academically to leave those walls and go forward to be one of the best nurses employed by any facility. I still think of myself as being unique because LHSN was an excellent beacon that provided me with the educational background to reach my goal as a registered nurse. In my heart Lincoln will always be the lighthouse that guides my morals, as well as my willingness to learn, to be loyal, and to use my knowledge to promote quality health education.

various professional journals. Celestine Maness (RN '58) shared some of her publication experience.

There were many accomplishments that I was blessed to have been at the forefront of at Hartford Hospital. One was writing and implementing standards of care for the patient with a latex allergy and providing a latex safe environment. This was copyrighted by Hartford Hospital. At the time, the Association of Critical Care Nurses was granted permission to post it on their Best Practice Network website. There were many, many calls from hospitals in the United States on how to develop a policy on providing a latex safe environment for their patients.

My biggest triumph, which gained national and international recognition, was having my article, "Bloodless Medicine and Surgery," published in the international *AORN Journal* in January 1998. This I was told "put our hospital on the map." The writing was and is all mine. I chose to invite a nurse, surgeon, and anesthesiologist to become a part of the article, although the chief of surgery at the time suggested that I didn't have to. However, the information contained in the article had so many nursing/health-care implications that I needed to include some of the surgical team players. Questions and consultations, both on-site and via telephone calls, about the bloodless medicine and surgery program were too numerous to count. Bloodless medicine and surgery is now a world-wide practice. C. P. Maness et al has been used as a reference for another publication entitled "Bloodless Medicine and Surgery in the OR and Beyond." I was also commissioned by the director of nursing service at Hartford Hospital to write an article entitled "On Being a Perioperative Nurse." It was published in the Connecticut nursing newspaper.

Lastly, Lincoln nurses are a spiritual group. Perhaps Carrie Stone Reavis, a 1965 graduate, captures the sentiments best: "God, I thank you for allowing me to become a Lincolnite. It is an honor and privilege to be a member of the Lincoln Angel of Mercy Sisterhood."

The Lincoln legacy is perhaps an unlikely one. Lincoln Hospital started with the idea of a monument dedicated to the descendants of slaves who served the Duke family during the Civil War. Now, Lincoln Hospital School of Nursing graduates are prepared to continue the legacy. In 2005 Gloria Taylor Cheek King, (RN '67) president of LHSN Alumni Association, spearheaded the brick marker initiative to perpetuate the name of Lincoln Hospital School of Nursing. This brick marker monument, along with the commemorative bricks, was placed on the front lawn of Lincoln Commu-

(continues on page 236)

Celestine Patricia Rascoe Maness, RN '58, BSN

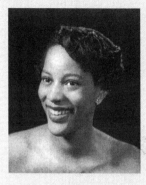

Lincoln Hospital School of Nursing (LHSN) in Durham, North Carolina, is where I began my educational journey into nursing and into what became a most rewarding profession in the healthcare world. However, before classes began, the world, especially the Black world, was shocked by the brutal murder of Emmett Till. The year was 1955. I remember that a couple of us incoming freshmen walked to the public library to read the newspapers' current account of the incident.

Reprinted from *The Nightingale*, 1958. Courtesy of Marion Glen Miles.

At the age of six, I knew that I wanted to be a nurse. Through the eyes of a six-year-old, there was something special about wearing the crisp white uniform and nursing cap. The nurse in our family physician's office, with her caring attitude and patience, was someone I admired. Many of my family members were educators in the public school system, one of them being my mother. I watched her correct papers many nights. Correcting papers was not what I wanted to do when I grew up. Because of a family connection, LHSN provided the opportunity for me to become what I really wanted to be: a nurse. As time unfolded, I did become a nurse educator; I had not as many papers to correct, but a myriad of papers to write.

Geraldine Butler, one of my nursing instructors, was my secret role model. She had a certain sophisticated presence and she exuded self-confidence and professionalism. I even wore nurse's shoes that had high heels because that's what she wore.

The diploma nursing curriculum consisted of classroom and clinical instructions. As we progressed from the pre-clinical stage to the clinical area, for me it became more about delivering compassionate care to another human being and not so much about the wearing of a white uniform. Student nurses supplemented the nursing staff. Under the watchful eye of nursing staff members, we began to develop our bedside nursing skills.

The extracurricular courses that we attended at North Carolina College, known as North Carolina Central University (NCCU) of course, broadened our knowledge base and provided the opportunity to interact with other students. It helped me to articulate my thoughts about events other than nursing.

Anatomy and Physiology and Drugs and Solutions were the courses that, for me, required more study time.

We received our pediatric and psychiatric education at off-campus sites. Our pediatric affiliation was conducted at Meharry Medical College in Nashville, Tennessee. It was in the heat of the summer. Dorm rooms were 90 degrees Fahrenheit at 5:00 a.m. Across the street from Meharry is Fisk University. Fisk is now listed as one of the historically Black universities.

In the fall, we traveled to the mental institution in Crownsville, Maryland, for our studies in psychiatry. What a contrast in weather; at one point, much of the area was blanketed by a heavy snowfall. Both affiliations provided both the theory and clinical academic requirements needed for graduation.

At Lincoln, to nurture our spiritual needs, many of us attended Sunday Church services. The challenge was to return to campus and the cafeteria before the last of the main Sunday dinner was served. Anyone remember ox tails?

My BSN was obtained from Central Connecticut State University (CCSU) and I enrolled in the MSN program at the University of Hartford. During my studies at Central I portrayed Mary Eliza Mahoney, the first Black nurse (1845–1926), at a statewide luncheon in honor and celebration of women's history month. Her life is an interesting story.

Surgery was my area of practice, and I was one of the first nurses on our staff to become certified in this clinical specialty by the Association of Operating Room Nurses (AORN).

My career has included assignments at Muhlenberg Hospital in Plainfield, New Jersey, and St. Mary's and Waterbury Hospitals in Waterbury, Connecticut. My long-term employment (twenty-six years) was at Hartford Hospital in Hartford, Connecticut. I began in the surgical area as a staff nurse and was promoted to supervisor of orthopedic surgery and later to the role of perioperative nurse educator, which I fulfilled for twenty of those twenty-six years.

As a perioperative educator I spent many hours in the classroom in the teaching/learning aspect of that role, which involved many health-care providers (nurses, surgical technologists, residents, physicians, support staff), as well as time in the intraoperative area. Other responsibilities included writing research-based Standards of Patient Centered Care, policies, and procedures; designing story boards; designing and implementing a specific program used for teaching ancillary (support) staff members;

and orienting new employees to their varied responsibilities. I developed and administered evaluation tools for several levels of operating room staff members and shared in the planning and presentation of weekly in-service educational programs.

In the surgical arena, technology and surgical techniques are constantly evolving to include minimally invasive and robotic techniques. It was part of my responsibility to help train staff and keep staff informed regarding their role in the use of new technology, as a surgical team member. As a perioperative nurse educator, I was also the laser nurse educator and nurse instructor for teaching nurses to operate the intraoperative autologous blood collection system using a "cell saver."

It was at LHSN that I received the basic knowledge and skills to become a professional nurse. It was at Lincoln that I became aware that a career in the healthcare field had many disciplines to choose from, thereby setting me on a path to further my education in the healthcare field. It was where I wanted to be.

As my nursing career continued to evolve, the many opportunities to learn in my chosen specialty area might have overwhelmed me had it not been so interesting.

I was given the opportunity to contribute to my profession through my writings and through sharing my clinical knowledge and experiences. I benefit from knowing that I shared my knowledge with others, including on an international scale. I feel rewarded for having done so. Thanks to those at LHSN who shared in "pouring and shaping the nursing mold," including my fellow classmates and schoolmates.

In retirement, I devote a lot of time to my family and church. I am an activist for HIV/AIDS and domestic violence and a member of both ministries at my church. I am invited to speak on these subjects at women's groups and youth and community gatherings. I also serve as the pianist for the Junior and Senior Choirs on the first, second, and third Sundays of the month.

I constantly encourage the youth, in our church community and beyond, to pursue a career in health care. The rewards can be endless. I have never regretted that my chosen educational path was in the healthcare field, especially in the surgical/perioperative arena. My career allowed me to witness unimaginable advancements in surgical techniques and those techniques used in anesthesiology.

nity Health Center among the grand oak trees that graced the lawn of the former Lincoln Hospital. The stately oak trees are the only permanent remnant of Lincoln Hospital. Community supporters, many of whose lives have been touched by Lincoln nurses, bought bricks in memory of loved ones, professional colleagues, and former employees of the hospital who interacted closely with Lincoln nurses. The unveiling of the monument was the highlight of the 2005 reunion. The ceremony was a community affair and was attended by city and county public officials. Student nurses from NCCU

Edwina S. Colbert, RN '59, FNP, MEd

I, Edwina S. Colbert, RN, FNP, MEd, was born in Charlottesville, Virginia, on February 24, 1938, to Edward and Phobe Sellers. My father, with a fourth-grade education, was a shoe repairer by day and a drummer on the weekends. My mother, who completed the eleventh grade, went from being a maid to opening her own beauty salon upon completing beauty school. My only sibling and twin finished Cortes Peters Business School. She retired from the Department of Defense in Alexandria, Virginia, and died shortly thereafter of lung cancer.

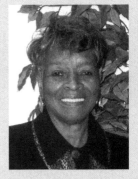

Courtesy of Edwina Sellers Colbert.

At the age of six, I told my parents that I wanted to be a nurse. Having been sick most of my childhood with severe asthma, I was hospitalized on numerous occasions. I fell in love with the uniforms worn by the nurses who took care of me. Focusing on education for their daughters was my parents' number one priority. The question was never "if you go" but "What school can we send you to?"

I attended Jackson P. Burley High School in Charlottesville, Virginia, which was located in a segregated urban environment. I tried my hand as a Thespian a few times. Unfortunately, I could not remember my lines. I participated in several extracurricular activities, including co-editing the high school paper called the *Burley Bulletin*, the A/B Honor Society, and serving as treasurer of the International Honorary Society for High School Journalists.

I worked as a nurse's aide prior to attending Morgan State University, just to test the waters and see if nursing was something I really wanted to pursue. As I also excelled in math, one of my instructors tried to get me to rethink my path. One day

participated, dressed in re-creations of the various uniforms students of the School of Nursing wore through the decades.

The City of Durham has prominently placed at the new downtown train station a mural depicting an LHSN graduation in honor of the legacy of Lincoln Hospital and Lincoln nurses. The hope is that, through the GlaxoSmithKline Endowment, LHSN monuments, and this book, nurses of future generations will continue to blaze new trails in the tradition of Lincoln nurses.

---

while talking with my cousin, she informed me about Lincoln Hospital School of Nursing (LHSN) located in Durham, North Carolina. I applied and was accepted in 1956 and graduated in October 1959.

My first job was at the University of Virginia Hospital from 1959 to 1961 as a staff and charge nurse in an open ward for African American females with every diagnosis from open heart surgery to minor medical conditions. It was extremely difficult working in a segregated environment where those of the opposite race would demonstrate disrespect regardless of your position. Because of my dedication and professionalism, I was asked by a team of physicians from the Neurology Department to join their unit.

From 1961 to 1967, I worked at Moses Cone Hospital as a staff nurse on a post-op surgical unit, ICU, and trained new White nurses on how to be in charge. Before I left, I had the opportunity to witness the integration of Black physicians at that site. Later, I accepted a position as a school nurse for the Department of Public Health in Guilford County.

Understanding the importance of education, I returned to North Carolina College (now North Carolina Central University) and obtained my BSN in May 1971 while maintaining a full-time job. In 1976, I attended the University of North Carolina at Chapel Hill for the nurse practitioner program and became certified as a family nurse practitioner by ANCC. Finally, in December 1985, I received my master's degree in education from A&T State University. For the next thirty-plus years, I worked as a family nurse practitioner in a clinical setting, providing care to children from birth to twenty-one years of age while focusing on neurological and adolescent health problems. Currently, I am a lab and clinical instructor for nursing assistants at Guilford Technical Community College.

I am a member of the American Nurses Association, the HIV/AIDS Board of Greensboro, a member of Sigma Theta Tau, Mu chapter, a volunteer at Hospice and an active participant in many church ministries. I am the mother of one daughter, and I have a son-in-law and three grandchildren.

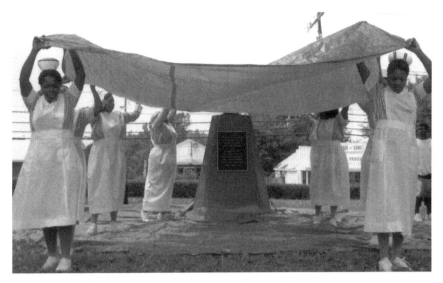

Unveiling of monument on grounds of old Lincoln Hospital by Keyna Anderson, Tina Taylor, Angela Williams, Sharon Davis, Temika Davis, Sonia White, Tashana Pettiford, and Andrea Page. These NCCU nursing students were dressed in uniforms depicting original school uniform and cap, 1907–1971. Uniform replicas created by Gloria Johnson Fulton. Courtesy of Lottie Fleming Hall.

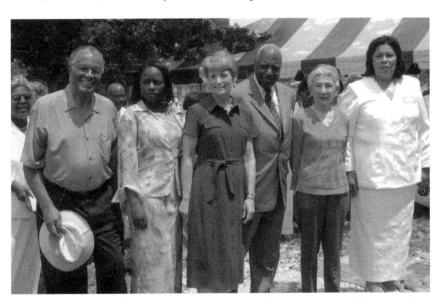

Officials at monument unveiling ceremony, 2005. Left to right: *Howard Clement III, Mayor pro tem; Angela Ray, CEO of Mahogany Dime; Ellen Reckhow, county commissioner; the Reverend Larnie G. Horton; Evelyn Schmidt, director of Lincoln Community Health Center; Gloria Taylor Cheek King, coordinator and mistress of ceremony.* Courtesy of Lottie Fleming Hall.

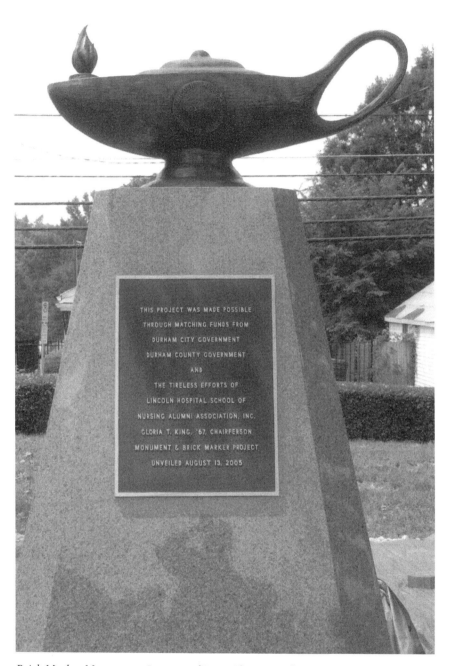

Brick Marker Monument. Courtesy of Lottie Fleming Hall.

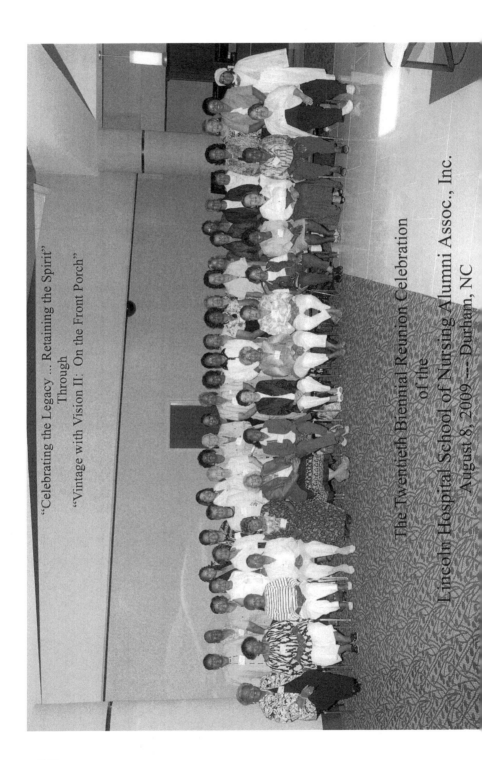

"Celebrating the Legacy ... Retaining the Spirit"
Through
"Vintage with Vision II: On the Front Porch"

The Twentieth Biennial Reunion Celebration
of the
Lincoln Hospital School of Nursing Alumni Assoc., Inc.
August 8, 2009 — Durham, NC

El Dora Laws, RN '54

I was born in Tommy Hawk, North Carolina, which is now Clinton. After graduating from LHSN, I worked in several staff nurse positions. My area of specialty was in pediatric nursing. I was expert in the care of babies, newborns, and premature babies needing special equipment such as the ventilator. I was night head nurse at Somerset Medical Center in Summerville, New Jersey, for approximately thirty years.

I have taken numerous continuing education courses to advance my practice. I am a member of the Lincoln Hospital School of Nursing Alumni Association.

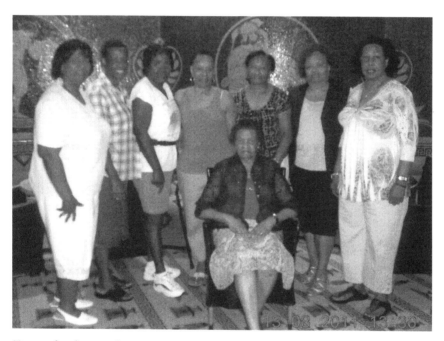

Twenty-first biannual reunion, August 2011, Carribean cruise. El Dora Laws seated in center surrounded by Lincoln sisters. Courtesy of Evelyn Booker Wicker.

facing page: *Twentieth biannual reunion, August 2009, Durham, N.C.* Courtesy of Ruby Jewel Bell Borden.

On November 12, 2011, LHSN Alumni Association, in the presence of community leaders and friends of Lincoln, participated in its inaugural historic preservation event at the Lincoln Community Health Center in Durham. Highlights of this memorable event included the return of the bust of Angier B. Duke and the signing of an archival agreement for storing historical documents at North Carolina Central University.

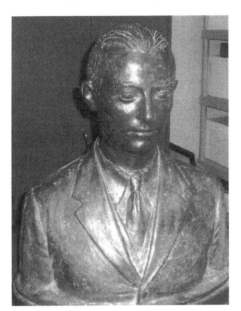

In 1937 a bust of Angier B. Duke was presented to the Angier B. Duke Nurses Home. The ceremony was opened by chairman Dr. Stanford Lee Warren and Mary Duke Biddle Trent Semans unveiled the bust. Charles Clinton Spaulding accepted the gift on behalf of the trustees of Lincoln Hospital and the citizens of Durham. The bust was prominently displayed on the elaborate breakfront in the foyer of the Angier B. Duke Nurses Home. Students were greeted by A. B. Duke as they entered the building.

Bust of Angier B. Duke, nurses' residence named in his honor.

Dr. Peggy Baker Walters, director of nursing, Watts Hospital School of Nursing, and Donna Rogers, archivist, Watts Hospital School of Nursing, present bust of Angier B. Duke to LHSNAA, Inc. Photo by Jerry Head.

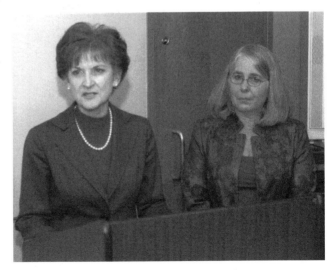

In 1971, upon the closure of the school, the bust was removed, after which it traced a circuitous route from Durham Regional Hospital to an antique shop, where Ms. Donna Rogers, Watts Hospital School of Nursing Archivist, discovered it, and moved it to a storage room at the Watts School of Nursing. On November 12, 2011, through the cooperation of Watts Hospital School of Nursing and the Lincoln Hospital School of Nursing Alumni Association, the bust was returned to the Lincoln Hospital School of Nursing alumni historical collection, which is maintained in North Carolina Central University's archives. In a moving ceremony in the presence of Lincoln alumni, Larry Suitt, the last administrator of Lincoln Hospital; Dr. Victor J. Dzau, MD, chancellor of Duke University Health Systems and president and CEO of Duke University Health Affairs; former instructors in the School of Nurs-

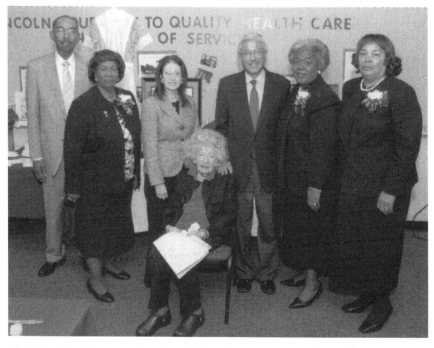

The Duke-Lincoln connection. Seated: *Mary D.B.T. Semans.* Left to right: *Larry Suitt, last administrator at Lincoln Hospital; Mary R. Baldwin, president of* LHSN *Alumni Association, Inc.; Ruth Dzau; Victor Dzau,* MD, *Chancellor for Health Affairs, President and* CEO *of Duke University Health System; Carolyn Evangeline Henderson, chair of* LHSN *Alumni Association, Inc., Historical Preservation Committee; Gloria Taylor Cheek King, corresponding secretary of* LHSN *Alumni Association, Inc., and member of Historical Preservation Committee.* Photo by Jerry Head.

ing; community leaders; and Mrs. Mary Duke Biddle Trent Semans, the bust was presented by Dr. Peggy Baker Walters, dean of Watts Hospital School of Nursing, and accepted by Mary Baldwin, then president of Lincoln Hospital School of Nursing Alumni Association, Inc.

Mrs. Semans, a niece of A. B. Duke, participated in the unveiling of the bust in an appropriate tribute to the Duke family. She stated, "Mother would be so pleased." She and her mother were steady contributors to the financial operation of Lincoln Hospital and Mrs. Semans enjoyed a long relationship with LHSN. This was probably one of the last public events she attended. She died shortly thereafter.

To ensure the preservation of all historical documents and artifacts related to Lincoln Hospital School of Nursing, an archival agreement was signed by Mary R. Baldwin, president of the Alumni Association (RN '66); Carolyn

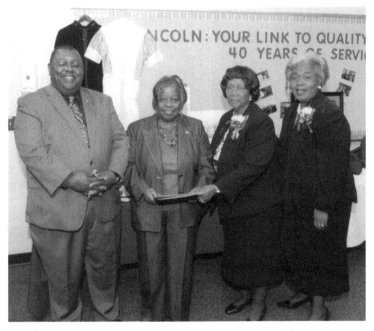

Lincoln alumni and NCCU archival agreement signing. Left to right: Andre Vann, coordinator of NCCU Archives; Dr. Theodosia Shields, director of library science at NCCU; Mary Richardson Baldwin, president of LHSNAA, Inc.; and Carolyn Evangeline Henderson, chair of LHSN Alumni Association, Inc., Historical Preservation Committee. Photo by Jerry Head.

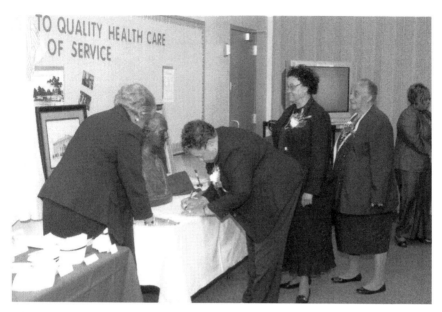

Alumni signing archival agreement with NCCU. *Left to right:* Carolyn Evangeline Henderson, Doris D. Smith, Valeretta Roberts Bell, Lula Cowan McNair. Photo by Jerry Head.

E. Henderson (RN '71), chair of the Historical Preservation Committee; Dr. Theodosia Shields, director of Library Science at NCCU; and André Vann, coordinator of university archives at NCCU. Members of the alumni signed as official witnesses to this historical agreement.

This historical preservation ceremony, which was followed by a brunch, enhanced the alumni's mission of maintaining the history of the School of Nursing and the Alumni Association.

IN CONCLUSION

Researching and writing this book has been a journey of anger and exhaustion, pleasure and frustration, sadness, joy, and enlightenment. This adventure started as a joint effort between two alumni sisters, myself and Ruby Jewel Bell Borden. In the course of our research, Ruby passed away. This has been a source of great sadness but also an inspiration to move forward and bring the project to fruition.

Although this book is by no means exhaustive, it is my hope that it will be a springboard for further research into Black schools of nursing, not only

(continues on page 247)

Carolyn Evangeline Henderson, RN '71, BS, MSN

I just retired as the Associate Director of Education Services at Durham Regional Hospital and Duke University Medical Health System. I am also Chair of the North Carolina Nurses Association Commission on Nursing Education. I grew up in eastern North Carolina.

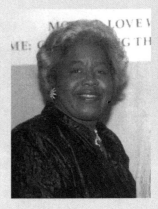

Nursing was an inevitable career for me. It was my father who solidified my decision to become a nurse. He was my first patient. Although my father wanted me to be a teacher because he considered it to be the female profession of choice during the fifties and sixties, his death, when I was only sixteen years old, convinced me that I wanted to become a nurse.

After my high school graduation in Kinston, North Carolina, I did not have the sudden urge to leave home as I continued to mourn the loss of my father.

Courtesy of Carolyn Evangeline Henderson.

So in 1965 I became employed at Lenoir Memorial Hospital in Kinston as an aide in the operating room. This was my second official job, in addition to my summer experiences of working on a tobacco farm and in the factory following graduation.

As an operating-room aide, my primary responsibilities were to prepare supplies and operating instruments for sterilization. At that time, operating gloves had to be washed, dried, powdered and sterilized, and labeled. Very few supplies were considered disposable. It was a challenge to learn all the instruments, and the supplies, procedures, and specifics for each surgeon's operation. However, within a year I had been promoted to the position of operating room technician, a position that I accepted with pride and that was based on achievements made as an operating room aide, observations from the operating room staff, and rare recommendations from the surgeons. I remember being given the dubious honor of working with the chief of the surgical staff who was fast and demanding on all of his operations. Not many staff relished the idea of working with him, but he was an excellent surgeon. Little did I know that he would have a role in my future as I aspired to be a nurse.

Having been an operating room technician for almost two years, I was encouraged by the nurses, physicians (including the chief of staff), and other technicians who supported my decision to continue my dream to become a nurse. So with much enthusiasm, I sent my application to Lenoir Memorial Hospital School of Nursing where I was denied entry during the segregated years of the sixties. Although disappointed, I was not discouraged. After a brief period of dismay, I was determined to continue my nursing pursuits. So, I sent two applications, rather than one this time, to Lincoln Hospital School of Nursing, a predominately Black nursing school in Durham, North Carolina, and Winston-Salem State Teachers College, also a

to capture their contributions and legacy but also to inspire people of color and others to fulfill the nursing call. African American females have an illustrious history in nursing and other careers, but documentation of their rich heritage has been limited. Recovering this ignored, devalued, unappreciated, and disrespected history is of paramount importance to African Americans and their descendants. I strongly believe that much more information is available than is reported here—it is incumbent on others to dig deeper. New technology can be helpful in this effort.

This book, true to its main title, "Voices," has attempted to establish the origin of LHSN, describe the joys and challenges of student life at Lincoln, and offer snapshots of some of the lives of its graduates. "Voices" of the current and past alumni presidents of our alumni chapters are here to chal-

---

Black institution (now Winston-Salem State University) in Winston-Salem, North Carolina.

The good news came when I was admitted to Lincoln Hospital School of Nursing, which closed in 1971. I was proud to be one of the fourteen graduates in the last class in 1971. In August 2003 the alumni celebrated in Durham, North Carolina, the 100th Anniversary of the School of Nursing.

Following my acceptance at Lincoln Hospital School of Nursing, I received my acceptance to Winston-Salem as well. I am proud of my choice to become a Lincoln nurse. I did not accomplish this dream alone. My Kinston extended family, foster parents, teachers, operating room nurses, physicians, and technicians gave me a heroic send off when I left for Durham to enter nursing school. Although I was not able to fulfill my nursing career in my hometown, it was my hometown's support, both Black and White, that packed a trunk of books, nursing paraphernalia, wrote letters of recommendation, and enhanced my courage to become a nurse. That is why I have chosen several personal mottos throughout my nursing profession and educational achievements. The mottos guided my transition from high school to nursing school—"behind us lies the barrier; before us comes the challenge"—and from nursing school to college/university—"wisdom is the principal thing, in all thy getting, get understanding."

Today, I'm grateful for my undergraduate degree in commerce and health administration from North Carolina Central University, my graduate degree in nursing administration and education from the University of North Carolina at Greensboro and my post-graduate and pre-doctoral studies at the North Carolina State University. Currently, my daily motto is "thank you, Lord," and this one has permeated my positions as an operating room nurse, a continuing education nurse educator, and an educational administrator.

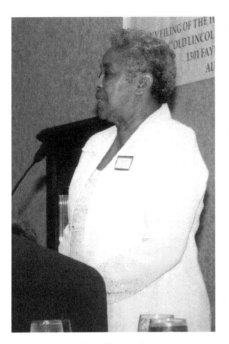

lenge young women and men to take up the "mantle" of assuring that the legacy of LHSN lives on.

Annie Lee Phillips (RN '52), former business manager of the New York chapter of the Alumni Association, has this advice for future nurses:

"Do good and look good doing it" is my message to you as you serve in the many roles and arenas in the nursing profession. Examples include the community; the ministry; political, family, civic organizations; art; or whatever. Our world is becoming more diverse each day, and I think that what little bit we can do for each other comes back to us.

Nellie (Ellis) Clemons-Green (RN '64), the last president of the Washington, D.C., chapter (see page 204 for picture), writes:

Annie Lee Phillips, former business manager of New York alumni chapter, at-large representative of LHSNAA, Inc.

Nursing, a universal profession, is practiced throughout the world. It offers satisfaction in a variety of opportunities, and is a profession that is open to men and women. Nursing education is comprehensive and offers so many choices such as hands-on caregiver, educator, administrator, policy maker, scientist, legal investigator, as well as astronaut. It is a career that is placed at the top of the list of professions. There are many paths to becoming a professional nurse; hospital schools of nursing, universities, and community colleges. Nursing gives you the opportunity to witness and impact all the individual changes along the life span, from the first breath of life to the last breath. Where else can you have such an intimate experience with humankind? How soon do you want to enter this exciting career?!

And lastly, Lottie Fleming Bolding Hall (RN '67), current president of the Alumni Association, expresses:

In 1961, I began my journey in nursing as a licensed practical nurse (LPN). During the winter of 1965, while performing private duty, I applied for admission to the Lincoln Hospital School of Nursing. In the spring of

1966, I was recruited to take a case at Lincoln Hospital. I was assigned to Dr. Clyde Donnell, who was chairman of the Board of Trustees at Lincoln Hospital. Dr. Donnell was an "inquisitive person" and began to ask me about my roots, my current status, and what I intended to do with "the rest of my life." I expressed my desire to become a registered nurse and told him I had applied to Lincoln Hospital for admission but that I had not received an answer. This interaction with a complete stranger gave me the opportunity to attend Lincoln Hospital School of Nursing, and I was the recipient of a student loan. This was the beginning

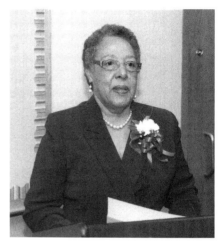

Lottie Fleming Hall, president, LHSNAA, *Inc.* Courtesy of Lottie Fleming Hall.

of my journey to the sisterhood of Lincoln Nursing. I am proud to continue the journey that began forty-eight years ago. It is a blessing to serve as president of Lincoln Hospital School of Nursing Alumni Association, Inc. This enhances my opportunity to assist others in pursuing their goals of nursing and giving back to the community. I say with pride that I am a "Lincoln Nurse" and part of the great legacy of Lincoln nurses. And I challenge you to be open to all kinds of experiences and people and to pursue all opportunities—maybe through a conversation with complete strangers or through exploring different health careers through health fairs, career fairs, volunteerism, and internships. Opportunities present themselves when you least expect them, so always present yourself in a positive light and be ready.

After 107 years, the question remains: What does it mean to be a Lincoln nurse? Spouse, mother, sister, friend. Strong, vibrant, compassionate, ambitious, self-directed, independent, innovative, creative, spiritual. These are all words that describe a Lincoln nurse. Students came to Lincoln with many of these traits and attributes already "in bud," and these individual characteristics were further developed and nurtured by the school's leaders as well as the Lincoln community of students, hospital staff, and the extended Lincoln family. Lincoln nurses have worked to maintain the spirit, love, and sisterhood they experienced in their school days throughout their professional careers. They initiate and execute service projects within the community and join together with other Lincoln graduates throughout the year, especially at

(continues on page 252)

Gloria Taylor Cheek King, RN '67, BSN, MSN

I was born in Wallace, North Carolina, on October 6, 1946, one of seven children. My father had a mechanical engineering degree and worked as a mechanical supervisor. He retired from Camp Lejuene, North Carolina. My mother had a high school diploma and was a wonderful housewife. My family members have made significant achievements: five of my seven siblings are college graduates, four are graduates of North Carolina Central University (NCCU), in Durham, North Carolina, and one served in the United States Air Force.

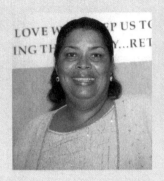

Courtesy of Lottie Fleming Hall.

I attended high school during the civil rights era when schools were segregated; it was also the beginning of civil unrest and civil rights marches. During my senior year of high school, President John F. Kennedy was assassinated. Later Dr. Martin Luther King Jr. was killed followed by Senator Robert (Bobby) Kennedy. This period was devastating to me. I attended Charity High School in Rose Hill, North Carolina, a rural town known for its tobacco farming, poultry- and pork-producing plants, and blueberry, strawberry, and vegetable farms. I was very active in high school. For example, I was a member of the Glee Club, as we called it, the student council, the 4-H Club, and the French Club. I was also a hall monitor and drove a school bus, for which I was paid. I was crowned Miss Debutante during my senior year, which was a pageant sponsored by the Home Economics Club.

I attended Lincoln Hospital School of Nursing (LHSN) from 1964 to 1967. When I came to Lincoln, Durham was in the midst of the civil rights marches and civil unrest. I remember the marches in downtown Durham and the setting of fires and burning down of major businesses during riots after the assassination of Martin Luther King. I am sure this period helped mold my thinking as it related to the workplace environment, the practice of hiring minorities in management positions, and the selection of students to attend college at predominately White institutions.

At Lincoln I sang in the choir and attempted to play basketball on the school league, but I was too blind without my glasses to be effective! The most disappointing experience for me was being skipped over for induction into the Santa Philomena Honor Society. The most rewarding was passing the nursing licensure board on the first try, and according to a letter sent to my parents by Mrs. Lucille Z. Williams, Nursing Director, I passed with some of the highest scores in the history of Lincoln. During that time we had to pass exams in five separate areas of nursing: Medicine, Surgery, Pediatrics, Psychiatry, and Obstetrics/Gynecology.

I attended White Rock Baptist Church during my training at Lincoln. White Rock was within walking distance of the school and it was also of my faith. I loved the Sanctuary Choir, and they also had a wonderful male chorus. The infamous Reverend Miles Mark Fisher was the pastor. His son, Rev. Miles M. Fisher III, was the chaplain for the nursing school and the basketball coach.

My first professional job was at Duke University Hospital (DUH), in Durham, North Carolina, on Campbell Ward, a gynecology unit with a head nurse from Lincoln, Mrs. Ethel McCullum (1947). Within ten months I was the first Afro-American nurse clinician hired to perform hemodialysis at Duke. Other employment experiences include being a staff nurse at the Veterans Administration Hospital in Durham, where I served for seven years, and a head nurse on the Psychiatric Service, also for seven years. I have been a clinical instructor in Psychiatry-Mental Health at NCCU, Vance Granville Community College, and in the Duke University Accelerated RN Program. I earned a master of science degree in nursing at the University of North Carolina, Chapel Hill, and hold ANA certifications in psychiatry–mental health and Nursing Administration.

My professional and extracurricular activities include a variety of board memberships, for example, the American Cancer Society, participation in a nursing sorority, serving as president of the Pi chapter of Chi Eta Phi Sorority, Inc., and as one of the founding members of Rho Phi chapter of Chi Eta Phi Sorority Inc., in Raleigh, and serving as president of the LHSN Alumni Association (LHSNAA). My most notable accomplishments during my tenure as president of the LHSNAA were doubling the membership, establishing a newsletter, and coordinating the 100-year celebration of Lincoln Hospital (in 2001), which resulted in the placement of a historic plaque on the old hospital grounds at 1301 Fayetteville Street. LHSNAA's receipt of 501(c)(3) status and the erection of a historic monument on the grounds honoring the School of Nursing and Lincoln Hospital were also in part due to my involvement. The monument is surrounded by bricks engraved with the names of all 600-plus nurses who graduated along with other names of individuals who were either born there, worked there, or supported Lincoln Hospital and the School of Nursing. Lincoln Community Health Center now operates on this site.

Mrs. L. Z. Williams, director of nursing at Lincoln Hospital and the School of Nursing, instilled in students the importance of professional participation. In addition to my membership in the sororities and the Alumni Association, I am a member of the North Carolina Nurses Association, the American Nurses Association, the Sigma Theta Tau National Honor Society, and Delta Sigma Theta Sorority, Inc. I love my community and have been honored for community service by receiving the Ebonette Service Award and the Mahogany Dime. For me, Lincoln and nursing are synonymous.

holiday time. The alumni make concerted efforts to maintain contact with one another, and at the time of death of a Lincoln grad or family member, they make special efforts to provide support. Lincoln nurses throughout the country are giving of themselves, their time, and their treasures—hard earned as they may be. They embody the spirit of Ralph Waldo Emerson's famous quote, "the greatest gift is a portion of thyself." What has kept Lincoln graduates committed to togetherness through the years is the familial bond of sisterhood they established and nurtured throughout their time at Lincoln.

Many of us came to Lincoln as naive, unsophisticated, frightened young women, unsure of what we were getting into but steadied by our passion for serving mankind. We came from homes in rural and urban communities alike, where our social, cultural, educational, and political experiences were limited. Most of us came from educational systems that prepared us to do our best despite the inequities. But the teaching, nurturing, caring, discipline, standards, expectations, and exposures we encountered while at Lincoln and beyond have created a whole new world for most of us. Many flames have been extinguished but not before they had shone their light of passion and service to mankind.

Perhaps future, young, African American women and men will view Lincoln nurses as role models and will choose to catch the torch, blaze new trails, take up the entrepreneurial spirit to provide nursing services and health care services to humankind. They will have the shoulders of Lincoln nurses as their launching pads, just as we had those of Mary Seacole, Mary Eliza Mahoney, Adele Thoms, Helen S. Miller, and others before us.

REFERENCES

Carolina Times (Durham, North Carolina). "Lincoln Hospital School of Nursing Graduates." June 4, 1938.

Constitution and By-Laws: Lincoln Hospital School of Nursing Alumni Association. Rev. December 1975. Lincoln Hospital School of Nursing Archives, Durham, N.C.

Constitution and By-Laws: Lincoln Hospital School of Nursing. Rev. 1963. Lincoln Hospital School of Nursing Archives, Durham, N.C.

Sullins, Della Mae Davison. Interview with Dorothy Esta Dennis Segars. June 12, 2010.

The Centennial Celebration of Lincoln Hospital School of Nursing, 1903–2003. August 2003. Lincoln Hospital School of Nursing Archives, Durham, N.C.

Epilogue

Reflections

So what has been the value of this book? We began with the basic observation that the story of Lincoln Hospital School of Nursing had not been told. The birth of the school was necessitated by the need of Lincoln Hospital. Not unlike parents and their children, the school and the hospital were inextricably linked until the demise of both. The hospital was established first, but without the school the hospital would not have survived. The founding fathers recognized the value of a training school for Negro nurses to care for the Negro citizens of Durham. As it happened, Lincoln Hospital served communities beyond that of Durham, its care extending to the surrounding counties and throughout the southeastern states. It developed a reputation as a solid community hospital despite always being poorly financed and funded. The community leaders, Negro and White, advocated for the establishment of two hospitals; the White population was cared for on one side of town and the Negro population on the other side of town. These were the days of segregation and Jim Crow in the South. Though segregated, the Durham medical and community leaders, both Negro and White, found ways to cooperate for the sake of addressing the health needs of the city's citizens. The end products were separate hospitals and nurse training schools for White and Negro citizens.

The value of this project lies in having a composite picture of the school as it developed and produced outstanding nurses while at the same time exemplifying support by people who lived the experience. This school of nursing and these graduates worked through hardships, poor elementary and secondary educational preparation, and an affiliation with a hospital that was always struggling financially to provide the necessary patient census (many patients were there on charity and therefore reimbursement was below what was needed). This census was required to provide the diversity necessary for student instruction and learning. All of these challenges were overcome so that students could have optimal learning experiences.

Many students, including me, were oblivious to the hardship the hospital was experiencing, a hardship that continued until the closure of the school in 1971. Our instructors and director always presented with such professionalism, strength, and upbeat attitudes that we didn't recognize or experience their burdens. Amazingly, despite these obstacles, the School of Nursing, thanks to its leadership, continued to promote student achievement and produce graduate nurses capable of competing in the ever changing world of health care. Lincoln nurses, in spite of obstacles of all kinds, demonstrated a determination and perseverance, scholarship, and commitment to patient care that has set them apart. They were able to maintain and achieve this through their relationship with God, the sisterhood bond, hard work, and an atmosphere filled with reverence for God.

The school and its students, from its beginning in 1903, experienced the isolation of the Jim Crow era, which although purportedly separate but equal, was in fact separate and really unequal. Even after Jim Crow was eliminated and integration legislated, Lincoln students continued to be goal oriented and approached change judiciously.

In the early years of the school's operation, the doctors were the only White individuals with whom Lincoln students interacted on a daily basis as they made rounds or taught a course. However students in the mid- to late 1960s participated in affiliations that were integrated. Following the rules and adhering to Lincoln's high standards made us the nurses we are today. It made us nurses who were sought after by institutions. We were the nurses who could do everything. There is a saying that goes like this: "Train a White nurse and she will be a nurse until she marries a doctor; train a Negro nurse and she will be a nurse forever." Such is the case with Lincoln nurses. Beyond retirement, most Lincoln graduates continue to work one-on-one with individuals needing care or assistance, be it in their own homes or in nursing homes. Such is the case with Gwendolyn C. J. Parham, whose special person is 101 years old and in a nursing home. Retired Lincoln nurses work in the community providing education and counseling and in churches providing health screenings for the congregation. They perform clinical supervision and teach allied health and other professional students, all the while imparting the values of integrity, commitment, high standards, a strong work ethic, and spirituality.

They also impart valuable truths to those they mentor. Among these truths is the fact that even though U.S. society is now integrated and we have an African American president, the playing field is still not level. Youth today seem not to cerebrate on that level. Not knowing their history, they cannot grasp the full implication of the early travails of pioneers. Racism still abounds, but where Lincoln students faced segregation until the late 1960s, the African American youth of today are not able to recognize the covert racism of "anything goes" attitudes or the subtleties of concepts such as "equality of opportunity" or platitudes like "all is well," and "that level of work is good for you." The philosophical perspective I propose to young African Americans is that they create a vision of where they want to go, explore what it will take to get them there, and, despite all the odds, barriers, and obstacles, persevere until they get there. If you present a positive, forward-moving persona, the sky can be your limit. There are those who will recognize your intellect, energy, enthusiasm, and motivation and will actively support you. My personal work ethic, which was ingrained in me from my family and nurtured at Lincoln, has been the foundation of my growth, development, and achievement. At this point in my life, I recognize the importance of mentors and sponsors. Mrs. Z's caution that you cannot afford to be casual and that you must always do your best were permanently etched on my brain. Casual to a then seventeen-year-old meant dress, but the meaning was broader than that. It includes your whole personhood, how you present yourself, how you speak, how you interact with others, and the respect you have for self and others. But foremost for me has been my strong abiding faith in God, which has deepened through this work and is the rock on which I have stood along with my family and Lincoln sisters to complete this book.

In the "voices" presented in the stories throughout these pages, Lincoln graduates express what was important to them and how those things helped to transform their lives and their careers. In the course of their practice as nurses, educators, and more, they faced racism, were treated as less than professional, and were not recognized for their roles and contributions because of their skin color. Despite these attitudes and behaviors, these graduates became outstanding, contributing members of the nursing and health-care communities. Their passion, tenacity, intelligence, and strength propelled them to unparalleled heights in all arenas across the health-care spectrum, from local to international. Then there were those graduates who because of their physical features could have passed for White and probably avoided the ostracism but chose not to out of their belief in themselves and their own

racial pride. There were those graduates who broke through the color barrier and the glass ceiling and achieved great things despite seemingly insurmountable odds.

And now, what does this mean to me? Nursing is my life's passion. A
former, highly respected colleague of mine frequently quoted this guiding
principle: "to be a nurse is to walk with God" (author unknown). As I have
matured and grown wiser, I have come to a deeper spirituality. As I go about
my daily routines, whether at work, on vacation, or just in the street, my eyes
are continuously opened to the needs of others. In other words, I live my
passion, my chosen career, as an ingrained part of all I continue to do in life.

For young African Americans, the challenge is to look at their social, economic, and political landscape and make some predictions about their future. I advise them to choose careers that will afford them the opportunity
and privilege to serve all members of society. This, I believe, is a high calling
and requires beliefs and attitudes other than those associated with the quest
for financial stability, which too often offers little chance to impact one's own
life and the lives of others in a fulfilling way. My personal belief, after working with young and middle-aged students today, is that their value systems
about what is important and what is ethical are somewhat warped (based on
materialism). Many of them choose to do what is expedient rather than what
is right. This is not to say that all young people are callous or misguided.
Rather, I believe these tendencies stem from the changing sociological and
capitalistic nature of the times, fueled by technology and the fast-paced, "get
it done" attitude that does not leave much room for forethought or reflection. I have seen changes in the value system, a lack of respect for authority,
a lack of caring for the needs of each other as people, and a lack of standards
or concern about quality in their performance, both in the workplace and in
the classroom. I realize there are generational differences at work and that I
am the product of a more conservative generation, but I believe the old ad-
age "don't throw the baby out with the bath water" is still relevant. There is
still a place for ethics, standards, and caring for others in a world that seems
to emphasize status and ask always "what's in it for me?"

I based my choice of nursing as a career on three factors: First, my mother
wanted to be a nurse and was not able to accomplish this goal, though she
did work as a lay midwife. Second, in the late 1950s and early 1960s the
choices for women were limited mostly to teaching and secretarial or domestic work. And, third, I was the baby sitter for all the small children, including cousins, in my family, which put me in the nurturing role. Upon
reflection, the choice was a good one. My career has taken me down many

paths—caregiver, administrator, educator—but they have all been directed toward helping others, which is my passion. This I share with my alumni sisters, and it has brought me much satisfaction and joy.

I, like my alumni sisters, have had to make choices and sacrifices to move my career forward. Most times they were consciously made; a few times they were imposed upon me. Having lived through the civil rights struggles and the wars that stretch from the 1950s to the current crisis in the Middle East, I am more deeply thoughtful, cognitively aware, and thankful for the experiences I have had, all of which have contributed to my personal and professional growth and development. The ostracism, the scrutiny, and the lack of respect, recognition, and acknowledgement did not prevent me from doing what was ethical and professional. Although this was hurtful at times, I had some whimsical moments. At sixty-nine, retired but working as a part-time educator, I am realizing more fully my personal power with my family and colleagues. I firmly believe that you are as broad or as narrow as your environment. I have tried to enlarge that environment for myself, my family, and the students I teach. I tell them stories about my nursing school days, my early experiences, and the challenges I have faced. I tell them stories about my early years on the farm, working in the tobacco fields, growing flowers, and appreciating nature. I challenge them to create memories for themselves and their families, as many of them are parents, struggling the second time around. And I tell the teenagers (aged seventeen and up) to look at themselves as givers and thinkers, not as takers waiting to be spoon-fed. Today, whether you're young, a career changer, a retiree, or laid off, your career options and opportunities are more plentiful than ever. I encourage you to explore nursing as a rich, challenging, and rewarding career. It offers you the privilege of experiencing the most intimate moments in the life of a person: their birth and their death. You can experience joy and excitement upon the birth of a baby and peace and thanksgiving upon the death of a patient. In the scheme of life, what is greater than that? Those who read this book and hear the voices herein hopefully will see the values, the work ethic, the resolve, the strength, and the passion that is the foundation for our work as Lincoln nurses.

Appendix 1

Leadership and Service Contributors

WE DEVELOPED the following summary of leadership and service contributions to express my deep appreciation and gratitude to the graduates of Lincoln Hospital School of Nursing and their family members for their personal stories and interviews. These personal narratives present a snapshot of the historical journey and major contributions of the graduates. The highlighted areas reflect this select group's pursuits in the fields of education, nursing practice, health-care research, and other related arenas on the local, state, national, and international levels.

Julia Simpson Armstrong, RN, Class of 1938
    Julia has more than forty-five years of nursing service as a night supervisor at Lincoln Hospital and Durham County General Hospital in Durham, N.C. Her prior nursing service involved working with the government in a rapid treatment center for syphilis.

Mary Richardson Baldwin, RN, BSN, MPH, Class of 1966
    Mary has worked for forty-two years in various positions in the health-care industry. Her work experiences include: staff nurse, Lincoln operating room/med-surgery; head nurse, general surgery, plastics and burns; clinical instructor for LPNs; assistant supervisor, ambulatory care; discharge planning and quality manager; and assistant to the director of surgery and director of nursing/quality manager, Lincoln Community Health Center. Mary has a North Carolina educator's license and has served as an occupational health instructor for Orange County, N.C., and an adjunct clinical faculty at North Carolina Central and Duke Universities.
    Her work experience and professional activities have earned Mary many accolades. She coordinated the first prostate screening clinic for Lincoln Community Health Center and assisted in writing over $600,000 in grant

monies for the Susan G. Komen for the Cure foundation and the NCCU Biotechnical Department for breast/prostate health screenings. Mary gave a presentation at the international educational seminar "Models of Nursing Practice: Paths to Success." Her professional memberships include: the National Black Nurses Association, the Central Carolina Black Nurses Council (CCBNC), and the American Nurses and North Carolina Nurses Association (NCNA), of which she has been a member for thirty-eight years. As a member of NCNA she served on the Commission on Service Committee and the Centennial Committee. Mary was elected chair and a member of the NCNA Board of Directors, who were instrumental in getting the North Carolina General Assembly to approve the "First in Nursing" license plate. She became the first president of the Triangle Region of the NCNA and served as treasurer for District 11. In addition, she served as president and treasurer for the CCBNC and the Lincoln Hospital School of Nursing Alumni Association.

Awards Mary has received include: the NCNA Nurse Manager of the Year; the N.C. Great Registered Nurse of Excellence for Durham County, Primary Healthcare Association; the CCBNC Outstanding Service and Distinguished Nurse award; the N.C. Distinguished Alumnus and Nurse of the Year awards from Lincoln Hospital School of Nursing; and the Most Inquisitive Nurse award from Lincoln Community Health Center.

Saundra Obie B. Clemmons, RN, BSN, MSN, FNP, Class of 1967
Saundra has worked as a certified clinical nurse specialist and as a national certified investigator. She served thirty-plus years in various roles, including quality improvement coordinator and clinical nurse specialist, at Person County Memorial Hospital in Roxboro, N.C. She also had a joint part-time appointment as a family nurse practitioner with Person Family Medical Center and Beckford Medical Center in Henderson, N.C. She has worked as a clinical instructor with Person County Memorial Hospital and Piedmont Community College in Roxboro, N.C. Saundra worked ten-plus years as an investigator for the N.C. Board of Nursing in Raleigh, N.C. She conducts investigations for various other boards such as the Medical Board, the Pharmacy Board, and State Bureau of Investigation.

Saundra's awards include a Robert Wood Johnson full scholarship to UNC-Chapel Hill, and an Allegra Ward award for perseverance. Her professional memberships include: the American Nurses Association, the N.C. Nurses Association (NCNA), Chi Eta Phi (XHO), and the Sigma Theta Tau honor society. She has held various offices at the district level in NCNA and at the chapter level in Chi Eta Phi, Rho Phi chapter. Her civic and church memberships include Prospect Hill Baptist Church, in Roxboro, N.C., where she participates in the usher ministry and the choir ministry and serves as the assistant financial secretary. She also provides oversight for the church's health ministry.

Lyda Ruth Flintall Betts, RN, BSN, Class of 1935

Lyda received a certificate in public health from St. Phillips Medical College in Richmond, Virginia. She is a certified public health nurse supervisor for the North Carolina State Board of Health.

Lyda served thirty-plus years in public health nursing as a staff nurse and supervisor. She provided public health nursing service at the Wayne County Health Department in Goldsboro, N.C., and at the Person County Health Department in Roxboro, N.C. She served as a supervisor at Lincoln Hospital in Durham, N.C. She was the first African American to be appointed supervisor in the Public Health Department in Durham County, Durham, N.C.

Lyda served as president of the Lincoln Hospital School of Nursing Alumni Association and is a member of the American Nurses Association and the North Carolina Nurses Association. She served on the board and as chairperson of the LHSN Alumni Association's bylaws committee. Lyda is a lifetime member of the North Carolina Public Health Association, served Chi Eta Phi sorority as the chapter's first anti basileus and as tamias for more than twelve years. She also served as tamiochus and chaired the Nominating and Finance Committees of Chi Eta Phi sorority, Inc., of which she is a life member. She served as the past treasurer of the southeast region.

She is a life member of the NAACP, and a member of the National Council of Negro Women, Inc., the Coordinating Council for Senior Citizens, and Women-In-Action for the Prevention of Violence. She is the secretary and a board member of the American Cancer Society (the Durham, N.C., unit) and secretary of the Patient Advocacy Committee of Durham County. She belongs to White Rock Baptist Church, in Durham, N.C., for which she has served as financial secretary and as chair of the bylaws and policy committee of the senior and sanctuary choirs. For several years, Lyda has been a leader and secretary for the church's College View District.

Minnie Williams-Beverly, RN, Lieutenant Colonel, USAF (Retired), Class of 1953

Minnie served for thirty-plus years in the field. She served three years as a psychiatric nurse at St. Elizabeth's Hospital in Washington, D.C.; five years in the USAF stationed at Gunter Air Force Base (AFB), Alabama, at

Wright-Patterson, Ohio, at Johnson Air Force Base, Japan, and at Travis Air Force Base, California. She completed active duty and joined the reserves.

Minnie was called back to active duty during the Cuban Crisis and served three years at Andrews Air Force Base in Maryland. She attended flight school and became a flight nurse. Minnie spent three years at Wiesbaden USAF Hospital in Wiesbaden, Germany. She also served one year as a nurse supervisor in the hospital in Cam Rahn Bay, Vietnam. She was stationed another two years at Andrews AFB in Maryland and then returned to Travis AFB, California, for a second tour. She worked for a year as a flight nurse bringing home prisoners of war (POWs) from Hanoi.

Minnie's awards and honors include: the Bronze Star Medal; the Meritorious Service Medal with one Oak Leaf Cluster; the Combat Air Crew Medal; the National Defense Medal; the Air Force Longevity Service Award with four Oak Leaf Clusters; the Vietnam Campaign Medal with four service stars; the Republic of Vietnam Medal with palm leaf; a City of Goldsboro Human Relations Award for notable achievement, in this case, her volunteer service with the Red Cross (twenty-one days in Baton Rouge and twenty-one days in New Orleans) in the aftermath of Hurricane Katrina. She received a certificate of appreciation from the Local Red Cross chapter. Minnie is a member of the Tuskegee Airman Inc. chapter, the Dillard/Goldsboro Alumni Association, and has served for several years on the Wayne County Nursing Home Advisory Board.

Patricia Martin Blue, RN, BSN, MPH, Class of 1965

Licensed as a nursing home administrator by the State of North Carolina, Patricia has forty-five years of service in administration and management in the community, long-term care, and hospital-based ambulatory care. In the course of her career, she has served in various nursing positions, including several pioneering roles. Patricia's work experience includes: charge nurse in maternal/child care at Lincoln and Duke Hospitals in Durham, N.C.; staff nurse in the Student Health Service at Duke University; and director of nursing at Lincoln Community Health Center. She was the first nurse director of center operations for Wake Health Services, in Raleigh, N.C., the first African American associate director for health services at Carol Woods Retirement Center in Chapel Hill, N.C., and the first African American director of clinic operations at Duke Family Medicine in Durham, N.C. Currently, she is working part-time as an adjunct faculty in the Department of Nursing at North Carolina Central University in Durham, N.C.

Patricia served as a delegate in the House of Representatives for the American Association of Homes for the Aging and is past president of the Nursing chapter of the NCCU Alumni Association. She has served on several boards including those of the Durham County Board of Health, in Durham, N.C., and the Adult Day Care and Home Health Advising Board in Chapel Hill and Durham, N.C. She is a volunteer with the AIDS Alliance of North Carolina and with the Substance Abuse and Mental Health services in Durham, N.C. Patricia has received numerous awards and recognitions from various employers and community groups.

Ruby Jewel Bell Borden, RN, BSN, Class of 1959

Ruby provided forty-plus years of nursing service in management and as a leader in medical informatics. Ruby started her career as a staff nurse and head nurse on the Clinical Research Unit at Duke University Hospital, in Durham, N.C. Ruby has thirty years of experience as an administrator, analyst, and project manager in medical informatics at Duke Hospital, in Durham. Her expertise in informatics (now known as management information or the electronic health record) led her to the executive role of director of information systems at Vanderbilt University Medical Center in Nashville, Tenn. Ruby presented papers on the use of technology in patient care. She received certifications in project management, facilitative leadership, and work redesign.

Ruby maintained membership in the Central Black Nurses Association, Inc., the North Carolina State Nurses Association, the Chi Eta Phi nursing sorority, and the Lincoln Hospital School of Nursing Alumni Association, Inc. In addition she held various offices in these organizations, from president and secretary to treasurer and chair of the bylaws and constitution and membership committees.

Peggy Christine Jones Butts, RN, Captain, USAF (Retired), Class of 1955

Christine served forty-plus years in the nursing field. She functioned as a staff nurse in the Veterans Hospital in Hampton, Va., for a brief period. Her primary service was in the USAF. She provided general duty nursing services on military assignments in Japan, the Andrews Air Force Base in Washington, D.C., and the Wichita Falls Station in Texas. Christine retired as a First Captain in the USAF.

Rebecca Mitchell Carter, RN, Class of 1966

Rebecca's twenty-nine-plus years of experience run the gamut of nursing positions, from staff nurse and assistant supervisor to assistant head nurse and head nurse. In addition, she is a certified nurse in the operating room and was employed as a clinical instructor and laser safety nurse officer in the Greater South East Hospital in Washington, D.C. Rebecca is a member of Chi Eta Pi sorority, Lambda Phi chapter.

Loretta Gail Flateau Chestnut, RN, BSN, Class of 1966
After graduating from Lincoln, Loretta continued her education and earned a bachelor of science degree in nursing. She worked for twenty-eight years as a head nurse and as the director of nursing for the South Carolina Department of Mental Health.

Yetta Hardy Clark, RN, CRNA, Class of 1968
Yetta has the honor of being the first Black nurse to graduate, in 1972, from Wake Forest University Baptist Hospital in the anesthesiology program, which is located in Winston-Salem, N.C.

Edwina Marie Sellers Colbert, RN, BSN, FNP, MEd, Class of 1959
Edwina has more than forty years of service as a staff nurse and charge nurse at the University of Virginia Hospital and Moses Cone Hospital. She also served as a school nurse for the Department of Public Health in Guilford County, Greensboro, N.C. Edwina received her certification as a family nurse practitioner from the American Nurses Credentialing Center (ANCC). Edwina is a member of several organizations, including the American Nurses Association, the HIV/AIDS Board of Greensboro, N.C., and the Sigma Theta Tau, Mu chapter. She also volunteers as a hospice nurse.

JoAnna Neal Dowling, RN, BHA, Class of 1962
Additional Education: Certified nephrology nurse
JoAnna has thirty-five years of service in the Dialysis and Kidney Transplant unit at Mt. Sinai Hospital in New York. Her other nursing experience includes head nurse in a long-term care hospital in New York and five years of service in a hospital in Bermuda. She returned to Mt. Sinai and worked in leadership and education roles. JoAnna's specialties in nursing include newborns, geriatrics, critical care, and ambulatory care.

Pauline Langston Edwards, RN, BSN, Class of 1966
After graduating from Lincoln, Pauline earned her bachelor of science degree in nursing. She spent thirty-four years in various positions, including staff nurse and nurse manager in ambulatory care at Memorial Hospital in Chapel Hill, N.C. She serves as a delegate to the Democratic Party for her precinct.

Thereasea Clark Elder, RN, MPH, Class of 1948
Additional Education: Howard University (Washington, D.C.); Freedom
Hospital School of Nursing (Washington, D.C.); University of North
Carolina, Chapel Hill (Chapel Hill, N.C.); Livingstone College (Salisbury,
N.C.); and Johnson C. Smith University (Charlotte, N.C.).

Thereasea served for forty-five years in nursing. She spent the first fourteen years at L. Richardson Hospital in Greensboro, N.C., and at Good Samaritan Hospital in Charlotte, N.C. She served thirty years as a Public Health Nurse.

Thereasea spearheaded the revitalization of the Rockwell neighborhood in Mecklenburg County. The Thereasea Clark Elder Park is so named to honor this work. She also founded the Charlotte-Mecklenburg Black Heritage Committee and the Greenville Community Historical Society.

Thereasea was responsible for the placement of special markers to commemorate Black achievements in Mecklenburg County. One is for Good Samaritan Hospital and another is a monument at the Pearl Street Park.

Thereasea served on several local, regional, national, and international boards and commissions including: the Mecklenburg County Human Relations Commission; the National Council of Negro Women; the National Association of Negro Business and Professional Women's Clubs; the League of Women Voters; the Mecklenburg County Cancer Prevention Coalition; and the Charlotte Housing Strategy Stakeholders Committee.

Her awards and honors include the Order of the Long Leaf Pine, North Carolina's highest civilian honor. Her life history is archived in the Smithsonian's National Museum of African American History & Culture as part of the StoryCorps oral history project. She also received the "Maya Angelou/Elizabeth Ross Dargan Lifetime Achievement Award" at the 2009 Maya Angelou Women Who Lead luncheon. Thereasea is a lifetime member of Second Calvary Missionary Baptist Church and serves as president of the missionary society, as chairperson of the ministry of health, and as chairperson of the building fund committee.

Clara Mae Cobb-Fraling, RN, BSN, MSN, PhD, Class of 1953
Clara is a certified elementary, middle, and high school principal. She is also a certified in science, math, and reading teacher and has taught at the college level. In addition to Clara's background as a secondary teacher, she served thirty-five-plus years in the field of nursing, primarily in administration and education.

Clara served in numerous roles in psychiatric and general hospital settings as a staff nurse and a supervisor. She is a member of Chi Eta Phi and

Phi Delta Gamma sororities, and Top Ladies of Distinction, Inc. (Baltimore chapter). Clara received the M. L. King's Citation from Pleasant Plains Elementary School. Her doctoral dissertation is housed in the Library of Congress in Washington, D.C.

Della Marie Harris Clemons, RN, BSN, Class of 1946

Della served for forty-plus years as a nurse. She provided nursing services as a staff nurse at St. Agnes Hospital in Raleigh, N.C. She was a school nurse for the Public Health Department in Raleigh and a supervisor in the Department of Corrections (later known as the Correctional School for Women), also in Raleigh. Della was the first nurse and first African American RN to work for Department of Corrections. She is a member of Chi Eta Phi, the National Association of University Women, and the Lincoln Hospital School of Nursing Alumni Association, Inc.

Nellie (Ellis) Clemons-Green, RN, BS, MS, Class of 1964

Nellie worked for thirty-six years in government service, primarily in health services nursing administration. Throughout these years, she has worked in several nursing positions, both nationally and internationally. Nellie served for two years as a staff nurse in a hospital intensive care unit in Charlotte, N.C., and for three years providing phlebotomy services by processing blood and supplying the local hospital and Kennedy Space Center in Orlando, Fla. A brief stint as a private duty contract nurse in Washington, D.C., led to a full-time position in occupational health nursing with the federal government at the U.S. State Department, which helped earn her the honor of being the first African American civil service nurse in the medical bureau. Working as a civil service nurse provided many experiences, from extensive overseas travel with the Secretary of State to meeting many dignitaries and prominent people, including Egyptian President Anwar Sadat, Israel's Prime Minister Golda Meir, General Colin Powell, as well as Pearl Bailey and Liza Minnelli.

Glenda Howard Harris, RN, Class of 1970

Glenda has served for forty-plus years in a variety of nursing roles, including staff nurse, surgical charge nurse, psychiatric nurse manager, hospice nurse, triage nurse, long-term care nurse, outpatient clinic nurse, high school nurse educator, and now as a medical-surgical telemetry nurse with oncology experience (locations and settings not provided).

Laura Hart Harrison, RN, Class of 1958

Laura has forty-plus years of service in nursing administration and education. She served as head nurse on the Recovery Surgical Unit at North Shore University Hospital in Manhasset, N.Y. She has also served in the following positions: head nurse, recovery room, Jamaica Hospital, Jamaica, N.Y.; nurse consultant, Division of Day Care, Department of Health (DOH), New York, N.Y.; and nurse supervisor and clinical manager in the Federal Cap Home Care Agency, New York, N.Y.

Laura planned, developed, and submitted curriculum for the Joint Partnership Training Act (JPTA) program to prepare home health aides (HHAs) for certification. In the program she trained and certified over 3,000 HHAs. Laura received the Nurse of Distinction award from the New York State Legislature, as nominated by the Federal Cap Home Care Agency. Nominees were honored at the National League for Nursing in New York City. She was cited by Fed Cap for twenty years of service.

Carolyn E. Henderson, RN, BS, MSN, Class of 1971

After graduating from Lincoln, Carolyn earned a bachelor's degree in commerce and health administration and a master's degree in nursing. She worked as the director of education services at Durham Regional Hospital and as the assistant director of education at Duke University Health Systems in Durham, N.C. Carolyn served as president of the LHSN Alumni Association Inc. and chaired the North Carolina Nurses Association Commission on Nursing Education.

Jocelyn Thompson Hodges, RN, BSN, BA (in sociology), Class of 1958
Additional Education: Certified in medical nursing

Jocelyn has forty-plus years in the medical, surgical, and neurological nursing areas. She served as a charge nurse on the midnight tour of duty with the Veterans Hospital system in Baltimore, Md. Her initial nursing roles include staff nurse at Cape Fear Valley Hospital in Fayetteville, N.C., and staff nurse at Michael Reese Hospital in Chicago, Ill. She has thirty years of service at the Veterans Hospital. She is a member of Chi Eta Phi sorority and received the Veterans Affairs award for excellence in nursing. She also received citations from President Clinton and Vice President Gore upon her retirement.

Mary Sara O'Lene Jinwright, RN, BA, Lt. Colonel, USAF (Retired),
Class of 1966
    Mary continued her education after graduating from Lincoln. She earned credentials as a certified registered nurse anesthetist (CRNA) and worked for more than thirty-five years as a staff nurse and nurse anesthetist. In addition to her nursing career, Mary served in the United States Air Force and was promoted to the rank of Lieutenant Colonel.

Gloria Taylor Cheek King, RN, BSN, MA, ANA, Class of 1967
    After graduating from LHSN, Gloria continued her education, earning a post-graduate degree and certification in psychiatry and nursing administration. She was employed as a clinical instructor at North Carolina Central University and in Duke University's accelerated RN program in Durham, N.C. Gloria has the honor of being the first African American nurse clinician in hemodialysis at Duke University Hospital. In addition, she served as president of Lincoln Hospital School of Nursing Alumni Association Inc. and helped to establish an endowed scholarship, the first of its kind in Historically Black Colleges and Universities in North Carolina, to support nursing student education at North Carolina Central University.

El Dora Laws, RN, Class of 1954
    El Dora served forty-plus years in the field of nursing. She functioned in several staff nurse positions in pediatrics. El Dora provided expert care of newborn and premature babies in the intensive care nursery. She also served as night head nurse at Somerset Medical Center in Summerville, N.J., for approximately thirty years.

Barbara Leathers, RN, Class of 1969
    Barbara served for more than forty years in direct patient care, working as a staff nurse and a head nurse on the Gynecology and Ear, Nose and Throat Units in ambulatory care at Duke Hospital, Durham, N.C. In both jobs, her managers, the head nurse Ethel McCullum and the supervisor Evelyn Wicker (also one of the authors), were fellow Lincoln graduates.

Norma Roberts Lipscomb, RN, BSN, MA, Class of 1963
    Norma was the first African American nurse educator at the Watts School of Nursing in Durham, N.C. She has twenty-three years of service as a nursing educator in a three-year nursing diploma program. She designed

and implemented a tutorial program to assist graduate nurses to successfully pass the North Carolina licensure examination.

Minnie Canarah Lyon, RN, Class of 1929

Minnie served thirty-plus years in the foreign mission fields of West Africa through the Lott Carey Foreign Mission Convention of the United States. In Brewerville, Liberia, West Africa, she helped pioneer the first mission station erected and maintained by Lott Carey and served as the instructor and nurse.

Minnie continued her education in public health at Harlem School of Nursing in New York, N.Y. She completed her undergraduate training at the Religious Training School at Chautauqua (later North Carolina College and now known as North Carolina Central University). She attended one semester at Spelman Seminary in Atlanta, Ga. Minnie traveled back and forth between Africa and North Carolina, eliciting financial support and recruiting young people to the foreign fields. Minnie was a lifetime member of the Women's Baptist Home and Foreign Mission Convention.

Celestine Patricia Rascoe Maness, RN, BSN, Class of 1958

Celestine was certified in surgical nursing by the Association of Operating Room Nurses. She served for more than forty years in the field and provided twenty-six years of service in supervisory nursing and staff nursing services at Muhlenberg Hospital in Plainfield, N.J., and at St. Mary's and Waterbury Hospitals in Hartford, Conn. She started as a staff nurse and then was promoted to supervisor of orthopedics and perioperative nurse educator at Harford Hospital in Hartford, Conn., spending twenty of those twenty-six years in the surgical area at Hartford Hospital. She made many contributions and educated staff as a perioperative nurse educator and a laser nurse educator on the uses of specialized equipment for blood collection and minimally invasive surgical and robotic techniques. She was at the forefront of writing and implementing standards of care for the patient with a latex allergy and providing a latex safe environment. This standard of care was copyrighted by Hartford Hospital. The Association of Critical Care Nurses granted permission to post it on their Best Practice Network website. Her greatest triumph, that won her national and international recognition, was having her article "Bloodless Medicine and Surgery" published in the international AORN *Journal*. Bloodless medicine and surgery is now a worldwide practice. She was commissioned by the director of nursing service at Hartford Hospital to write an article entitled "On Being a Perioperative Nurse," which was published in the Connecticut Nursing newspaper. In her retirement, she is an activist for HIV/AIDS and domestic violence. She is also a member of Grace Baptist Church in Woodbury, Conn., and serves as pianist for the junior and senior choirs at church.

Joan Miller Martin Jones Mathews, RN, BSN, MSN, EdD, Class of 1962
Joan's career in nursing began after she passed the N.C. Board of Nursing licensure examination in 1962 and received commendation from the board for being one of two students with the highest score on the obstetrics portion of the exam. She worked in nursing for more than thirty years, and as the profession evolved she continued her education and earned a doctorate in curriculum and teaching. Her experiences in nursing include working as a public health nurse for the N.C. Department of Health, as a staff nurse in the Medical-Surgical and Gynecological Units at Duke, Watts, and Lincoln Hospitals in Durham, N.C., and as a private duty nurse for Duke Hospital. In addition, Joan worked as a nurse educator at several institutions including NCCU as an assistant professor in nursing, Lincoln Hospital School of Nursing as an instructor of medical-surgical nursing, and the University of North Carolina at Greensboro (UNCG) as a visiting assistant professor in nursing. She retired in 1999 from UNCG as a clinical associate professor.

Joan embraced Lincoln Hospital School of Nursing's emphasis on participation in civic, professional, and community activities and organizations for students. She demonstrated these values by serving on several organizations including the N.C. A&T State University School of Nursing Advisory Committee, the North Carolina Association of County Boards of Social Services, and the Guilford County Board of Social Services for two terms. In addition she is a member of the American Nurses Association; the Sigma Theta Tau National Nursing Honor Society, Gamma Zeta chapter; the Lincoln Hospital School of Nursing Alumni Association (1964 president; 1976 Ms. Lincoln Alumni); and the Chi Eta Phi Nursing sorority. She is also a life member of the NAACP.

Joan has held a variety of leadership positions in these organizations such as president and committee chairperson. Moreover she sponsors the Woodrow Jones nursing scholarship at NCCU, has published articles in several journals, and has been recognized for her service. Awards she has received include educational scholarships, academic achievement awards, induction into the Golden Chain and Santa Filomena Honor Societies, citizenship awards, the Nurse of the Year award for District 11 from the North Carolina

Nurses Association, the Soror of the Year award from the South East Region of Chi Eta Phi sorority, and a nomination for a Martin Luther King Jr. Award for Excellence in Service.

Josephine Demmons Mcbride, RN, Class of 1936

Josephine served more than twenty years in management. She functioned as a head nurse and supervisor for a short time at Lincoln Hospital in Durham, N.C. For a number of years, she served as head nurse, supervisor, and director of nursing at Norfolk Community Hospital in Norfolk, Va.

Josephine is a member of Bate Street First Baptist Church and a recipient of a number of awards and honors for counseling high school and nursing students and for mentoring students at her church. Other honors include awards from Chi Eta Phi, Inc. and the National Civic League, and the Hattie McDaniel Award. Additionally, Josephine completed the Citizen's Police Academy program in 2010 and was named an honorary deputy sheriff for the City of Norfolk.

Alice Jean McClain, RN, BA, Class of 1966

Alice worked a total of thirty years as a nurse manager at Richmond Memorial Hospital and as the director of student health services at Virginia Union University in Richmond, Va. She continues to mentor pre-teens and provide them with scholarships to Virginia Union University.

Ethel Brown McCullum, RN, Class of 1947

Ethel served twenty-five years as head nurse in gynecology at Duke University Hospital, Durham, N.C. She has the distinction of being the first African American head nurse at Duke Hospital, which ranks as one of the twenty-five U.S. News Best Hospitals.

Carlita LaVerne Hall Merritt, RN, Class of 1964

Carlita served thirty-five years with the federal government. She was the first African American nurse in the Medical Surgical Unit in Arlington Hospital, in Arlington, Va. She was a staff nurse at the Veterans Hospital in Washington, D.C., and a head nurse at Freedman's Hospital in Washington, D.C. Carlita was also the first African American nurse promoted to nurse manager at the Parklawn Building, which has over 11,000 employees. Carlita helped to pioneer a number of first health-care initiatives in the system. She was the first to organize a comprehensive lactation program, the first to set up an AIDS screening program in partnership with the Public Health

Service of Montgomery County, Md., and the first to implement a pilot program for practical nurses. Her last assignment was with the United States Attorney's Office in Washington, D.C.

Marion Glen Miles, RN, Class of 1954

Marion has more than forty years of nursing service as a staff nurse, head nurse, and nurse supervisor at Lincoln Hospital in Durham, N.C. She also served as a managing nurse at IBM in Research Triangle Park in Durham. She continues to volunteer in various health and community organizations.

Marion has received several honors and awards including Nurse of the Year from the Lincoln Hospital School of Nursing Alumni Association Inc., Leadership Recognition from the National Council of Negro Women, Inc., and auxiliary membership in the Durham Academy of Medicine, Dentistry, and Pharmacy. She is an honoree for the Committee on the Affairs of Black People and was presented with the Order of the Long Leaf Pine. She is a member of Chi Eta Phi, Inc. and the Occupational Health Nurse Association, has been treasurer of the New Hope and Durham Missionary Association for thirty years, and is the chairperson for the Central Children's Home in Oxford, N.C.

Mary Lee Mills, RN, BSN, MSN, MPH, CNM, Captain, USPHS (Retired), Class of 1934
Additional Education: Certified nurse midwife; public health nursing; and a graduate certificate in health-care administration.

Mary has fifty-plus years of local, national, and international service in public health nursing and health-care management, in both the military and civilian life. She was an outstanding humanitarian. Mary served as a public nurse and a nurse midwife in New York City. She returned to Durham, N.C., to direct the public health nursing certificate program at the Historically Black College North Carolina College (now North Carolina Central University). During this time, she was commissioned as Chief Nursing Officer for the United States Public Health Services (USPHS) in the Office of International Health. She was also assigned to Monrovia, Liberia, in West Africa.

In Liberia, she initiated a national public health library, advocated for legislation to strengthen nursing as a profession, and created some of the country's first health education campaigns. Mary helped organize and establish the Franklin D. Roosevelt Memorial Children's Ward at the government hospital. She was instrumental in organizing the Tubman National School of Nursing. Liberia invested Mills as Knight Official of the Liberian Human Order of African Redemption.

Mary saw promotions from the rank of Major to Lieutenant Colonel, to Colonel, and finally to Captain. Captain Mills was proficient in several languages: Arabic, French, Cambodian, and several African dialects. She served in Beirut, Lebanon, to establish Lebanon's first school of nursing, for which Captain Mills earned the National Order of the Cedar, one of the country's highest service awards. A nursing dormitory at the school was named in her honor.

Mary served as a nursing consultant in the migrant health program in the U.S. Department of Health Education and Welfare (HEW), which is now the Department of Health and Human Services. In this role, she studied the national health-care systems of Finland, Germany, and Denmark. She also represented the United States at international nursing, midwifery, and other conferences in Mexico, Canada, Germany, Australia, Italy, and Sweden.

Mary's memberships include the American College of Nurses-Midwives, the National League for Nursing, the Frontier Nursing Service, the American Public Health Association, the American Nurses Association, the North Carolina Nurses Association (District 11), and the National Association for the Advancement of Colored People (NAACP). Other awards and honors include a USPHS Distinguished Service Award, Princeton University's Rockefeller Public Service Award, the American Nurses Association's Mary Mahoney Award, and the Long Leaf Pine Award (North Carolina's highest honor). She was awarded an honorary doctorate of science degree from Tuskegee University and an honorary doctorate of laws degree from Seton Hall University. She was selected by the Harmon Foundation for her distinguished service in public health to have an oil portrait painted by Betty Braves Reyneau. This portrait is a permanent part of the Harmon Collection at the Smithsonian Institution in Washington, D.C. Ms. Mills was posthumously inducted into the American Nurses Association Hall of Fame in 2012.

Janie Lee Canty-Mitchell, RN, BSN, MSN, PhD, Class of 1971

Janie served forty-plus years in nursing leadership and education. Her years of nursing service include roles in psychiatric/mental health, public health, supervision and administration, teaching, and research. She taught in the schools of nursing at Florida International University, University of Miami, Indiana University, and the University of Florida. Janie served as associate dean/director of research at the University of North Carolina-Wilmington. She has delivered fifty-five podium speeches at local, regional, national, and international conferences and published twenty peer-reviewed articles and book chapters. Janie was a charter member and nurse consultant for the National Institute of Health (NIH), in the Children and Families section of the Center for Scientific Review. She was one of twenty nurses to be accepted into the Robert Wood Johnson Executive Nurse Fellow program in 2009.

Edna Martel Jones Moore, RN, BSN, Class of 1947

Edna has thirty-seven years of service in nursing as a staff nurse, assistant head nurse, and head nurse at the Veterans Administration in Tuskegee, Alabama, and the Bronx, New York. She is a member of the Tuskegee University Nurses Alumni Association, the National Coalition of 100 Black Women, the Alabama Nurses Association, the American Nurses Association, and Chi Eta Phi Nursing sorority. She is a life member of Delta Sigma Theta sorority and is active with the Cancer Research Foundation. Her awards and recognitions include: Chi Eta Phi, Epsilon chapter's Sisterhood and Nurse of the Year award, a Habitat for Humanity Angel award, and several appreciation awards from Tuskegee University. In addition, Edna was a special guest at Harvard University's graduate exercise in recognition of her inclusion in a dissertation titled "Professional Commitment and Activism in the Lives of Five Southern African American Nurses." The dissertation was published as a book, and an article titled "Nurses Making a Difference" appeared in the February 2001 edition of the *American Journal of Nursing.*

Lois Smith Morris, RN, Class of 1947

Lois served in the field for twenty-five years as a school and staff nurse at various hospitals and schools. Upon graduating from Lincoln Hospital School of Nursing, she worked as a staff nurse at Brooklyn Jewish Hospital in labor and delivery and at Jamaica Hospital, both in New York. During this time, Negro nurses had begun integrating into mainstream hospitals.

After her tenure in New York, she moved to Craven County in North Carolina where she continued to serve and enhance the school nurse positions in secondary schools. She was influential in starting a training program for school nurses. She supervised three nurses who later went on to become school nurses. One of her most loved projects was working to get all students in Craven County immunized. This project occurred right on the cusp of legislation mandating immunization for all children.

Nora Kendall Noble, RN, Primary Nurse Practitioner, Colonel, USAF (Retired), Class of 1957

Colonel Noble completed twenty-seven years of consecutive military service. She served as a First Lieutenant at Dyess AFB in Abilene, Tex. She was promoted to Captain and stationed between Wiesbaden, Germany, and the Dow AFB in Bangor, Maine. She completed flight nursing school in San Antonio, Tex. She became a flight nurse in Rhine-Main, Germany, and then was promoted to standardization evaluation flight nurse and was responsible for administering flight nurse qualification exams.

Noble received an early promotion to Captain and volunteered as a flight nurse in Vietnam. She completed the bachelor of science degree at the Air Force Institute of Technology via Catholic University of America in Washington, D.C. She became a primary nurse practitioner and was promoted to the position of Lieutenant Colonel. After her promotion she went to Denver, Co., as the chief nurse of the Air Force Reserve Nurses.

While in Denver, Noble was promoted to full Colonel and was deployed to Elmendorf AFB in Anchorage, Alaska. In Alaska, she was dual rated as the Alaskan Air Command nurse and as chief nurse of the Elmendorf Medical Center. Colonel Noble was the first female Base Commander of the Newark Air Force Station in Newark, Ohio. She remained in this role until her retirement in 1987. In 1996 Colonel Nora Kendall Noble was inducted into the Ohio Veterans Hall of Fame.

Gwendolyn C. Jones Parham, RN, BSN, MSN, Class of 1958
Additional Education: Pre-doctoral studies, North Carolina State University, Raleigh, N.C.

Gwendolyn has twenty-plus years of nursing service, primarily in education. She served as a staff nurse at Duke University Hospital, an industrial health nurse at Liggett Myers Tobacco Company, and a staff nurse at Lincoln Community Health Center (LCHC), all located in Durham, N.C. She also served as a nurse educator at Durham Technical Community College and as a tenured assistant professor and assistant chair in the Department of Nursing at North Carolina Central University, Durham, N.C.

Her professional affiliations include: the American Nurses Association, the National League for Nursing, the National Black Nurses Association, the North Carolina Nurse Association, Sigma Theta Tau sorority (Duke University chapter) and Delta Sigma Theta sorority (Durham Alumni Association chapter).

Gwendolyn's most valued honors include her meritorious evaluations by students and the North Carolina Central University for teaching excellence, her service as a university marshal, and her leadership roles in the faculty senate.

Mary Louise Williams Pointer, RN, Class of 1959
Additional Education: Parish nurse, Duke Divinity School, Durham, N.C.
Mary has forty-plus years of service in various nursing leadership roles including head nurse, clinician, and nurse manager at the VA Medical Center in Durham, N.C. She was the manager for the Cancer Detection Center at Lincoln Community Health Center in Durham, N.C. Mary collaborated and worked in research at Duke Medical Center and with Operation Breakthrough to procure funding from the American Cancer Society, Susan G. Komen for the Cure, and the Duke Endowment.

Carrie Stone Reavis, RN, Nurse Anesthetist, Class of 1965
Carrie was the first African American to graduate from the MCV School of Nurse Anesthesiology in Richmond, Va. She has thirty years of service as a chief nurse anesthetist. Carrie served thirteen years as a staff nurse anesthetist and seventeen years as a chief nurse anesthetist. She is a member of Chi Eta Phi sorority, Inc., for which she serves as historian of the northeast region, and the Zeta chapter, for which she serves as president; the American Association of Nurse Anesthetists; and the Saint Paul Baptist Church usher board.

Dorothy Esta Mae Dennis Segars, RN, BSN, Class of 1968
Esta is certified in Medicaid Personal Care Services. Her health care practice spans 30 years from 1968–1998. She practiced in psychiatry at Duke University Medical Center (DUMC), Veterans Administration Medical Center, and John Umstead Hospital, Butner, N.C. Positions ranged from charge nurse, head nurse, and night supervisor. At DUMC Esta also worked as administrative nursing supervisor (ADN). In the Department of Medicine (Hematology) she was nurse clinician with the Duke Comprehensive Sickle Cell Center. She also worked as nurse discharge coordinator with the Department of Social Work at DUMC. At North Carolina Central University Department of Nursing, she held the position of counselor/tutor.

Elaine Richardson Smith, RN, BA, BS, MA, Class of 1963
Elaine provided over twenty-two years of service to the people she cared for. She continued her education and earned a master's degree in counseling psychology. Her employment includes one year of service as a psychological counselor for Family Consultation Services, in Jacksonville, Fl., and twelve years of service as a project coordinator in the Women's Center in Jacksonville, where she developed the Department of Employment and Training to help place individuals in full-time high-wage jobs. In 1980 Elaine was promoted to director of resource development in the Department of Institutional Advancement at Florida Community College. Five years prior to retirement she worked as a counselor in student affairs and taught faculty at the college.

Marian (Smith) Smith, RN, BSN, Class of 1957
Marian served as a nurse for over forty-five years in a variety of roles and settings. She functioned as a staff nurse in the Old Emergency Hospital in Washington, D.C. (now Washington Hospital Center), and as a staff nurse in the operating room at Children's Hospital in Washington, D.C. Marian also served for thirteen years as a private duty nurse at all of the major hospitals in Washington. She was employed with the Washington, D.C., Department of Corrections for eight years and then moved to forensic psychiatry at John Howard's Pavilion at St. Elizabeth Hospital. Marian retired from the Washington, D.C., Department of Corrections. She was recognized and honored by the Sigma Theta International Society of Nursing as one of "100 Extraordinary Nurses."

Aquilla Watkins Stanfield, RN, Lieutenant Colonel, U.S. Army (Retired), Class of 1958
Aquila Watkins Stanfield was the first married student to attend Lincoln. After graduation she served for twenty-three years in the U.S. Army where she earned many accolades. Her tours of duty include head nurse positions at Walter Reed Army Medical Center and Fort Indiantown Gap and area coordinator positions at Fort Dix and Fort Drum. In addition, she served at the Walter Reed Army Medical Center as the Assistant Chief Nurse of the 229oth U.S. Army Reserves Unit during Desert Storm. Aquilla received the Army Service Ribbon, National and Defense Service Medals, Army Achievement Medals and two Oak Leaf Cluster Armed Forces Medals. She is a member of Chi Eta Phi sorority.

Alice Harrell Young Tharrington, RN, BS, Class of 1968
Certified in teaching non-nursing personnel how to deliver medication, basic life support, cardiopulmonary resuscitation, and first-aid medical care and as an apheresis practitioner, Alice has more than thirty years in health care. She has twenty-five years of service at the American Red Cross with twenty-two years as supervisor of the apheresis lab. Her service also includes eight years in a hospital setting as well as entrepreneurial endeavors in CPR and first aid. She organized the first community project for the Alston Heights Community in Health Education at North Carolina Central University, in Durham, N.C. Edna is a member of the Chi Eta Phi nursing sorority.

Elsie Long Waddell, RN, Class of 1939
Elsie served for thirteen years in hospitals as a staff nurse, charge nurse, and private duty nurse. Her initial service began at Community Hospital in Wilmington, N.C. She also worked as a staff nurse at Brooklyn Children's Hospital in Brooklyn, N.Y., a staff nurse at James Walker Hospital in Wilmington, N.C., and a charge nurse (evening and night) at Seaview Hospital in New York. Prior to her retirement in 1952, Elsie provided private duty service at Staten Island Hospital, Staten Island, N.Y.

Dellamar Inez Davis Washington, RN, Class of 1966
Dellamar has worked more than thirty-two years in the nursing field. She has been employed as an intensive care nurse, surgical nurse, and cardiovascular recovery room assistant head nurse. Since her retirement she has continued to practice nursing as a hospice admissions nurse. Dellamar continues to pay it forward by giving scholarships to high school students and participating in the Susan B. Komen for the Cure walk for breast cancer and in other walks for Alzheimer's disease and AIDS.

Evelyn Pearl Booker Wicker, RN, BSN, MPH, EdD, Class of 1963
Evelyn served in the health and medical field for more than forty-five years. Her work experiences include serving as a staff nurse at Moses Cone Hospital in Greensboro, N.C., Memorial Hospital (now UNC Hospital) in Chapel Hill, N.C., and Duke Hospital (now Duke University Health System); a head nurse at Rogers Memorial Hospital in Washington, D.C.; supervisor of ambulatory care at Duke Hospital; director of nursing at Duke South Hospital; director of nursing for Women's and Children's Health at Duke

Hospital; and director of hospital career development in human resources at Duke University Medical Center.

Evelyn has also served as an educator in the health services field at several institutions: North Carolina Central University, St. Augustine's College in Raleigh, N.C., Wake Technical Community College in Raleigh, N.C., and Duke University's School of Nursing. She has also served as a consultant for home care agencies.

Evelyn has been a member of several professional and community organizations. She is a longtime member of the North Carolina Nursing Association, serving as home care board member; the American Nurses Association, serving as a board member in District 11; the Central Carolina Black Nurses Council; Chi Eta Phi, Inc.; Sigma Theta Tau; Duke University; and NCCU. She also has served on the YMCA Board of Directors and was the first nurse to serve on the Board of Health for the Durham County Health Department. Evelyn has given numerous presentations on nursing, leadership, and mentorship at national conferences, before the state government, and at Duke Medical Center. In her community, she was instrumental in the establishment of the Cultural Arts Society of Fuquay Varina, serving as a charter member of the organization. Among her many honors and awards, she was named a YMCA Woman of Achievement and as a Robert Wood Johnson Executive Nurse Fellow by the Wharton School of Business at the University of Pennsylvania.

Linda Lofton Woodson, RN, BSN, MEd, Class of 1966

After graduating from Lincoln, Linda went onto pursue her BSN and MEd degrees. She worked for thirty-two years as an instructor in obstetrics and gynecology at Orlando Technical Education Center and provided mission service to the nursing homes and community in the Orlando area. She continues to facilitate couples' and singles' ministry and teaches adult Sunday school.

Appendix 2

Historical Roster

1907

Katie E. Creasman
Elizabeth Devane
Marie Antonette Gray
Cora Lee Hines
Elizabeth Spruell
Theda Eleanor Williams

1908

Addie Ernestine Largin
Pearl Lee Moore

1909

Mattie M. Graves
Willie F. Jones
Nellie McKenzie Saunders
Nannie P. Watkins

1910

Bettie A. Coles
Clara Lockhart

1911

Pearl Henderson
Mary E. Jeffreys
Emma Richardson

1912

Minnie Hackney
Ora Hamilton
Laura Logan
Ethel Powell
Emma Salmon

1913

Eliza M. Cauley
Carrie Clark
Mary E. Hampton
Margaret Hicks
Maud Smith Knox

1914

Marjorie D. Alston
Clarissa E. Dukes
Anna E. Hill
Cornelia E. Lewis
Gertrude L. Patterson

1915

Jessie Birdsall Bolding
Josie Wilson Harvey
Willie Martin
Girley Jones Strickland
Daisy Bell Teer

1916

Lizzie Newell Blanks
Katie T. Corbett
Sadie Price

1917

No graduates; end of two-year
   program

1918

Arneta Breeden
Annie D. Clark Evans
Ula Hagan
Luvesta Marable
Pattie Nichols
Beauford Pickens
Majorie Pickens
Willette Freeland Bailey Price

1919

Eula M. Julia David
Beulah Hudson
Minnie T. Williams

1920

Helen King

1921

Mary E. Grant Diggs
Mary E. Henry
Henrietta Easter Foster Mebane
Claudia E. Tucker

1922

Adelia D. Compton
Minella Dewey Shoffner Jones
Ella Louise Mason
Priscilla Alma Newby

Alberta Lofton Snipes
Fannie Lee Toliver Padget

1923

Zera A. Spann

1924

Etta Imes Farmer
Madeline Ragan
Carrie Lillie Stowe
Catherine Young

1925

Dora Burchette
Elizabeth Jackson
Nannie Gibson Jordan
Carolyne McIlwain
Beatrice Freeman Moss

1926

Soulee Graham
Ida M. Hairston
Ollie B. Love Hendrick
Pearl Frances Jones Trulove

1927

Edna Bradsher
Annie Bynum
Doris Y. Evans
Ruby Glaspy Farmer
Elizabeth Lee Hackney
Nannie B. Herbin
Lorena Hill
Annie Strickland
Naomi Swails
Clara Payton Williams

1928

Lee Ila Blount
Gertrude Carter Foreman
Lillie Mae Greene Gray
Bessie M. Goss
Ethel Colston Harrison
Annie Dorothy Jeffers
Eleanor Frances Jones
Elizabeth L. Johns
Sallie M. Smitherman
Creola Juanita Stradford
Nettie Marie Thomas
Nadine R. Williams
Naomi Savanna Williams

1929

Manna Beaman
Minnie Brown
Alice Inez Crawley
Caroline E. Allen Dunn
Adelaide Jenkins
Vergie Lee Coleman Keys
Minnie Canarah Lyons
Mattie Peace
Maggie Prince
Nettie M. Thomas

1930

Ruth Ellison Alexander (Bibby)
Hallie Louise Bryd
Janeta Bell Gatling
Bertha Elizabeth Grier Green
Eliza M. Clements Patterson
Blanche Sowell
Lillian Wallace

1931

Hannah Odell Barfield
Annie Mabel Brown
Anna Cladwell
Willie Clark
Bettie Freeman
Edith Gray
Addie Jones
Willie McKnight
Clara Maxwell
Tommie Smith
Vaughn Smith
Mary E. Spencer
Gwendolyn Sykes-Corney

1932

Sallie Benjamin
Annie Bennett
Lowenia B?
Ethel Clark
Lula Durham
Eunice Hamilton
Mildred Haywood
Marie B. Jones
Ruth Jones (Ruby)
Eva Christine Lunsford
Mamie Batchelor Maddox
Prilly C. Raeford

1933

Nannie Franscena Blue
Charlotte Bryant
Cora Stevenson Clanton
Eleanor Harris
Lula McCoy Harris
Mary Lee Mills
Irma Elizabeth Whitaker Mock
Desdamonia Witby
Mabel DeZella Wright Young
Susie Frances Wright

1934

Mary Sue Archer
Helen Dillahunt Brown
Mamie Dirton (?)
Roseanna Cameron Hall
Emma Bell Hampton
Jessie Leach
Katie Mae Long
Viella Margarette Mitchell
Dymphia Sadler
Lillian Amanda Jenkins Shute

1935

Lydia Ruth Flintal Betts
Pearl E. Griffin
Helen Hogan
Margaret Howard
Helen Howell
Frances Derr Martin
Mattie Pearl Wallace

1936

Mary Adams
Dympha Brown
Phloy Freison
Nala Harrington
Gertrude Bullock Henry
Terri B. Isler
Evelyn Jeffreys
Josephine LaFranz Demmons
    McBride
Mary McNeil
Ruth F. Reed
Pattie Scott
Jimmie D. Trammell
Pearl Winbush

1937

Della Raney Jackson
Lucille Jones
Della Mae Davison Sullins

1938

Julia Marie Simpson Armstrong
Carrie M. Henderson
Catherine B. Dixon Reeves

1939

Lucille Alford
Dellah Allen
Dorothy Dixon
Ruth Faulkner
Bessie Glymph Gray
Julia M. Hogan
Odessa Hoover Jones
Jessie B. Keys
Mildred Jordan Luter
Eva Barnes McPhail
Catherine Perry
Ruth Spruell Ridley
Frances Sutton
Mason Thompson
Elsie Long Waddell
Julia White

1940

Irma Harris Balfour
Helen Blair
Mildred Crisps
Emily Culmers
Helen Curry
Willie Edwards
Louise Gay
Blanche Beatrice Meadows
Pearl Roberts

Lucretia Taylor Thomas
Eula Brown Wilborn
Dessie J. Williams Young

1941

Pauline Chambers
Mary Frances Durensell
Frances Exum
Ella Ferguson Hargraves
Lucille Howard
Rosetta Edmonds James
Janet Mullens
Thelma P (sp)?
Frances Roberts
Naomi Taggert Clark
Lydia Walls

1942

Jolsie Curry
Lillian Grace Currie
Edna Harris
Alice Patterson Hayes
Ida J. James Howe
Mamie Jemison
Gertrude Lassiter
Ruth Murchinson
Vivian Savage Nealy
Sarah McKoy Rhynie
Alice Perry Walker
Alice Hazel Harrison Waller
Alice White

1943

Gladys Williams Britt
Susie Virginia Carrington Buie
Janie Goodman Cooke
Lillian F. Cuffie
Doris Dicks
Ida Bliss Griffin
Cornelia Jackson Hardie
Nellie Nelson
Pearl Parks
Vivian Rudd Parks
Mariam Walden Smith

1944

Marion Holmes Bass
Clara Bates Collins
Reva Exum
Roberta Vaughn Griffin
Elizabeth Jones
(?) Simon
Shirley Reid Tyler
Callie Smith Upperman

1945

Ruth Parlor Amey
Audrey Green McCoy Beavers
Mollie Jones Clark
Clara Josephine Miller Harris
Clara Lancaster
Carrie M. Baker Lingard
Doris M. Peters
Eva Richardson
Bertha Walker
Mildred Watkins

1946

Ruth Bazemore
Dossie Jones Blue
Georgia M. Bristol
Della Marie Harris Clemons
Beatrice Fellers Coleman
Bernice Dix
Helen Tate Harvey
Helen Neal Webb Jones
Blanche Gillispie Keene
Annie Blyther Lenix
Louise Mahone
Emma Jane McArthur Myles
Wilhelmena Murphy
Norma Chestnut Peddy
Gloria Campbell Richardson
Marion Elizabeth Sanders
    DeGreffread Rogers
Theresa Bassard Taylor

1947

Lula Bell Woods Bolding
Rosa Lucille Brown
Lee Ruth Crowe
Margaret Evans
Edith Celia Wade Lee
Ethel Marie Brown McCullum
Deloris Bessie Bettes McNeil
Edna Martel Jones Moore
Lois Smith Morris
Willie Lee Alexander Parker
Pearlie Mae Williams Price
Lola Royall Robinson
Lucy Ardellie Thompson
Gail Hancock Traylor
Nannie Thomasine McDaniels
    Wigfall

1948

Rosebud Roderick Beverly
Helen Jaunita Black
Annie B. Coley Boyd
Lillian Brown
Muriel Harris Daniels
Thereasea D. Clark Elder
Dorothy A. Farley
Margaret Davis Reeder
Zella Perry Thomspon
Elizabeth Williams Thorpe
Mary Lois Clements Brown Thorpe
Corona McClary Umstead
Alice Williams
Othello Cave Williams
Mary B. Worley

1949

Emma Crow
Annie Evans (Cotton)
Dorothy Scurlock Hampton
Geraldine Jackson
Georgia Majors
Madeline Gardner Matthews
Eloise McKeithan
Alease Woods Mosely
Carrie Ray
Eleanor Matthewson Ruffin
Ida Ree Smith Sanders
Edith Gray Tankersley
Evelana Saunders Woods

1950

Ovelia Dowdy Barnes
Jodie Carson
Mary Craft
Donnie Davis
Louise Davis

Elizabeth Bailey Foushee
Elizabeth Funny
Carrie Minor Hill
Fannie Randolph Johnson
Stella Reeves McLean
Lelia Thompson Miller
Effie Smith Pounders
Selena Boykins Reid
Clara Savage Sutton
Ruth Harrell Wade
Lula Barnes Rowland Williams

1951

Josephine White Baylan
Helen Hargraves (Best)
Willie Mae Brown
Lessie Edwards Futrell
Harriett Green
Mary Hall Knight
Juanita Moore
Emma McArthur Myles
Ercelle O'Neil
Goldie Saunders Richardson
Hattie Royall
Martha Wooten

1952

Nellie Ferguson Faison Collins
Elfreda Crawford-Fassett
Christine Haywood Foust
Mary Gillard
Annie Lee Phillips
Mary Frances Shorts
Sylvia McNeal Stapleton
Etta Young Wallace
Mildred Paige White
Margaret Holloway Wigfall
Joyce Young

1953

Minnie Williams-Beverly
Ora Ruth Davis
Clara Cobb-Fraling
Annie Anderson Dunnigan French
Bertha Hardy Gavins
Mary Hall Knight
Lula Crown McNair
Mildred Deer Parkinson
Berta Williams Pinckney
Dorothy Bolton Rodgers
Geneva Smith Wade
Irene Dawson Young

1954

Joyce Clarke Armour
Frances Hawkins Benson
Hazel L. Best
Louise Best Cooke
Evelyn Nelson Dicks
Frances Godhigh
Elizabeth Kearney Grubbs
Queen Esther Alexander Campbell
  Hamby
Dora Highsmith
Johnnie Odessa Autry Hill
El Dora Shaw Laws
Nora Lee Matthews
Marion Glen Miles
Laura Halsey Moseley
Sylvia Carver Pointer
Bernice Dawson Robinson
Aljurie Cozart Spivey
Clorene McGhee Taylor
Jerlean Graves Utley
Beulah Tidline Wade
Doshia Melvin Walker
Dorothy Spiller Williams
Evelyn Ferguson Williamson

1955

Dorothy P. Addison
Pearl Credle Bell
Peggy C. Jones Butts
Eleanor R. Dawson
Rosetta Clyburn Dudley
Mary Jane Hall
Lucy Ingram
Annie L. Josey
Alice E. Hopkins Lindsey
Thelma Smith Mayberry
Rosa Coleman McNeil
Doris Bonner Odom
Annie Ruth Carter Simon
Alma Simmons
Julia Foye Thompson

1956

Delores Craighead Chatman
Mable Ray Easter
Virginia D. McAllister Fauntleroy
Gloria Johnson Fulton
Carrie E. Cunningham Hayes
Dorothy Lee Davidson Johnson
Sylvia Annette Johnson
Jean Carolyn Cherry Brown Jordan
Sarah Lee Saunders McCloud
Laura Bell Britton Nixon
Doris Wright Patterson
Emily Lee Watson Price
Elsie Payne Boyd Queen
Dorothy Collins Rhodes
Dora Robbins
Mattie Beatrice Stanton

1957

Marie Catherine Divers
Wilhelmina Matthews Dixon

Mary Helen Yancey Fuller
Velma Cooper Foskey
Saundra Shamburger Harris
Carolyn L. Jones
Flossie R. Johnson
Katherine Whiteside Jordan
Nora Lee Kendall Noble
Marian Smith Smith
Clarine Delores Armstrong Spratley
Cassie L. Nixon Stansburg

1958

Delores Rae Wiggs Artis
Cynthia Marie Coulter Houston
  Brickey
Mary Deneice Harris Carpenter
Laura Lee Hart Harrison
Fannie Mae Jackson Henderson
Jocelyn LaGrant Thompson Hodges
Eileen Howard
Annie Lucille Thomas Lawrence
Celestine Patricia Rascoe Maness
Gwendolyn Melba Cooper Jones
  Parham
Margaret Aquilla Watkins Stanfield
Leatha Alease Joyner Stokes
Darlease Hodges Wormack

1959

Ruby Jewel Bell Borden
Edwina Marie Sellers Colbert
Cleo Marie Dunn Bell
Bobbie Jean Hightower Fair
Rosa Lee Outerbridge Harrell
Mary Louise Williams Pointer
Valeretta Roberts Bell
Margaret Louise Wilson Smith
Maurice Otelia Blount Snead

1960

Aleatha Mae Anderson
Mary Agnes Clark
Rosetta Marie Logan Clarke
Patricia Jean Wells Cousins
Grace LaVerne Green
Ethelrine (Ethel) Pettiford
    Hennessee
Florine Stevenson Jackson
Vertabell Exum Lee
Sallie Elizabeth McAdoo
Ernestine Mayhue Scott
Doris Daye Smith
Shirley Bryant Southerland
Alice Juanita Trayham

1961

Gloria Atkinson Armstrong
Shirley Jean Long Bethel
Christine Coleman Calhoun
Ola Ruth Putman Davis
Margaret Elda Parker Elliott
Betty Jean Talford Fisher
Eva Johnson Geer
Evangeline Boone Harrell Rickman
Helen Taylor
Ernestine Smith Thomas Westbrook
Marion Patricia Godley Wilson

1962

Jennie Louise Adams
Ann Perry Allen
Altamease Ridley Arnold
Eugenia Inman Brown
Emily Jean Carrington
JoAnna Neal Dowling
Josephine Marie Woods-Green
Esther Jones Grissom

Della Ann Johnson
Maggie Lee Ledbetter
Anna Gertrude Brown Lubatkin
Joan Miller Martin Jones Mathews
Geraldine Richardson
Mattie Bell Fisher Rouse
Mary M. Bass Satterwhite
Attemerell Smith
Otelia Blanks Smith

1963

Miron A. Anderson
Mary Lassiter Howell
Norma R. Roberts Lipscomb
Gertrude Carson Meadows
Elaine Richardson Smith
Yvonne Golsby Spencer
Jeannie Woodard Slade
Thelma Hayes Thornton
Evelyn Pearl Booker Wicker
Irene Wright
Mary Davis Wright

1964

Margaret Kindred Hunt Capehart
Nellie Olivia Ellis Clemons-Green
Ann Gooding Davis
Joyce Williamson Goings
Carolyn Levister Harris
Barbara Hemans Hayes
Florida Jones
Carlita Laverne Hall Merritt
Lila B. Millard
Geneva Armstead Monroe
Betty Riddick

1965

Patricia Ann Martin Blue
Betty Evelyn Dalton Brown
Penny L. Davis
Geneva Earline Vann Dees
Marion Christine Henderson
    Groover
Jeronica Williams Hardison
JoAnn Moore
Jimmie Ruth Gore Persley
Carrie Essie Stone Reavis
Shirley Ann Oliver Scott

1966

Mary Lee Richardson Baldwin
Rebecca Mitchell Carter
Loretta Gail Flateau Chestnut
Pauline Langston Edwards
Mary Sarah O'lene Jinwright
Alice Jean McClain
Dellamar Inez Davis Washington
Linda Gayle Lofton Woodson

1967

Saundra Obie Best Clemmons
Melvina Cochran
Lenora Graham Gerald
Beverly Miller Harris
Carolyn Williams Jones
Gloria Taylor Cheek King
Reatha Young Knighton
Mary Ruth Lemmon-Black
Polly Colclough Pringle
Thelma Witherspoon Waller
Eula Pullium Winston

1968

Theresa Fields Andrews
Mary Ellen Price Britton
Yetta Hardy Clark
Linda Floyd Hill
Myrna Lynn Watson Hughes
Carolyn Beatrice Martin
Dorothy Esta Mae Dennis Segars
Brenda Joy Howell Shephard
Alice C. Harrell Young Tharrington

1969

Queen Brown Graves Browne
Gwendolyn Underwood Thomas
    Colvin
Joyce Bell Garner
Shirley Vareen Gore
Lottie Flemning Bolding Hall
Barbara Anderson Leathers
Connie Brown Webster
Ellen Webster Wells
Lillian Crannell Willis

1970

Phyllis McCoy Barbour
Lonnie LeVane Donnell
Vivian Barnes Green
Caroline Gore Hankins
Glenda Howard Kirkland Harris
Geraldine Vareen Hayes
Edith May Claudette Lindsey
Jacqueline Vivian Hicks Murphy
Allegra Ward

1971

Shirley Wallace Speight Alexander
Janie Lee Canty-Mitchell
Mary Esther Carmichael
Barbara Jean Davis-Porter
Ava Gail Edwards
Cordelia Louise Quarles Edwards
Diana Otis Felton
Carolyn Evangeline Henderson
Ruth Elizabeth Foy Holliday
Carol Ann Russell Johnson
Dorothy Mae Terry Justice
LeMona Carilla McCoy
Jerris Cobb Wells
Geraldine G.Whitley

Sources

1. Classes 1907 verified by 1931 *Bulletin* of Lincoln Hospital School of Nursing, Durham, North Carolina archived in the University of North Carolina at Chapel Hill Library, Cp610.73 L73b 1931.

2. Classes 1932 through 1971: North Carolina State Archives, *The Scalpel* and *Nightingale* Yearbooks, Reunion listings of alumni (every two years) since 1950s, personal submission of graduates, memorabilia, employees and friends of Lincoln.

3. Student nurse records now stored at Watts Hospital School of Nursing, Durham, North Carolina.

4. State Archives listing of all Black Licensed Registered Nurses in the State of North Carolina and schools attended.

5. 1912, no listing of nurse graduates for year 1912 in the 1931 Bulletin of the School of Nursing (number 1 above). Historical Roster compiled by Dorothy Esta Dennis Segars (RN '68), LHSNAA, Inc., Recording Secretary, 2003–2012.

List of Supporters

IN MEMORIAM OF	DONOR
Pearl L. Adams	Dr. and Mrs. James D. Ballard
Jessie and Margaret Austin	Carolyn A. Wilkins and Austin Sisters
David Baldwin	Gwendolyn B. Thornton
Arthur Banks	Wayne and Donna Hubert
Rev. J. W. Barnes	John and Jean Croslan
Lydia F. Betts	Margo F. Garrett
Calvin Blue Jr.	Calvin A. Blue III
Cleopatra Blue	Patricia B. Bingham
Elijah Booker Jr.	Elijah L. Booker
	Lisa Booker
	Towanda Booker
K. B. and Ethel Booker	Brenton and JoAnn Booker
	Harold and Linda Booker
	James and Dorothy Killan
Ralph K. Booker	Mary E. Booker
Fredrick L. Boone	Franklin D.Boone Sr. and Lois D. Boone
Ruby Jewel Bell Borden	Ann Y. Borden
	Shirley D. Brown
	Mr. and Mrs. Charles Bynum
	Gerri Cummings
	Etheldreda Guion
	Eva D. Scott
	Dorothy Slade
	Dr. William W. and Mrs. Janet M. Stead
	Delores Taylor
	Dr. Bernadette G. Watts
Eartha C. Bridges	Arvis D. Bridges-Epps
Mark Browne	Etienne Thomas

IN MEMORIAM OF	DONOR
Patricia "Pattie" Carter	Dr. Howard M. Fitts
Janie Lee Geter Canty	Dr. Janie Lee Canty-Mitchell
Rosetta Logan Clark	John H. Clark Jr.
Dr. William A. Cleland	John and Ellen Amy
Ruth D. Collier, '55, LHSN	Peggy J. Butts
Mr. and Mrs. Terry Cooper	Gwendolyn Cooper Jones Parham
Inez Novella Brown Dennis	Dorothy Esta Dennis Segars
Virginia Kathryn Drane	Ronald and Standra K. Patterson
Margaret Kennedy Goodwin	Sylvia and Fred Black
	Marsha G. Kee
	Dr. and Mrs. Cecil Lloyd Patterson
Torian Leondras Graves	Helen K. S. Williams
Bill Hennessee	Ethelrine P. Hennessee
Susie Mae Hickman	Montena and Ruth Terrell
Eddie Verdis Hood	Barbara J. Hood
Frankie E. Johnson	Tiffany D. Johnson
Rufus H. Jones	Jacqueline McKinney
Raymond H. Lassiter	Dr. Ernestine Lassiter
Robert A. and Annie M. Leach	Robert and Jennie Leach
Norma Roberts Lipscomb	Carolyn R. Gill
	Robert L. and Priscilla W. Hoover
	Reginald Lipscomb
	Alfred M. Roberts
Willie and Evelyn Lovett	Tracy Lovett
Anna Brown Lubatkin	JoAnna Neal Dowling
Minnie Lyon	Mable Butler
	Ernestine D. Lyon
Margie Marsh	James A. Marsh
Dr. Joan Miller Martin Jones Mathews	Lt. Col. Elmontenal C. Allens
	Norris Burton
	Ernest J. Grant
	Linda L. Hester
	Dr. Joseph H. Martin Jr.
	Linda F. Rouse

IN MEMORIAM OF	DONOR
Clarence and Corine Mayo	Wanda Adams
Lonnie McAllister	Lonnie and Paulette McAllister
Julia McAllister	Marla D. McAllister
Carl McCree	Cletus and Sue Gill
Pearl C. Miller	Dr. Joan Miller Martin Jones Mathews
Dr. Donald T. Moore	Dr. Charles B. Hammond
Bernard and Chestina Obie	Saundra Obie Clemmons
Ashley "Ash" and Annie Bell Overton	Sylvia Overton Richardson
Edith Richardson Pearson, RN	Elaine Richardson Smith
	Crawford C. Richardson Jr.
Willie Mae Peterson	Maxine Peterson
Mr. and Mrs. John Price	Lois Brooks
Kevin B. Pringle	Polly Colclough Pringle
Lois Sebastian	Diane Cardamone
Willie Mae Sanders	Barbara Vinson Burt
Phoebe Sellers	Edwina S. Colbert
Cleo Solomon	Marla D. McAllister
Paul Solomon	Lonnie and Paulette McAllister
Elma Thompson	Jocelyn Thompson Hodges
L. B. Thompson	Marian Smith
Cleon Umphrey Sr.	Cleon and Veronica Umphrey
Bennie and Levonia Wicker	Dr. Ingrid Wicker McCree
	Floyd W. Wicker
James and Suferia Wicker	Felicia W. Campbell
Lucille Zimmerman Williams	Minnie M. Beverly, Lt. Col. Ret., USAF
Ken M. Wormack	Darlease Hodges Wormack
Lena Young	Jesse J. and Ann M. Dunn

IN HONOR OF	DONOR
All members of Pi Chapter who graduated from LHSN	Pi Chapter of Chi Eta Phi Sorority, Inc.
Virginia Brown	Vince Brown
Bridgette Brown Bynum	Douglas and Beatrice Brown
Josie Cates	Jim and Val McLean
Sue and Cletus Gill	Geno McCree
Mabel McLean	Jim and Val McLean
Glossie P. Johnson	Diann Johnson
Ermateen Horton Rogers	Patricia A. Jones
Lee Doris Thomas	Tiffany D. Johnson
Tom and Thelma Thornton	Thelma Hayes Thornton
Dr. Evelyn Wicker	Dr. H. Keith H. Brodie

SUPPORTERS

Wanda Adams
Kwesi Aggrey and Deborah
  Hamlin-Aggrey
Lt. Col. Elmontenal C. Allens
John and Ellen Amey
Terrell R. Amos
Annie's Nursing Services
Julia S. Armstrong
Mary R. Baldwin
Edward H. and Jocelyn E. Bailey
Dr. and Mrs. James D. Ballard
Laquetta and John Barbee
Dr. Iris Barrett
William V. Bell
Minnie M. Beverly, Lt. Col. Ret., USAF
Patricia B. Bingham
Sylvia and Fred Black
Calvin A. Blue III
Patricia M. Blue
Ronald Boney
Austin Booker
Brenton and JoAnn Booker
Elijah L. Booker
Harold and Linda Booker
Jacqueline Booker
Lee W. and Evelyn S. Booker
Lisa Booker
Mary E. Booker
Towanda Booker
Franklin D. and Lois D. Boone Sr.
Ann Y. Borden
Betty K. Borden
Mary Jones Boykin
Elester L. Brandon
Dr. Cheryl Brewer
Arvis D. Bridges-Epps
Dr. H. Keith H. Brodie
Lois Brooks
Tanisha Brooks

Douglas and Beatrice Brown
Shirley D. Brown
Vince Brown
Barbara Vinson Burt
Norris Burton
Mable Butler
Peggy J. Butts
Mr. and Mrs. Charles E. Bynum
Tera Caldwell
Felicia W. Campbell
Janie Lee Canty-Mitchell
Diane Cardamone
Care One Nursing Services, Inc.
  (Kuburat Ganiyu)
Michael J. Carpenter
Mary T. Champagne
Helen Chavious
John H. Clark Jr.
Saundra Obie Clemmons
Nellie Clemons-Green
Dr. Clara Mae Cobb-Fraling
Edwina S. Colbert
Community Baptist Church (Pastor
  Percy Chase)
Joan A. Cozart
John and Jean Croslan
Gerri Cummings
Ann Daves
Barbara Davis-Porter
Purvis Jesse and Toshie Dennis
Barbara Donegan
Joanna Neal Dowling
Duke University Health System
Jesse J. and Annie M. Dunn
EBO Consulting/Evelyn S. Booker
Pauline Langston Edwards
Thereasea C. Elder
Delores W. Estes
Betty H. Faucette

Virginia M. Fauntleroy
Dr. Howard M. Fitts
Dr. Millicent B. Ford
Gloria J. Fulton
Fuquay Consolidated Alumni
    Association
Margo F. Garrett
Carolyn R. Gill
Cletus and Sue Gill
Dr. Louise J. Gooche
Ernest J. Grant
Dr. George Talmadge Grigsby Jr.
Etheldreda Guion
Lottie Fleming Hall
Dr. Charles B. Hammond
Annie B. Hargett
Drs. Sampson E. and Lizzie J. Harrell
Glenda Howard Harris
Laura Hart Harrison
Carolyn E. Henderson
Dr. Lana T. Henderson
Ethelrine P. Hennessee
Linda L. Hester
Susan L. Hester
Jacqueline Hicks
Jocelyn Thompson Hodges
Sandra G. Hodges
Kevin M. and Lauretta H. Holloway
Barbara J. Hood
Robert L. and Priscilla W. Hoover
Wayne and Donna Hubert
James Hudson
Kathleen A. Huffman
Oeglaire Ingram
Dr. Charles Johnson
Diann T. Johnson
Hannah J. Johnson
Tiffany D. Johnson
Patricia A. Jones
Reverend Percy R. Jones

Dorothy T. Justice
Marsha G. Kee
James and Dorothy Killian
Erma and Wilbert King
Gloria T. King
Dr. Ernestine Lassiter
Robert and Jennie Leach
Virginia Leach
Barbara A. Leathers
Richard J. Liekweg
Lincoln Hospital School of Nursing
    Alumni Association, Inc.
Reginald Lipscomb
Willie and Evelyn Lovett
Ernestine D. Lyon
Carlton T. Mack
James A. Marsh
Dr. Joseph H. Martin Jr.
Mary Duke Biddle Foundation
Iva Mason
Dr. Joan Miller Martin Jones Mathews
Lonnie and Paulette McAllister
Marla D. McAllister
Josephine D. McBride
Walter and Grace McClamb
Dr. Ingrid Wicker McCree
Janet and Sam McCullers
Ethel McCullum
Dr. William H. McDougal
Jacqueline McKinney
Jim and Val McLean
Natalie Booker McMillian
Carlita H. Merritt
Marion Glen Miles
Vicki Booker Miller
Arthur and Carolyn Mims
Lonette Mims
Edna Martel Jones Moore
Lois Smith Morris
Delma D. Murdock

JoAnna Neal Dowling
Dr. Charlie Nelms
Brenda M. Nevidjon
New Providence Missionary Baptist
  Church (Rev. Dr. Nathaniel Wood)
Orlean B. Newton
Patricia Ann Nicholson
Dr. Nora M. K. Noble, Col. Ret. USAF
Gwendolyn Cooper Jones Parham
Mona Parks
Dr. and Mrs. Cecil Lloyd Patterson
Ronald and Standra K. Patterson
Dr. Dwight Perry
Dr. Mary Ann Peter
Maxine Peterson
Eulonda Booker Pfister
Pi Chapter of Chi Eta Phi Sorority, Inc.
Polly Colclough Pringle
Priscilla Ramseur
Carrie Stone Reavis
Dr. Bobbie K. Reddick
Crawford C. Richardson Jr.
Sylvia Overton Richardson
Alfred M. Roberts
Valeretta Roberts
Janet Pines Robinson
Carolyn Rogers-McMillan
Paul and Brenna Rouse
Linda F. Rouse
Vivia K. Scales
Carolyn Scavella
Eva D. Scott
Dorothy Esta Dennis Segars
John William Segars
Randolph William Segars
Dorothy Slade
Thenia and Joseph Small
William and Rosa Small
Elaine Richardson Smith
Mr. John N. and Dr. Laura Smith

Marian Smith
Michelle H. Smith
Lt. Col. Margaret A. W. Stanfield
Dr. William W. and Mrs. Janet M. Stead
Rosa Marie Steele
Larry T. and Gwendolyn C. Suitt
Linda Jones Sutton
Dr. Latoya Tate
Ted and Peggy Tatum
Delores Taylor
Vanessa Taylor
Montena and Ruth Terrell
Donald and Kay Thomas
Etienne Thomas
Geraldine H. Thompson
Gwendolyn B. Thornton
Thelma Hayes Thornton
Marion Jean Tucker
Cleon and Veronica Umphrey
Veronica J. Walker
Dr. Bernadette G. Watts
Fred and Julie Webb
Lauriette West-Hoff
White Rock Baptist Church
Bennie and Arneta Wicker
Dr. Benita Wicker
Floyd W. Wicker Sr.
Floyd Wicker Jr.
Michelle Wicker
Norris and Gwen Wicker
Carolyn A. Wilkins and Austin Sisters
Bertha R. Williams
Edna Andrews Williams
Helen K. S. Williams
Kinston D. Williams
Larry and Arnita Williams
Michelle Williams
Juanita M. Wilson
Veronica W. Woodruff
Darlease Hodges Wormack

References

A Tradition of Excellence: Pictorial History of Watts School of Nursing. Durham, N.C.: Watts School of Nursing, 2006.

Annual Report Lincoln Hospital and Nurse Training School. 1924. Durham Regional Hospital Archives, Durham, N.C.

Annual Report of Lincoln Hospital. 1927. Durham, North Carolina. Lillian Green Gray (RN '28) and Cornelia Jackson Hardie (RN '43) Collection. Information compiled by Gloria King, April 2004.

Board of Nursing Communication to Lincoln Hospital, L. Z. Williams, RN. June 23, 1969. p. 10. Duke University Archives, Durham, N.C.

Boyd, W. K. *Chapter XI Health Philanthropy and Relief: The Real Story of Durham, City of the New South.* Durham, N.C.: Duke University Press, 1927.

Bulletin. 1931. Lincoln Hospital of the School of Nursing. University of North Carolina at Chapel Hill Library Cp610.73 L73b 1931.

Carol, Edith, and Edna Scott. "Jubilee Hospital Department of Nursing." Henderson, N.C.: Henderson Institute Historical Museum, June 2012.

Carolina Times (Durham, North Carolina). "Lincoln Hospital School of Nursing Graduates." June 4, 1938.

Certification of Amendment to the Charter of Trustees of Lincoln Hospital. 1901. Durham Regional Hospital Archives, Durham, N.C.

Certification of Incorporation of the Trustees of Lincoln Hospital. 1901. Durham Regional Hospital Archives, Durham, N.C.

Constitution and By-Laws: Lincoln Hospital School of Nursing Alumni Association. Rev. December 1975. Lincoln Hospital School of Nursing Archives, Durham, N.C.

Constitution and By-Laws: Lincoln Hospital School of Nursing. Rev. 1963. Lincoln Hospital School of Nursing Archives, Durham, N.C.

Highlights in Nursing in North Carolina, 1935–1976. 1977. A 75th Anniversary Project. North Carolina Nurses Association, Raleigh, N.C.

Johnson, G. "Nursing as a Profession." *Davis Nursing Survey* 17, no. 4 (April 1953): 101.

Laws of 1907. 1907. North Carolina Board of Nurse Examiners. North Carolina State Archives, Raleigh, N.C.

Legislation in North Carolina Brief Summary of the Nursing Laws Including Amendments and Revisions Public Laws of North Carolina, 1903. 1903. Section 1-10, Chapter 359, pp. 586–88, North Carolina State Archives, Raleigh, N.C.

Letter to all Departments from Lincoln Hospital Directors. April 10, 1970. Duke University Archives, Durham, N.C.

Lincoln Hospital Annual Financial Statement. 1933. Durham Regional Hospital Archives, Durham, N.C.

Lincoln Hospital Annual Report of Hospital Operations, January 1–December 31, 1916. 1916. Durham Regional Hospital Archives, Durham, N.C.

Lincoln Hospital Report of Operations to the Durham City Alderman, 1914. 1914. Durham City Records and Archives, Durham, N.C.

Lincoln Hospital School of Nursing Application for National League of Nursing Accreditation. 1957. Lincoln Hospital School of Nursing Archives, Durham, N.C.

Lincoln Hospital Trustees Hold Annual Meeting. 1948. Administrative office files publicity periodicals, 1948–1956. Duke University Archives, Durham, N.C.

Lincoln Hospital, Durham, North Carolina, Report of Hospital Operations: Financial Report, January 1 to December 31, 1923. 1923. Durham Regional Hospital Archives, Durham, N.C.

"Mary Seacole Biography." Last accessed October 2011. http://www.biography.com/people/mary-seacole-39430

McCall, Michael. "Lincoln Hospital School of Nursing Graduates: The Last Class." *Durham (N.C.) Morning Herald*, August 22, 1971.

Medical Examination Questions. 1919. North Carolina Board of Nurse Examiners. North Carolina State Archives, Raleigh, N.C.

"Medical History." *Journal of National Medical Association* 57, no. 2 (1965).

Miller, H. S., and E. D. Mason. *Contemporary Minority Leaders in Nursing: Afro-American, Hispanic, Native American Perspectives*. New York: American Nurses Association, 1983.

Minutes of Meeting of North Carolina Association of Colored Graduate Nurses. 1941. North Carolina State Archives, Raleigh, N.C.

Notes on North Carolina Board of Nursing Consultant Visit to Lincoln Hospital Between 1967 and 1968. p. 9. Duke University Archives, Durham, N.C.

Nurses Licensed in North Carolina by Waiver. 1919. North Carolina State Archives, Raleigh, N.C.

"Original Lincoln Hospital." Endangered Durham. http://endangereddurham .blogspot.com/2008/12/original-lincoln-hospital.html.

"Philosophy of Lincoln Hospital School of Nursing." *Bulletin.* 1959. Lincoln Hospital School of Nursing. Lincoln Hospital School of Nursing Archives, Durham, N.C.

Public Law 74: The Bolton Act Highlights in Nursing in North Carolina, 1935–1976. March 1977. A 75th Anniversary Project of North Carolina Nurses Association.

Regulations for Schools of Nursing in North Carolina. 1948. Joint Committee on Standardization. North Carolina State Archives, Raleigh, N.C.

Report of Attrition. 1960. Excerpts from the Board of Nursing to Lincoln Hospital School of Nursing. Duke University Archives, Durham, N.C.

Resolution of Board of Trustees of Lincoln Hospital. 1901. Private Laws of North Carolina, Session 1901, Chapter 133. Durham Regional Hospital Archives, Durham, N.C.

Some Laws Controlling Hospitals in North Carolina in 1917. 1917. North Carolina Board of Nurse Examiners. North Carolina State Archives, Raleigh, N.C.

Some Laws Controlling Hospitals in North Carolina in 1917. 1917. North Carolina Board of Medical Examiners. North Carolina State Archives, Raleigh, N.C.

Some Laws Controlling Hospitals in North Carolina in 1919. 1919. North Carolina Board of Nurse Examiners. North Carolina State Archives, Raleigh, N.C.

The Centennial Celebration of Lincoln Hospital School of Nursing, 1903–2003. August 2003. Lincoln Hospital School of Nursing Archives, Durham, N.C.

The Dispatch 2, no. 2 (1960). Lincoln Hospital School of Nursing Archives, Durham, N.C.

The Grading of Nurse Training Schools in North Carolina. 1928. North Carolina State Archives, Raleigh, N.C.

The Scalpel. 1946. Lincoln Hospital School of Nursing yearbook. Lois Smith Morris, Durham, N.C.

The Scalpel. 1948. Lincoln Hospital School of Nursing yearbook. Lincoln Hospital School of Nursing Archives, Durham, N.C.

The Scalpel. 1963. Lincoln Hospital School of Nursing yearbook. Lincoln Hospital School of Nursing Archives, Durham, N.C.

They Caught the Torch, Milwaukee: Will Ross, Inc., 1939.

Thirty-Eighth Annual Report Lincoln Hospital. 1938. Stanford L. Warren Library, Durham, N.C.

Wilson, E. H., and S. Mullally. *Hope and Dignity: Older Black Women of the South.* 1933. Reprint, Philadelphia, Penn.: Temple University Press, 1983.

Wyche, M. L. *Early North Carolina Hospitals: History of Nursing in North Carolina.* Chapel Hill, N.C.: University of North Carolina Press, 1938.

Wyche, M. L. *The Establishment of Negro Hospitals and the Progress of the Negro Nurses: History of Nursing in North Carolina.* Chapel Hill, N.C.: University of North Carolina Press, 1938.

Interviews

NOTE: Tapes, transcripts, or notes from most interviews may be found in the Lincoln Hospital School of Nursing Archives, Durham, North Carolina.

Clemons, Della Marie Harris. Interview with the author. October 21, 2010.

Gordon, Elizabeth. Interview with the author. June 2011.

Harris, Clara J. M. Interview with the author. 1998.

Harris, Clara J. M. Interview with the author. August 1998.

Jones, Patricia. Interview with the author. May 12, 2012.

Lawrence, Lucille. Interview with the author. September 29, 2012.

Lyons, Minnie Caranah. Interview with the authors. March 1971.

Maddox, Mamie B. Interview with the authors. October 1972.

McBride, Josephine D. Interview with the author. August 2010.

McCullum, Ethel B. Interview with Dorothy Esta Dennis Segars and the author. March 13, 2011.

McCullum, Ethel B. Interview with the author. August 25, 2011.

McCullum, Ethel B. Interview with Dorothy Esta Dennis Segars and the author. March 25, 2012.

Morris, Lois S. Interview with the author. August 2011.

Morris, Lois S. Interview with the author. March 25, 2012.

Oliver, Julia. Interview with the author. March 2011.

Rhynie, Sarah M. Interview with Dorothy Esta Dennis Segars and the author. March 2, 2011.

Richardson, Sylvia O. Interview with the author. September 2011.

Sullins, Della Mae Davison. Interview with Dorothy Esta Dennis Segars. June 12, 2010.

Sullins, Della Mae Davison. Interview with Dorothy Esta Dennis Segars. October 2011.

Thorpe, Elizabeth W. Interview with the authors. March 1971.

Index

Page numbers in *italics* indicate a photograph.
Page numbers in **boldface** indicate a personal recollection.

A. B. Duke Nurses Home, *38, 39, 73,*
73–74, 242; demolishing of, 206
Act to Provide for State Registration
for Trained Nurses in North
Carolina (1903), 14; amendments
to, 16
Adams, Jennie Louise, 74, *127*
Adams, Mary, 35, *59*
Admassu, Lidya, 224
African Americans, 252, 256; as
advocates of professional nursing,
6–7; and nursing organizations,
xvi; as nursing students, xv–xvi;
training of African American
nurses in North Carolina, 7–9;
views of hospitalization, ix
American Medical Association
(AMA), 89
American Nurses Association (ANA),
7, 94, 141
Amey, Ruth E. Parlor, 107, *107,* 200
Ammons, James H., *223*
Anderson, Kenya, *238*
Andrews, Mary Linda, 222, *223*
Andrews, Theresa Fields, *61*
Angier B. Duke Nurses Home. *See*
A. B. Dukes Nurses Home
Armstrong, Gloria Atkinson, *67*
Armstrong, Julia Marie Simpson,
88, 107, *107,* **172–73,** *192,* 200;

leadership and service contribu-
tions of, 259
Armstrong, W. H., 9–10
Arnold, Altamease Riley, *105, 127*

Baker, Peggy, *see* Peggy Baker Walters
Baldwin, Charles, *148*
Baldwin, Mary Lee Richardson, xiv,
68, 140, 141, *148,* **162–63,** 176, *208,*
210, 218, 219, 220, 225, *243, 244, 244;*
leadership and service contribu-
tions of, 259–60; as recipient of the
NCCU Alumnus of the Year Award,
221
Banks, Manice P., 104, *105*
Bannister, Michael, 224
Barham, Martha, 214, 216
Barnes, Ophelia Dowdy, 155
Barnes, Vivian, *149*
Bell, Cleo Marie Dunn, *142, 207*
Bell, Valeretta Roberts, 200, *245*
Bell, William V. "Bill," 218, 222
Bethel, Shirley Jean Long, *67*
Betts, Lydia Ruth Flintal, 89, **90–91,**
140, 200; leadership and service
contributions of, 261–62
Beverly, Rosebud Roderick, *60, 97,* 143
Big Sister Program, 74, 133–34, 135–36
Birdland Social Club, 156
Black, Helen J., *60, 97*

Blue, Patricia Martin, xii, xiv, *60*, 74, 117–18, *132*, 132–33, 160, 176, **177–79,** *208*, 210, 220, 222, 225; leadership and service contributions of, 263–64

Blue Cross/Blue Shield of North Carolina, 222, 223

Board of Examiners of Nurse Training Schools for North Carolina, 14, 23; name change of, 42

Board of Nursing Examiners of North Carolina, 42, 53, 89; board standards of, 111; clinical experience plan of, *112*; increasingly high standards of, 102–4, 129; influence of, 42–44; letters of to Lincoln Hospital School of Nursing (LHSN), *168–69, 171. See also* Board of Nursing Examiners of North Carolina, Standardization Board of

Board of Nursing Examiners of North Carolina, Standardization Board of, 13, 45, 102, 114, 166; establishment of, 42

Booker, Evelyn Smith, xiv

Borden, Ruby Jewell Bell, v–vi, ix, xii, xiv, 1, 136, *142*, 161, 198, 200, *207*, 222, 223; illness of, xiii; leadership and service contributions of, 263; work ethic of, xiii

Bowen, Dr., 156

Boyd, Annie B. Coley, 97

Brawley, Benjamin, 17

Britt, Gladys Williams, *150*

Britton, Mary Ellen Price, *61*

Broadfoot, Carrie Early, 8

Brown, Betty Evelyn Dalton, *60*, 74

Brown, Connie, 100

Brown, Dympha I., 35, *59*

Brown, E. E., 43

Brown, Lillian, *60*, 97

Brown, Rose Butler, *143*, 143–44

Brown, Slappy, 109

Brown, Thelma, 176

Brown, Viola, 48

Bryant, R. Kelly, xiv

Buie, Susie Virginia Carrington, *150*

Bullock, Gertrude, 36, 77, *99*, 99, 184

Burgess, Bessie, 47

Burgess, Marie Louise, 7–8

Butler, Geraldine C., 85, 109, *110, 233*

Butts, Mr., 109

Butts, Peggy Christine Jones, **40,** 41; leadership and service contributions of, 263

Cadet Nurse Corps. *See* United States Cadet Nurse Corps

Calhoun, Christine Coleman, *67*

Callahan, Shirley, 91

Cannon, Reverend, 155

Canty-Mitchell, Janie Lee, 68, **116–17;** leadership and service contributions of, 273–74

"Capping, The" (Mortenson), 66

Carmichael, Mary, 68, 131, 151, 160

Carr, Albert G., 9–10

Carrington, Emily, *74*, 74

Carter, Catherine, *60*

Carter, Hawkins W., 21

Carter, Patricia "Pattie" Hawkins, 21, *21*, 30, 36, 173; leadership of, 41, 46–47, 216; salary of, 41

Carter, Rebecca Mitchell, *140*, 263–64

Central Carolina Black Nurses Council, Inc., vi, 199, 220

Champagne, Mary T., 217–18

Chestnut, Loretta Gail Flateau, *140*, *157*; leadership and service contributions of, 264

Chi Eta Phi Sorority, 183, 184, *186*, 220, 229
Children's Hospital of South Philadelphia, 53
Choates, Fannie, *60*
Civil Rights Act (1965), 170
Civil Rights Movement, xvii, 74, 75, 95, 167
Civilian Conservation Corps Camp Clinic (cccc Clinic), 88
Clark, Yetta Hardy, *61*, **187**; leadership and service contributions of, 264
Clarke, Lee, 109
Clarke, Vernon, 109
Cleland, James, 52, *52*, 156
Clement, Howard, III, *238*
Clemmons, Saundra Obie Best, **137–39,** 140, 200, *208*, 210, 223; leadership and service contributions of, 260–61
Clemons, Della Marie Harris, **126,** 128, 129–30, 151; leadership and service contributions of, 266
Clemons-Green, Nellie Ellis, 204, **204–5,** 214, 248; leadership and service contributions of, 266
Club 55, 134
Cobb-Fraling, Clara Mae, **230–31;** leadership and service contributions of, 265–66
Colbert, Edwina Marie Sellers, *142*, **236–37;** leadership and service contributions of, 264
Coleman, Beatrice, 79
Coles, Bettie A., 20
Coley, Annie, *60*
College Inn, 134, 156–57
Collins, Geneva Sitrena, 8
Collins, Nellie F., 201

Colored Nurses of North Carolina Organization, 136
Connors, Marsha, 222
Contemporary Minority Leaders in Nursing: Afro-American, Hispanic, Native American Perspectives (H. Miller and E. Mason), 229
Cooke, D. B., 156
Cooke, Janie Goodman, *150*, 184, 185, *186*
Cooke, Mrs., 109
Craig, Thenia, 74
Creasman, Kate E., 19
Crisp, A. Mildred, 104, *105*
Crockett, Leona, 109, *110*
Crownsville Mental Hospital, 164
Cuban Missile Crisis, 83, 95, 167, 262
Cuffie, Lillian F., *150*

Daniels, Muriel Harris, *60*, 97
Darden, K. C., 109
Davis, Margaret, *60*
Davis, Mary Ida, 35
Davis, Ola Ruth Putnam, *67*
Davis, Penny L., *60, 132*
Davis, Sammy, Jr., 201
Davis, Sharon, *238*
Davis, Temika, *238*
Dawson, Robert E., 156
Dejarmon, Mrs., 109
Dennis, Betty P., 216–17
Dert, Mildred, *150*
Dispatch, The, 118, 154
Dixon, Catherine B., 192
Donnell, Clyde, 249
Dowling, JoAnna Neal, *105, 127,* 143–44, **145–46**; leadership and service contributions of, 264
Drew, Charles, 130
Duke, Angier B., 37; bust of, *242,* 242–44

Duke, B. N., 37
Duke, J. B., 37
Duke, Washington, ix, *11*, 37
Duke Health System, 223
Duke Hospital, ix, 88, 133, 160, 167, 176;
    establishment of (1930), 166
Duke School of Nursing, 152, 161
Duke University, x, 109, 166, 223
Duke University Medical Center, 210
Dukes family, 9–10
Dunn, Caroline Allen, 192, 200
Durham, North Carolina, x, xi, 31,
    170, 223, 237, 253–54; businesses of,
    156–57; churches of, 155; environ-
    mental conditions in, 9; Hayti area
    of, 156; poor health conditions in, 9
Durham County General Hospital,
    174, 176
Durham County Hospital
    Corporation, 174, 176
Durham County Public Health
    Department, 199
Durham Historical Preservation
    Society, 221
Durham Regional Hospital (DRH),
    175–76
Dwane, Elizabeth, 19
Dzau, Ruth, *243*
Dzau, Victor J., *243*, 243

Easley, Mike F., 214
Eastern State Hospital, 53
Edwards, Pauline Langston, *140*,
    198, 222; leadership and service
    contributions of, 264
Elder, Thereasea D. Clark, *60*, 97,
    188–89; leadership and service
    contributions of, 265
Elliott, Mary, 8
Elliott, Roberta, *67*

Elmino Castle, *209*
Emerson, Ralph Waldo, 252
Ender, Clara Adams, 221
Ethengane, Elizabeth, 35, 36, 184
Evans, Mrs. Addie, 10

Fabiola, 6
Fair, Bobbie Jean Hightower, *142*
Farley, Dorothy A., *60*, 97
Fisher, Betty Jean Talford, *67*, *122*
Fisher, Miles Mark, 47, 251
Fisher, Miles Mark, III, *78*, *140*, 251
Fitts, Howard, xiv
Florence Nightingale Pledge, 69
Forrest, Henrietta, 37, 47
Forsyth Hospital School of Nursing,
    8, 170
Foy, Ruth, 68
Franklin D. Roosevelt Memorial
    Children's Ward, 4
Freedman's Hospital, 89, 129, 190, 271
Frieson, Phloy, 36
Fulton, Gloria Johnson, *124*, 222, *238*

Garrett's Pharmacy, 156
Geer, Eva Johnson, *67*
General Convention of the Episcopal
    Church, 7
Gerald, Lenora Graham, *140*
GlaxoSmithKlien, 222–23
Good Samaritan Hospital School of
    Nursing, xv, 8, 170, 265
Goodwill Club, 134
Goodwin, Margaret Kennedy, 29, 85,
    194–95
Gordon, Elizabeth Robin, 104, 106, *106*
Graves, Mattie M., 20
Gray, Marie Antonette, 19
Gray, Mary, 47, 48
"Great 100 Nurses" program, 141

Great Depression, 88, 167
Groover, Christine Henderson, *60*
Groves, Anna A., 8
Guidelines for Nursing Education in North Carolina, 166

Haidermoto, Murtaza, 224
Hale House, 201
Hall, Lottie Fleming Bolding, 100, *136*, 149, 184, 185, *186*, 200, 222, 248–49, *249*
Hamilton, Jake, v
Hamilton, Lula Mae, v
Hardie, Cornelia Jackson, *150*
Hardison, Jeronica Williams, *60*, *132*, *208*
Hargrave, Ella Ferguson, 109, *110*
Harrell, Rose Lee Outerbridge, *142*
Harriet Cooke Carter Lectureship, 220
Harrington, Nola, 36
Harris, Beverly Miller, *140*
Harris, Clara Josephine Miller, 26, 48, 50–51, 88, 155; as winner of the Nurse of the Century Award, 198, *200*
Harris, Cora L., 19
Harris, Glenda Howard, 100–101; leadership and service contributions of, 266
Harris, Lorna, *223*
Harrison, Laura Hart, **98–99**; leadership and service contributions of, 267
Helen S. Miller Lectureship, 220–21
Henderson, Carolyn Evangeline, xiv, 68, 131, 140, 176, 198, 200, 222, *223*, 223, 225, *243*, *244*, 244–45, *245*, **246–47**; leadership and service contributions of, 267

Henderson, Carrie M., 192
Henderson, Pearl, 20
Hennessee, Etherline "Ethel" Pettiford, 200, *201*
Henry, Gertrude Bullock, *59*
Hicks, Mrs. L., 43
Hill, John Sprunt, 32
Hill, Linda Floyd, *61*
Hill-Burton Act (1947), 165, 166
Himes, J., 109
Historically Black Colleges and Universities (HBCU), 219, 220
Hodges, Jocelyn Thompson, **159–60**; leadership and service contributions of, 267
Holmes, —, *150*
Hopper, Mr. (laundry orderly), 157, 160
Hopper, S. (nutrition instructor), 109
Horton, Larnie G., *238*
Houston, L. H., 109, *110*, *150*
Howell, Mary Lassiter, *114*, *154*
Hubbard Hospital, 164
Hughes, Myrna Watson, *61*, *136*, *149*

Isler, Terri B., 35, *59*

Jackson, Beulah Porter, 47–48, 136
Jackson, Della Raney (Rainey), 79, *81*, 81–83; as the first African American woman commissioned as a lieutenant in the Army Nurse Corps, 82; as part of the Tuskegee Airmen, 82–83
Jackson, Mrs. B. E., 43
Jackson, Phyllon, xiv
Jeffreys, Evelyn, 35, *59*
Jeffreys, Mary E., 20
Jim Crow era, 3, 253, 254
Jinwright, Mary Sara O'Lene, 268

John's Diner, 156
Johnson, Carol Ann Russell, 200, 205, 220, *220*, 224
Johnson, Diann, xii, xiv
Johnson, Dr. Charles, *140*
Johnson, Marion, *114*
Johnson, Mary P. "Polly," 217
Johnson, Tiffany Deana, xiv
Jones, Helen Neal Webb, 49, 79, 108, *108*, *207*, 224
Jones, Mary L. Thicklin, 85, 104, *105*
Jones, Willie F., 20
Jubilee Hospital, 8
Jubilee Nurse Training School, 8–9, 170
Justice, Dorothy Terry, 68

Kate Biting Reynolds Hospital, 8
Kate Biting Reynolds Memorial School of Nursing, xv, 8, 170
Kayescott, Allyson, 224
Kennedy, Alice C., 109, *110*
Kennedy, John F., 250
Kennedy, Robert F., 250
Kindred, Mildred, *149*
King, Dr. Robert E., 156
King, Gloria Taylor Cheek, xiv, 140, 155, 184, *186*, 200, 214, 220, 222, *223*, 223, 225, 232, *238*, *243*, **250–51**; leadership and service contributions of, 268; as recipient of the NCCU Alumnus of the Year Award, 221
King, Martin Luther, Jr., 250
Knighton, Reatha Young, *140*

L. Richardson Memorial Hospital School of Nursing, xv, 8, 172
Largin, Addie Ernestine, 20
Laryea, Joan, *208*, 210
Latta, Julia, 10, 12, *12*, 19, 21

Lauray, Daniel, 54, 56
Lawrence, Lucille Thomas, 85, **175,** 175–76
Laws, El Dora, **241;** leadership and service contributions of, 268
Leathers, Barbara Anderson, 72, *72*; leadership and service contributions of, 268
Ledbetter, Maggie Lee, *105*, *127*
Leonard Hospital, 7
Liberia, 3–4, 17
Lincoln Angel of Mercy Sisterhood, 232
Lincoln Community Health Center, 174, 176, 199, 206, 222, 232, 242
Lincoln Hospital, x, xvi, xvii, *31*, 31–32, 38, 253; challenges of and changes to, 164–67; collaboration with Duke Hospitals, 167; demolishing of, 206; deteriorating physical facilities of, 94; incorporation of, 9; and integration, 166; lack of psychiatric services in, 52, 53; leasing of from the County of Durham, 165; new facilities of (1920s), 37, 39, 41; new facilities of (1951–1953), 165; original charter of, 10; pediatric services of, 52–53; relationship with Lincoln Hospital Nurse Training School, 13–14; rules of governing student training, 44–48; Well Baby Clinic of, 89
Lincoln Hospital Board of Trustees, 111
Lincoln Hospital Nurse Training School (Durham), 8; admission standards of, 23–24, 45; application form of, *25*; clinical training provided by, 28, 30; commencement exercise of (1914), 22; costs of attending, 26, *27*, 28;

curriculum and training standards of, 24, 26; diploma of (1914), 23; earliest graduates of, 19–20; first graduation class of (1907), 20, 21; graduating class of (1914), 22; long hours put in by students, 28, 30; name change of, 89; origins of, 9–10, 12; relationship with Lincoln Hospital, 13–14

Lincoln Hospital School of Nursing (LHSN), ix, x–xi, xv, xvi, xvii, 174; academic standards of, 118–19; admission requirements of, 115; admissions and recruitment at, 19, 101–2, 113–18; affiliations of, 52–53, 129–33, 132, 164; attrition at, 122–23, 170; "Big Sisters" program of for new students, 74, 133–34, 135–36; bulletin of (1931), 46, 46, 52, 61–62; challenges faced by, 164–65; challenges and conflicts of with the Board of Nursing, 167, 168–69, 170–71, 171, 172–75; class poem of (1948), 93–94; class schedule of (1927), 44; clinical experience practices of, 48–52, 126, 128–33; closing of, 170, 171, 172–74; community surrounding, 88–89; curriculum of, 113, 125; daily routines of a student at, 50–51, 160–61, 164; difficulties faced by students not passing the board examinations, 103–4, 115–17; extended support and family of LHSN students, 156–57, 160; graduating ceremony of, 68; leadership role of the superintendent in, 43–44; legacy of, vi, 1, 176, 194, 214, 218, 232, 236–37, 247–49, 252; and the National League of Nursing (NLN) accreditation, 166; nurse instructors and grading

requirements of, 43; nursing capes of, 60, 61; nursing caps of, 62–63, 65, 65–66, 67; nursing pin of, 68–69, 72; nursing station of, 50; nursing ward routine of, 51, 51–52; objectives of, 125–26; patient care procedures of, 127, 128; pediatrics rotation and affiliation of, 129–31, 164; philosophy and guiding principles of, 123–25; placement of historical marker of LHSN on the former grounds of Lincoln Hospital, 221–22, 238, 239; political events affecting students of, 78–79, 81–83, 88; post-graduate careers of representative nurses, 185, 187–89, 191; problems of in attaining affiliation agreements, 168, 170; professional development activities at, 135–36, 140–41; psychiatry affiliations of and training in, 52, 53, 128, 132, 133; student attire and ceremonies, 58, 58–59, 59, 61–62, 66, 68–69, 72; Student Council of, 135, 135; success of because of collaboration between Whites and Blacks, 174–75; superintendents of, 46–48; transition of nurses from LHSN to DRH, 175–76; value of to students, 54; wards of, 50. *See also* Lincoln Hospital School of Nursing (LHSN), dorms and dormitory life at; Lincoln Hospital School of Nursing (LHSN), faculty of; Lincoln Hospital School of Nursing (LHSN), graduating classes of; Lincoln Hospital School of Nursing (LHSN), student activities of; Lincoln Hospital School of Nursing Alumni Association (LHSNAA)

Lincoln Hospital School of Nursing
(LHSN), dorms and dormitory life
at, 30, 72–75, 77; dormitory directors, 72; dormitory housemothers,
74–75, *75*, 77; dormitory kitchen,
73, 74; job description for dorm
directors, *76*
Lincoln Hospital School of Nursing
(LHSN), faculty of, 102–4, *105–8*,
106–9, *110*; continuing education
of, 109; and the difficulties faced
by students not passing the board
examination, 103–4; faculty
support of students' emotional
and spiritual development, 103; the
only White faculty member, 104
Lincoln Hospital School of Nursing
(LHSN), graduating classes of:
(1936), *59*; (1948), *60*, 97; (1959 ["The
Big Nine"]), 146; (1965), *60*; (1968),
61
Lincoln Hospital School of Nursing
(LHSN), student activities of, 77–78,
133–35, *136*; basketball, 154; choir,
152, *152*, *153*; Choral Communion,
152, 152; coronations, proms, and
dances, 144, 146, *148–50*; outdoor
activities, 150–51; religious activities, 77–78, 155–56; student awards,
68; student yearbook (*The Scalpel*,
later *The Nightingale*), 141–43, *142*;
tea time, 143–44, *144*
Lincoln Hospital School of Nursing
Alumni Association (LHSNAA),
xiv, 141, 170; alumni trip to West
Africa, 206, *208*, *209*, 209–10;
archival agreement of with NCCU,
244, 244–45, *245*; centennial
celebration of LHSN, 214, *215*,
216–19; constitution and bylaws of,

192–93; development of, 192–96;
Durham Chapter of, 196, 198–200;
founding of (1938), 192; inaugural
historic preservation event of,
242–45; incorporation of (1976),
193, *194*; membership composition,
196; membership dues, 196; and the
Miss Lincoln contest, 200; New
York Chapter of, 200–201, *202*,
203; Nurse of the Century Award
of, 198, *200*; original chapters
of, 196; and the Parade of Stars
procession and video, 218–19;
proposal to revise the constitution,
194, 196; reunions of, 205–6, *206–9*,
209–10, *240*, *241*; Washington, D.C.
Chapter of, 204
Lincoln Hospital Training School
(New York), 8, 21
Lincoln Scholars, 223–24
Lipscomb, Norma R. Roberts, *114*,
225; leadership and service
contributions of, 268–69
Lockhart, Clara, 20
Lott Carey Foreign Mission
Convention of the United States,
17, 18, 19
Lubatkin, Anna Gertrude Brown,
127
Lucas, Jeanne H., 218
Lyon, Minnie Canarah, **17–18,** 19, 28;
leadership and service contribu-
tions of, 268
Lyons, Jesse, 85

Maddox, Mamie B., 46, *207*
Mahoney, Mary Eliza, 7
Major, Georgia, *60*
Maness, Celestine Patricia Rascoe,
136, **233–35;** leadership and service

contributions of, 269–70; publications of, 232

Martin, Carolyn Beatrice, *61*, 197, *201*

Mary Duke Biddle Foundation, xiv

Mason, Albertine, 74, *75*, 85

Mason, Ernest D., 229

Mathews, Joan Miller Martin Jones, 104, 106, *106*, *122*, 140, *208*, 210, **211–13**, 223, 224; as recipient of the NCCU Alumnus of the Year Award, 221; leadership and service contributions of, 270–71

McBride, Josephine Demmons, xvi, 26, 35, 39, 41, 47, *59*, 72, 77, 183–85, **184**, *186*, 187; leadership and service contributions of, 271; recollections of the class of 1936 (1933–1936), 35–37

McCarthy, Eugene, 29

McClain, Alice Jean, *140*, 271

McCree, Ingrid Wicker, xiv

McCree, Sydney Lorraine, 184–85, *186*

McCullum, Ethel Brown, 48, 89, *128*, 128–29; leadership and service contributions of, 271

McDaniel, Norcy, *67*

McGill, Lavette Steele, 210, 224

McKenzie, Neil S., 20

McLaurin, Miss, 35, 36

McNair, Lula Cowan, 63, **63–64,** 108, *245*

McNeill, Mary, 36

Meadows, Gertrude Carson, 102, *114*

Medical Care Commission. *See* North Carolina Care Commission

Meharry Medical College, 164, 234

Merrick, John, ix–x, 10, *11*, 21, 30

Merritt, Carlita LaVerne Hall, **190–91;** leadership and service contributions of, 271–72

Michaux, H. M., Jr., 218

Miles, Marion Glen, 41, 85, 107, *107*, 198, **198–99,** *207*; leadership and service contributions of, 272

Miller, Helen S., 91, 172–73, 219, 229; lectureship established in honor of, 220–21

Miller, Lelia, 85

Mills, Betsy, 47

Mills, Jack Dallas, 3

Mills, Joseph Napoleon Bonaparte, *13*, 28

Mills, Margaret Ann, 3

Mills, Mary Lee, 1, 2, **3–5,** 219; awards bestowed upon, 5; leadership and service contributions of, 272–73; portrait of, *2*

Moore, Aaron M., 10, *11*, 17, 21, 30; death of, 32

Moore, Beatrice, 74, *75*

Moore, Edna Martel Jones, **80–81;** leadership and service contributions of, 274

Moore, JoAnn, *xviii, 60*

Moore, Pearl, 20

Moore, Washington, ix

Morris, Lois Smith, 48, *149*; leadership and service contributions of, 274

Mortenson, Alice Hansche, 66

Moss, Beatrice Freeman, *206*, 206

Munger, Claude, 165

National Association for Colored Graduate Nurses (NACGN), 7

National League of Nursing (NLN), 95, 166, 167; accreditation expense and application of, 133

National Nurses Association, 192

Nealy, Vivian Savage, 201

New Deal, 88

New England Hospital for Women
and Children, 7
Nightingale, Florence, 6. *See also*
Florence Nightingale Pledge
"Nightingale Lamp Poem" (Kendall),
67
Noble, Nora Kendall, 83, **86–87;**
leadership and service contribu-
tions of, 275
Nobles, Josephine McBride, 183
North Carolina Agricultural and
Technical University (A&T), xv, 166
North Carolina Alumni and Friends
Coalition, 219
North Carolina Board of Examiners
for Trained Nurses, 12, 13, 14;
revision of its standards, 16; sample
examination questions of, *15*
North Carolina Board of Examiners
of Training Schools for Nurses, 39
North Carolina Board of Nursing
Examiners, 41
North Carolina Care Commission,
28, 165
North Carolina Central University
(NCCU), 233, 236–37, 242;
Department of Nursing, xv;
involvement of LHSN alumni in,
224–25; relationship with LHSN,
219–24. *See also* North Carolina
Central University (NCCU) Alumni
Association
North Carolina Central University
(NCCU) Alumni Association,
220–21; establishment of the
Distinguished Alumni Award,
221; establishment of the Lincoln
Scholars Scholarship, 222–24;
financial support of for NCCU's
Department of Nursing, 221–22
North Carolina College (now North

Carolina Central University
[NCCU]), 46, 173, 219
North Carolina Grading Committee,
43
North Carolina Lincoln Hospital. *See*
Lincoln Hospital
North Carolina Medical Care Com-
mission, 165
North Carolina Nursing Practice Act
(1965), 166
North Carolina State Association of
Colored Registered Nurses, Inc.,
xvi
North Carolina State Association of
Negro Registered Nurses, Inc., 140,
229
North Carolina State Nurses Association (NCSNA), 140, 192, 229
North Carolina State Sanatorium, 8,
36
North Carolina State Student Nursing
Association, 136
Nurse Training School Committee,
44; members of, 47
nursing, xv, 248; background and
development of nurse training
in North Carolina, 14, 16, 19–21;
history of, 6–7; political and world
events that challenged professional
nursing, 95; progressive nature
of, 94–97, 99, 101–2; training of
African American nurses in North
Carolina, 7–9
nursing schools, 244, 247; accreditation of throughout the United
States, 42–43; in North Carolina,
166, 219; survival of black nursing
programs in North Carolina,
219–20; transition of nurses from
LHSN to DRH, 175–76
Nycum, Harry E., 47

Oliver, Julia, xiv, 104, 106, *106*

Page, Andrea, *238*
Pages Store, 156
"Parade of Stars: Capturing the
    Legacy" (LHSNAA video), 219
Parham, Gwendolyn Melba Cooper
    Jones, xii, xiv, 136, 176, 224, **226–28,**
    254; experience of as a "little sister"
    at LHSN, 134; leadership and service
    contributions of, 275–76
Parker, Margaret Elda, *67*
Parks, Pearl, 48
Parks, Vivian, *150*
"Pathways to Leadership" conference,
    210
Pattie H. Carter Nurses Club, 21
Peach, Helen S., 48
penicillin, 88
Persley, Jimmie Ruth Gore, 53, *60, 66,*
    132
Pettiford, Tashana, *238*
Phillips, Annie Lee, 200–201, 222,
    248, 248
Plummer, Josephine, 108, *108*
Pointer, Mary Williams, 146, **147–48,**
    148, 160–61, 164, *207*; leadership
    and service contributions of, 276
Pollitt, Phoebe, xiv
Porter, Barbara Davis, 68
Price, Emily, 224
Price, Freeland Bailey, 48
P&W Pub, 134

racial designations, changes in,
    xvi–xvii
racial discrimination, 253–56
racism, 189, 255
Randolph, Emma Lee, 48
Randolph, Robert P., 47
Ray, Angela, *238*

Reavis, Carrie Stone, *60*, 69, **70–71,**
    156, *201*, 232; leadership and service
    contributions of, 276
Reckhow, Ellen W., 218, *238*
Redding, Claretta, 8
Reed, Ruth F., *59*
Reeder, Margaret Davis, 97
Regal Theater, 156
Reid, Ethel, 35
Rex Hospital, 7
Rhodes, Dot Collins, 85
Rhynie, Sarah McKoy, 129, **130**
Rich, William, 47, 109
Richardson, Emma, 20
Richardson, Geraldine, *127*
Richardson, Lyn, xiv
Richardson, Sylvia Overton, 104, *105,*
    109, *110*, 113, *122*
Rickman, Evangeline Boone Harrell,
    67, 204
Ricks, Miss, 74, *75*
Riddick, Fostine, 184
Robinson, Laura, 108, *108*
Rogers, Donna, *242, 243*
Rogers, Marion G. Elizabeth Sanders
    DeGreffread, 106, *106*
Roland, E. Joyce Simmons, xi, 104,
    105
Roosevelt, Franklin D., 56, 88
Rudolph, Wilma, 164
Ruff, Andre Doris, 134–35
Ruffin, Eleanor Matthewson, 184, 185,
    186
Rush, Ruth, 47

Santa Filomena Student Nurse Honor
    Society, *140*, 141
Satterwhite, Mary Bass, *105, 127*
Saunders, Gloria K., 109
Schmidt, Evelyn, 176, 206, 218, *238*
Scott, Frank, *149*

Scott, Polly, 36
Scott, Shirley Ann Oliver, *60*, 132
Seacole, Mary, 6–7, 252
Segars, Dorothy Esta Dennis, xii, xiv,
    47, 53, *61*, 78, 118–19, **120–21,** 129,
    184, *186*, 192, *221*, 222, 225; grade
    sheet of, *119*; leadership and service
    contributions of, 276
Semans, Mary Duke Biddle Trent,
    242, *243*, 244
Shaw University Medical
    Department, 7, 21
Shepard, Charles, 10, *12*, 21, 41, 43, 47
Shepard, James E., 17, 47, 221–22
Shephard, Brenda Howell, *61*
Shields, Theodosia, *244*, 245
Sigma Theta Tau Sorority, 229
Slade, Jennie Woodard, *114*
Smith, Attemerell, *105*
Smith, Doris Day, 225, *245*
Smith, Elaine Richardson, 54, **55–57,**
    114; leadership and service contri-
    butions of, 277
Smith, Laura, *221*
Smith, M. L., 106, *106*
Smith, Margaret Louise Wilson, *142*,
    207
Smith, Marian Smith, 29; leadership
    and service contributions of, 277
Smith, Marian Walden, *150*
Smith, Otelia Blanks, *105*
Snead, Maurice Otelia Blount, *142*
Social Security Act (1935), 165
Southerland, Shirley Bryant, 184, *186*
Spaulding, Charles Clinton, 242
Speed, Joseph A., 47
Spencer, Yvonne Goolsby, *78*, 102, 103,
    114, 224
Spruell, Elizabeth, 19
St. Agnes Hospital, 7, 21

St. Agnes Hospital School of Nursing,
    xv, 7–8, 170
St. Augustine College (now St.
    Augustine University), 7
Stahl, Mr., 109
Standardization Board. *See* Board
    of Nursing Examiners of North
    Carolina, Standardization Board of
Stanfield, Margaret Aquilla Watkins,
    83, **84–85,** *102*; leadership and
    service contributions of, 277
Stanford L. Warren Library, 156
Steele, Edith, 47
Steele, Rosa S., xiv, 219
Stephens, Cora, 47
Stephens, Ophelia White, 85
Stokes, Christine, *157*
Stokes Nurses Home, *39*, 39
Suitt, Larry T., 170, 176, 243, *243*
Sullins, Della Mae Davison, 47, 192,
    193
Swift, Leroy R., 88, 156

Taylor, James, 109
Taylor, Salome, 8
Taylor, Tina, *238*
Tennessee State University, 164
Tharrington, Alice Harrell Young, *61*,
    136, 196, **197;** leadership and service
    contributions of, 278
Tharrington, George, 155
Thomas, Ernestine Smith, 67
Thomas, Lucretia T., 201
Thomas, Mrs. William H., 17
Thomas, William H., 17
Thompson, L., *114*
Thompspon, Lelia B. Miller, 29, 107,
    107, 109
Thompson, Lelia P., 106, *106*
Thompson, Zella Perry, *60*, 97

Thoms, Adah B., 7
Thornton, Thelma Hayes, 102, **103,** *114*
Thorpe, Elizabeth Williams, *60*, 85, *97*, 97, 107, 109
Thorpe, Mary Lois Clements Brown, xiv, 21, 59, *60*, 79, 97, 108, *108*; fundraising of for the student yearbook, 141–42; on her first day of school at LHSN, 142–43
Titus, Harold, 29
Training School for Nurses, The (Board of Nursing), 46
Trammell, Jimmie, 35, *59*
Tubman National School of Nursing, 4
Turner, I. E., 44
Tyson, Elsie Boyd, *208*

Umstead, Corona McClary, *60*, 97, 107, *107*
United States Cadet Nurse Corps, 79, 79, 81–82
United States Public Health Service (USPHS), 3, 4
University of Ghana, 210
University of North Carolina Board of Governors, 219–20
University of North Carolina (UNC) at Chapel Hill, 166

Vann, Andre, xiv, *244*
Vann Dees, Geneva, *60*, *148*
venereal disease, 88
Vereen, Shirley, *149*
Vietnam War, 95, 167

W. D. Hill Recreation Center, 156
Waddell, Amber M., 224
Wade, Dalisha, 210, 224
Wade, Geneva Smith, 204

Wade, Ruth Harrell, 201, 214
Wadell, Elsie Long, 278
Walker, Laura, 104, *105*
Walker, Leroy T., 109, 161
Walters, Peggy Baker, 216, *242*, 244
Warren, Stanford Lee, x, 10, *11*, 21, 47, 242
Washington, Dellamar Inez Davis, *157*; leadership and service contributions of, 278
Watkins, Nannie P., 20
Watts, Charles, 156, 176
Watts Hospital, 9, 165; and integration, 166
Watts Hospital School of Nursing, 133, 152, 161, 170, 173; success of because of collaboration between Whites and Blacks, 174–75
Watts Hospital Training School for Nurses, 9
Weaver's Dry Cleaners, 156
Webster, Ellen, 100
White, Beatrice "Mama Bea," 40, 74, *75*, 85
White, Sonia, 224, *224*, *238*
Wicker, Evelyn Pearl Booker, ix, *114*, 140, 173, *184*, *186*, 189, 191, *207*, *208*, 210, 220, 222, 224–25; on the challenge for young African Americans, 256; leadership and service contributions of, 278–79; reasons for her choice of a nursing career, 256–57; as recipient of the NCCU Alumnus of the Year Award, 221
Wicker, Floyd, xiv
Wicker, Floyd, Jr., xiv
Wilkerson, Mary K., *67*, 109, *110*
Wilkerson, Miron Andrews, *78*, *114*, 136

Wilkins, Willie Mae, 35, 36
Williams, Alice, *60*, 97, 143
Williams, Angela, *223*, 223–24, *238*
Williams, Frances, 29, 85
Williams, Lucille Zimmerman, *66*,
   67, 85, 95–97, *96*, 98, 109, 138, *140*,
   143, 170, 187, 198, *207*, 216, 250, 251;
   admonition of to always do one's
   best, 255; changes made under her
   administration of LHSN, 101; and
   the "L. Z. Era" at LHSN, 95; and the
   student yearbook, 141
Williams, Othello Cave, *60*, 97, 143
Williams, Theda Elenor, 19
Williams-Beverly, Minnie Mae,
   82–83; leadership and service
   contributions of, 261
Wilson, Margaret, 109
Wilson, Marion Patricia Godley, *67*

Wilson, Raya S., 224
Winbush, Pearl, 35, *59*, 184
Wingate, Mr., 157
Winston, Sharon D., 85
Winston-Salem State Teachers
   College, 166
Winston-Salem State University
   School of Nursing (WSSU), xv
Wood, Josephine, *122*
Woodson, Linda Lofton, *201*; leader-
   ship and service contributions of,
   279
World War I, 167
World War II, 78–79
Worley, Mary B., 97
Wright, Irene, *114*
Wright, Mary Davis, *114*

Yarboro Dees Pool Hall, 156

About the Author

EVELYN PEARL BOOKER WICKER, RN, BSN, MPH, EDD

Evelyn Pearl Booker Wicker was born on April 21, 1943, on the family farm in Fuquay Varina, North Carolina, the fifth in a family of seven children. Her parents were deeply religious, had a phenomenal work ethic, and strongly believed in the value of education.

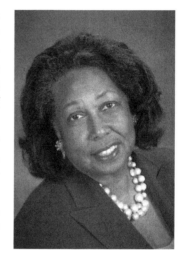

Her mother was a lay midwife, delivering and attending many of the births in the area. She really wanted to be a nurse and transferred that desire to Evelyn. Additionally, Evelyn, having grown up on a farm, had always been the caretaker for her brothers and other small cousins. Eventually, these two factors helped her to conclude that nursing was the career choice for her.

Throughout elementary and high school, Evelyn excelled. Her academic achievements in high school contributed to her success on the Lincoln Hospital School of Nursing (LHSN) entrance exam and acceptance into LHSN in 1960. While at Lincoln, exposure to the educational system and camaraderie at North Carolina College (now North Carolina Central University) provided Evelyn with the foundation and inspiration to pursue advanced education. This proved to be a valuable asset, allowing her to achieve career mobility in nursing leadership. She earned a bachelor of science degree in nursing from North Carolina Central University, Durham, North Carolina, in 1972, a master's degree in public health from the University of North Carolina at Chapel Hill, North Carolina, in 1973, and a doctorate in adult education from North Carolina State University in Raleigh, North Carolina, in 1995. Today, though retired, Evelyn is teaching nursing assistant courses to adult learners, many of whom are on track to enter professional nursing programs.

Evelyn has 40-plus years of professional nursing experience, which include clinical, administrative, educational, and career development roles in health care and human resources. She devoted the major part of her nursing career to nursing management at the executive level. In this role, Evelyn was able to influence decisions about and help chart the course for nursing services and patient care. She has served in a number of community and professional leadership roles at local and state levels and has received many certificates and awards. She was the first nurse elected to serve on the Board of Health in Durham County, and she was a longtime member of the board of directors of the Durham YMCA. Additionally, she had the opportunity to become a Fellow in the international Wharton Nursing Leaders Program at the University of Pennsylvania. Evelyn continues to reside on the family farm in North Carolina.